DATE DUE

Cognitive Effects of
Early Brain Injury

The Johns Hopkins Series in Psychiatry and Neuroscience

Paul R. McHugh, M.D., and Richard T. Johnson, M.D.,
Consulting Editors

Also of Interest in This Series:

The Neurobiology of Autism, edited by Margaret L. Bauman, M.D., and
Thomas L. Kemper, M.D.

Dementia: Presentations, Differential Diagnosis, and Nosology, edited by V.
Olga B. Emery, Ph.D., and Thomas E. Oxman, M.D.

Psychiatric Epidemiology: Assessment Concepts and Methods, edited by Juan
E. Mezzich, M.D., Ph.D., Miguel R. Jorge, M.D., Ph.D., and
Ihsan M. Salloum, M.D., M.P.H.

The Prevention of Depression: Research and Practice, Ricardo F. Munoz
and Yu-Wen Ying

Philosophical Perspectives on Psychiatric Diagnostic Classification, edited by
John Z. Sadler, M.D., Osborne P. Wiggins, Ph.D., and Michael A.
Schwartz, M.D.

Depression in Neurologic Disease, edited by Sergio E. Starkstein, M.D.,
and Robert G. Robinson, M.D.

Cognitive Effects of Early Brain Injury

CASEY DORMAN and BILHA KATZIR

Department of Psychology and Family Studies
United States International University San Diego, California

The Johns Hopkins University Press
Baltimore and London

©1994 The Johns Hopkins University Press
All rights reserved. Published 1994
Printed in the United States of America on acid-free paper
03 02 01 00 99 98 97 96 95 94   5 4 3 2 1

The Johns Hopkins University Press
2715 North Charles Street, Baltimore, Maryland 21218-4319
The Johns Hopkins Press Ltd., London

ISBN 0-8018-4856-3

Contents

Preface

Many people associate the field of neuropsychology with traumatic head injury. But the pediatric neuropsychologist, pediatric psychologist, pediatric neurologist, pediatrician, and special education professional may typically encounter children whose brain injury has been present since birth. These children have genetic disorders, perinatal injury, or a congenital malformation syndrome. Such disorders, which are usually not progressive, often result in intellectual impairment or, at least, learning disabilities. These problems become the focus of treatment and rehabilitation efforts.

As clinicians and researchers, we are acutely aware of the lack of any organized source of information on the cognitive effects to be expected in children with early brain injury. Because of this, we have gathered and synthesized the available findings on the cognitive effects of genetic disorders, malformation syndromes, infections, toxic influences, and perinatal brain injury. In each case, we have attempted to relate what is known about the pathophysiology of the disorder and its cognitive sequelae. As part of this effort, we include an introductory chapter dealing with brain development and the mechanisms of injury.

This is a book for both clinicians and researchers. The former may simply use it as a reference. Each chapter contains the most recent findings regarding the development of cognitive and academic skills in each of the disorders covered. Particularly useful should be the sections that discuss fairly common syndromes (such as Down syndrome, fetal alcohol syndrome, spina bifida, and AIDS) and the effects of premature birth. The final chapter deals exclusively with learning disabilities, especially in the area of reading. We have included new data from our own studies on both arithmetic and reading disabilities in chapters 6 and 8.

The researcher interested in early brain injury may be interested in such practical issues as the prediction of intellectual and academic skill deficits from birth histories or in such theoretical issues as the ability of the brain to reorganize, functionally, after injuries at different ages. In chapter 6 we offer new data regarding the prediction of intellectual and academic abilities from a knowledge of factors related to birth injury. In chapter 7, we reexamine the existing data concerning plasticity in the development of cognitive functions after early focal injury. Throughout the book, we have highlighted the relevance of findings to current neurodevelopmental theories.

As a specialized volume that deals with brain disorder occurring in a circumscribed period (i.e., genetic, prenatal, and perinatal), this book may be a useful supplementary text for courses on cognitive development, biological psychology, or learning disabilities. It may serve as a suitable primary text for graduate-level courses in child neuropsychology, developmental pediatrics, or developmental neurology.

Cognitive Effects of
Early Brain Injury

1

Normal and Abnormal Development of the Nervous System

Cognitive development involves an interaction between biological and environmental factors. Any attempt to focus on either of these domains by itself involves an abstraction. At the same time, there is enough regularity in the development of the nervous system, and even in some areas of its pathology, to allow us to portray a coherent picture.

The aim of this chapter is to acquaint the reader with the normal process of development of the central nervous system and to identify the major points of vulnerability to the kinds of damage that are later discussed in terms of their implications for cognitive development.

The Embryonic Period

The major event that initiates the development of the central nervous system is *primary neurulation.* The process of neurulation takes place during the third and fourth weeks of gestation, initiated by the formation of the *neural plate.* The neural plate is a layer of tissue that becomes differentiated on the dorsal surface of the embryo, apparently by a process of induction from the underlying notochord (Lemire et al. 1975). The edges of the neural plate develop into the neural folds that close around the central canal. The fusion of the neural folds occurs from anterior to posterior. As the closure proceeds, neural crest cells are formed caudally beneath the overlying

1

ectoderm. The cells of the neural crest give rise to the developing dorsal root ganglia, sensory ganglia of the cranial nerves, autonomic ganglia, Schwann cells, and cells of the pia and arachnoid layers (Volpe 1987).

Within days after the neural tube begins to form from the fusion of the neural folds, the rostral portion begins to differentiate to form the structures of the forebrain. Although the closure proceeds both rostrally and caudally, the anterior neuropore, which is the site of closure rostrally, is fused before the caudal portion of the neural tube is fused. The anterior neuropore early develops distortions related to the development of the primordia of the thalamus and corpus striatum and the optic evaginations (Lemire et al. 1975). The closure of the posterior end of the neural tube occurs about two days after the closure of the anterior neuropore (Volpe 1987).

The lower lumbar, sacral, and coccygeal segments of the neural tube form by successive processes called *canalization* and *retrogressive differentiation*. After the conclusion of primary neurulation (around twenty-six days gestation), a mass of undifferentiated cells at the caudal end of the neural tube develops small vacuoles in the next two to four days. These vacuoles come together to form a larger canal, which makes contact with the central canal of the neural tube. This process continues until about seven weeks gestation, when the additional caudal tube structure formed by canalization begins to degenerate. This process is called *retrogressive degeneration,* and it continues until sometime after birth (Lemire et al. 1975; Volpe 1987). The net result is that much of the lower portion of the cord disappears, leaving the ventriculus terminalis and filum terminale. This whole process has received popular discussion in terms of its appearance of first the formation and later the disappearance of an embryonic "tail."

The vast majority of disorders originating during the period of primary neurulation involve a failure of closure of the neural tube. Such disorders may range from a complete failure of closure along the length of the neural tube (cranioraschisis totalis) to myelomeningocele, which is related to a failure of closure of the posterior neural tube but may occur at various vertebral levels. By far, the majority of cases in which a failure of primary neurulation is compatible with life involve myelomeningocele. However, some children with encephalocele, a disorder of anterior neural tube closure, survive and some exhibit normal intelligence.

Myelomeningocele occurs in the lumbar region in approximately 80 percent of cases (Volpe 1987). The neural tissue is displaced dorsally, so it usually protrudes from the back. A typical myelomeningocele includes the protruding spinal cord and vascular network, covered by a layer of epithelial tissue. The Arnold-Chiari malformation, which involves a caudal displacement of a number of brain structures, including the medulla, pons, fourth ventricle, and cerebellum, occurs in nearly every case of myelomeningocele. Hydrocephalus, often related to complications from the Arnold-Chiari malformation, occurs in 60–90 percent of cases (Lorber 1961).

Encephalocele usually occurs in the occipital region, although frontal encephaloceles are not uncommon. The typical occipital encephalocele involves a protrusion of occipital brain tissue.

Volpe (1987) included a number of disorders involving the failure of development of forebrain, facial, and olfactory structures within the category of disorders due to a disorganization of the process of induction of forebrain development by the prechordal mesoderm in the fifth and sixth weeks of gestation. The majority of conditions usually grouped together under the rubric of *holoprosencephaly* are not compatible with life. Less severe facial deformities may result from similar but milder developmental failures (e.g., moderate ocular hypotelorism, median cleft lip and palate). The impairment of brain development is often less severe, with milder facial deformities, but this is not always the case.

Volpe cited two events that occur at approximately six weeks gestation as important to brain and cognitive development: the perforation of the roof of the fourth ventricle and the formation of the subarachnoid spaces. Both are particularly important with regard to potential causes of congenital hydrocephalus.

Cell Proliferation and Differentiation

After the initial division of the fertilized egg into blastomeres, the processes of gastrulation and, particularly, neurulation primarily involve changes in the shape of cells, rather than an increase in their number. Further development involves the production of cells through cell division (proliferation) and the differentiation of cells into types.

The process of cellular differentiation is far from understood completely. At present, it seems to be related to both intrinsic and extrinsic factors. Both neural and glial cells arise from the same population of epithelial cells. However, glial fibrillary acidic protein, a marker for glial cells, is present in recently divided cells in the proliferative zone around the ventricles before cell migration (Levitt and Rakic 1980).

Neural cells can be distinguished along a number of dimensions. Among these are the type of neurotransmitter synthesized by the cell, the form of the cell in terms of its dendritic branching pattern, and the pattern of connections with other cells. The presence of migratory errors in neural cell positioning, as well as the overproduction of cells and, perhaps, increased survival of some misplaced cells as a result of damage to others, makes the timing of differentiation important to an explanation of abnormally functioning nervous systems. In other words, if cell differentiation is largely a matter of postmigration positional influences, then a great deal of plasticity is built into the nervous system, and it can respond to early damage with this plasticity.

Few of these issues are settled at this time. Certainly, no overall answer is clear. Neurotransmitter "choice" seems to be fairly plastic and susceptible to the influences of the immediate environment. Experiments with cultured sympathetic ganglion cells have shown them to be able to change from adrenergic to cholinergic transmission, depending on the medium in which they are cultured (Furshpan et al. 1976; Potter, Landis, and Furshpan 1980). The medium in this case consisted of cardiac cells, strongly suggesting that the transmitter choice of neurons (albeit outside of the central nervous system) is influenced by the target cells that they innervate (Purves and Lichtman 1985).

The time at which neurons become programmed to develop their characteristic branching patterns, which are used to classify cell "types" in classic architectonic studies (Cajal 1911), is quite important. There is ample evidence that neurons contain some of the information that determines dendritic pattern irrespective of the surrounding environment. Banker and Cowan (1979), for instance, grew isolated hippocampal pyramidal neurons from fetal rats in tissue culture and compared them to those that developed in intact rats by four days after birth. The typical pyramidal cell morphology was present in the culture-grown cells, including a triangular soma, a large apical dendrite, and several basal dendrites. (Dendritic branching will be discussed more fully later.)

Purves and Lichtman (1985) cited the presence of variety in specific structure of dendritic patterns in genetically identical organisms as evidence of extrinsic factors affecting cellular development. Rakic (1975) was able to show that the presence of granule cells was a necessary condition for the specific arborization pattern of Purkinje cell dendrites in a strain of mutant mice that lack cerebellar granule cells. Typical numbers of dendrites were present, but the typical pattern was not. This would implicate both intrinsic and extrinsic factors in determining neural cell form.

Cell proliferation, or the production of new cells by cell division, is only one of the ways in which the brain "grows." The growth of cell processes (axons and dendrites, in the case of neurons) is another. In fact, the brain continues to grow long after the neural cells have ceased to be produced. The myelinization of cell fibers may continue well into adulthood.

Cell division occurs primarily in the two so-called proliferative zones lining the walls of the ventricles: the ventricular zone, immediately adjacent to the ventricles, and the subventricular zone, adjacent to it. Nowakowski (1987) speculated that the latter is a more phylogenetically recent development, since the majority of cortical cells come from the subventricular zone, whereas the ventricular zone contributes more substantially to such "older" cortical structures as the hippocampus (Nowakowski and Rakic 1981).

According to Dobbing and Sands (1973), the division of cells into neurons is essentially complete by around eighteen weeks gestation. The proliferation of neural cells generally precedes that of glial cells or at least terminates earlier. Glial cells continue to be produced, through mitosis in the germinal matrix layer surrounding the lateral ventricle, until around birth, although the production of new cells slows rapidly at twenty-six to twenty-eight weeks of gestation (Jammes and Gilles 1983). Dobbing and Sands's (1973) data indicated a continuous, albeit attenuated, increase in cell number in forebrain structures nearly to two postnatal years. Although it has long been known that cell density decreases with age, more recent evidence (discussed below) indicates that the number of neurons also decreases (Hamburger 1958, 1975; Hamburger and Oppenheim 1982; Janowsky and Finlay 1986). Despite this, the brain grows at a quite rapid rate, with the largest growth spurt occurring roughly from birth to two years of age (Dobbing and Sands 1973). The chief sources of this growth seem to be the development of neural processes and myelinization.

Cell Migration

It is not known how structural brain damage in the immature brain affects cell migration. Although defects in migration are becoming increasingly identified as sources of behavioral and cognitive abnormalities, these are generally thought to be due to genetic aberrations. For instance, cells that have migrated inappropriately have been found in the cortex, and particularly in the left hemisphere, of people with dyslexia (Galaburda, Sherman, and Geschwind 1983; Kemper 1984). Similar anomalies have been identified in mutant mice

(Sherman, Galaburda, and Geschwind 1985). Heterotopic, or mis-placed, cells have also been identified in the hippocampi of schizo-phrenic people (Kovelman and Scheibel 1983). However, it is quite clear that nongenetic factors such as exposure to alcohol can also influence cell migration (Miller 1985).

Cell migration from the initial proliferative zone around the ventri-cles takes place in either of two ways (Nowakowski 1987; Rakic 1990). Cells in subcortical structures such as the thalamus, hypothalamus, and dentate gyrus of the hippocampus migrate by what Nowakowski (1987) called *passive displacement.* That is, they migrate only a short distance from the proliferative zone, and cells that originate later more or less push them further peripherally. Cortical cells, on the other hand, show a much more active migratory pattern. They move by making adhesive contacts with a particular type of glial cell called *radial glia,* essentially pulling themselves along the glial path (Purves and Lichtman 1985). Unlike passive displacement, those cells that migrate earliest terminate their migration closest to their point of origin and later migrating cells move past them to reach their more peripheral locations.

By a mechanism not entirely known, neurons seem to recognize when their migration should stop. However, this process can err and neurons may end their migration too early or too late. In either case, they are not in their normal position and the groundwork is laid for abnormal connections between these and other cells. Rakic (1975) detailed how migratory failures of granule cells may alter the growth of dendritic patterns in their target Purkinje cells in the cerebella of mutant mice.

Nowakowski (1987) described four possibilities related to the fate of abnormally migrating cells: (1) axons of other cells that are in their normal positions will follow their usual path and *fail to make contact* with their normal target because it is out of position; (2) axons of other cells that are in their normal positions will follow an abnormal path to *make contact* with their abnormally positioned target; (3) axons from the cells that have migrated to the wrong position will follow an abnor-mal path to *make contact* with their normal targets; and (4) axons from the abnormally positioned neurons will *fail to find their normal targets.*

To the extent that any of the above possibilities occurs, the result-ing neural interconnectedness will approximate normal or abnormal "wiring" of the nervous system. It is interesting to speculate how early brain damage might interact with the possibilities outlined by Nowakowski. In the first place, there is good evidence that, when neurons migrate to the wrong position, both they and their target cells may make abnormal connections when the normal ones do not occur (Nowakowski and Davis 1985). It is also not known how often such migratory errors occur. Presumably, however, from all that is known regarding the role of competition for synaptic sites in determining cell or axon survival, the absence of competitive neurons because of early damage might allow the connections from abnormally positioned sites to survive. The likelihood of such an occurrence would be related to the timing of the migration and of the brain insult. Cortical cells originate last and migrate last, but generally before the time of birth (Rakic et al. 1974). The germinal matrix tissue where cortical cells proliferate is nearly exhausted by thirty weeks gestation, and those that are being produced during the range of premature birth are mostly glial cells (Wigglesworth 1988). Thus, damage at earlier fetal ages is most likely to influence the fate of migratory errors. There is some evidence that the proliferation and migration of cells destined for the cerebral cortex is most vulnerable from about the eighth to the fifteenth weeks of gestation in humans. Infants exposed in utero to the intense radiation from the atomic blasts in Japan during World War II were much more likely to develop mental retardation if the exposure was at eight to fifteen weeks gestation than if it was earlier or later (Otake and Schull 1984). This is considerably earlier than the timing for the kinds of damage related to postnatal complications of premature birth but not necessarily for the damage related to intrauterine complications or to the presence of toxic influences.

Dendritic Growth

The pattern of connectivity of neurons in the brain depends on not only the presence of neural cells and their axonal connections but also the pattern and viability of dendrites. After cell proliferation and migration to their eventual sites, neurons develop characteristic patterns of dendritic branches. Since these dendrites are the most typical site of connection with the axons of other neurons, alterations in dendritic patterns might have a profound effect on the ability of the brain to support normal cognitive functioning. Scheibel et al. (1985, 1990) and Simonds and Scheibel (1988) postulated that the degree of complexity in dendritic branching in a particular cortical area is related to the degree of behavioral complexity related to activities mediated by that area. The left posterior frontal area of the cortex (Broca's area), for instance, has more complex dendritic branching than the homologous area on the right (Scheibel et al. 1985). Furthermore, periods of increase in dendritic branching complexity of the language areas in the left hemisphere roughly correspond to periods of increase in language and motor development during early childhood (Simonds and Scheibel 1988). Cortical areas that mediate hand and finger dexterity show greater dendritic complexity than do those that mediate trunk sensation. However, there is no clear-cut difference between the dendritic complexity in the frontal and parietal association areas and that in the trunk area (Scheibel et al. 1990).

Purpura (1975) examined the growth of pyramid cell dendritic spines in the human fetal hippocampus and cortex. Dendritic growth of pyramidal neurons in both the hippocampus and the motor cortex reaches its peak at eighteen to twenty-four weeks gestation. The visual cortex, on the other hand, matures later, showing maximal dendritic growth of its pyramidal neurons about four to six weeks later. The development of spines on the dendrites of both granule cells and pyramidal cells in the hippocampus and cerebellum is also related to the time of origin of the cells. On cells that originate earlier, the dendritic spines develop earlier and more rapidly (Purpura 1975; Rakic 1975).

Afferent innervation from the axons of other neurons seems to be involved in dendritic growth. Rakic (1975) examined the role of afferent innervation from granule cells on the dendritic growth of Purkinje cells in the cerebellar cortex in the mouse. Although the timing of Purkinje cell dendritic growth coincides with the ingrowth of afferents from granule cells, experiments with mutant mice that have an absence of granule cells indicate that Purkinje cell dendrites grow at the same time, even in the absence of granule cells (Rakic and Sidman 1973). The particular pattern of dendritic growth, which is quite characteristic in the Purkinje cell, depends on the presence of granule cell afferents. Innervation from the normal parallel fibers from the granule cells seems to be necessary to guide the normal patterning of dendritic arbors (Rakic 1975).

The interdependence between afferent innervation and dendritic differentiation would imply that dendritic growth in even intact cells can be affected by genetic or traumatic alterations of other portions of the brain. The growth of dendritic spines can also be affected by early damage. In pyramidal neurons of the motor cortex, there is a progression in the development of apical dendritic spines from thin or long and thin spines early in development to short, stubby spines at later ages (Marin-Padilla 1972). Purpura (1975) reported that older children with severe mental retardation of unknown cause showed dendritic spines that were long and thin, like those of a normal preterm fetus. Also, the number of spines was reduced. In prematurely born infants with respiratory distress, both advanced development of dendritic spines and underdevelopment of dendritic spines were observed (Purpura 1975).

The development of dendritic spines continues well beyond birth (Marin-Padilla 1972). Branching patterns of dendrites continue to be modified throughout life (Scheibel et al. 1990). As Scheibel et al. (1990) pointed out, it seems logical to assume a relationship between dendritic complexity and the computational capacity of a particular area of the brain. Since dendritic growth is highly sensitive to a variety of influences, it may be a prime target for impairment by early brain injury.

Simonds and Scheibel (1988) conducted a fairly detailed investigation of dendritic development in the motor speech areas (Broca's area) and the orofacial zones of the left and right hemispheres. Their study was limited by using only seventeen cases covering a wide age range (three to seventy-two months) and looking only at pyramidal neurons in layer 5, rather than at more superficial cortical layers. With regard to dendritic growth itself, they found that the process is dynamic. There is a reciprocal relationship between proximal and distal branches, which may be continually changing. Maximal proximal growth is related to more limited growth of distal segments, and vice versa. Even after the more distal dendritic branches have developed, there is still active proximal growth or contraction, leaving the evolving dendritic system considerably plastic. The usual developmental pattern is that proximal branches exceed distal branches in both length and number early in development. As development continues, this pattern becomes reversed; by the second year of life, distal branches are longer and more numerous than are proximal ones.

In the first year, dendritic development is greater in the orofacial motor areas than in the motor speech zones in both hemispheres. After two years, this relationship has been reversed in both hemispheres. Of particular importance for laterality theorizing is the progressive alteration in the extent of dendritic development in the left versus the right hemisphere. Initially, the right hemisphere has more numerous and more lengthy dendritic branches. During the second year this pattern changes and the left hemisphere begins to "catch up" and eventually (by forty-two to seventy-two months) to exceed the right, primarily because of greater growth in the length of distal segments on the left side. Notably, however, the total distal segment length in the right motor speech area continues to exceed that of the left homologous area, even at older ages (forty-two to seventy-two months), a relationship that would presumably be reversed at even later ages.

Neuron Loss and Axon Retraction

Janowsky and Finlay (1986) reviewed the literature on normal neuron loss and axon retraction in the developing brain with the aim of speculating as to how perinatal brain damage might interact with such a process. There is a large literature on early neuronal death related to the development of the spinal cord and the spinal ganglia. It is clear that the typical pattern of muscular innervation is from multiple neurons and that, with the onset of muscle innervation, the majority of neurons die, leaving a single axon to innervate a single muscle fiber (Purves and Lichtman 1980). Presumably, neurons compete for synaptic sites (or for a trophic factor related to the synaptic site). Only a limited number of neurons can survive. However, the survival rate can be altered. For instance, depriving the motoneurons of target tissue results in rapid neuron loss (Hamburger and Oppenheim 1982). On the other hand, adding limb muscles reduces neuron loss (Hollyday and Hamburger 1976). Reduction of the neuronal population by artificial means results in increased survival of the remaining neurons (Pilar, Landmesser, and Burstein 1980).

Neural cell loss in spinal innervation of the musculature occurs early in development and results in the normal adult pattern of innervation. There seems to be much redundancy involved in initial multiple innervation, and serious errors in the pattern of innervation are not what is being corrected. In the brain, however, the initial pattern of connectivity, before cell loss, is much more diffuse and, in several instances, bears little resemblance to the adult pattern. For instance, the pattern of connectivity in the lateral geniculate of the adult primate is such that there are layers of distinct types of cell with an alternating arrangement related to each eye. In the fetus, however, there is no layering, and the cell types and projections from either eye are intermixed (Rakic 1976). Point-to-point callosal connections reciprocally connect only midline portions of the somatosensory or visual fields in the adult, but projections go to the entire somatosensory or visual cortex in early development (Innocenti 1981; Ivey and Killackey 1982). Even the laterality of projections is not specific early in development. Nasal retinal projections are contralateral in adult mammals but bilateral initially (Land and Lund 1979).

In most of the cases cited above, axon retraction is as important as cell death. Purves and Lichtman (1985) pointed out that, in many of these instances, there is no evidence of actual neuron loss, and they preferred the more inclusive term *synapse elimination* to cover both cell loss and axon retraction. Many neurons in the central nervous system show extensive axonal branching. The loss of terminals on such axons need not result in cell death (Jacobson 1978). Axon retraction begins late in fetal development, usually during the third trimester, and in the cortex and cerebellum may extend for several years postnatally (Janowsky and Finlay 1986).

Janowsky and Finlay (1986) referred to neuron death and axon retraction in terms of functions that are labeled *population matching, error correction,* and *sculpting.* The primary limiting factor in cell and axon survival is competition for terminal sites. Initial projections do not survive if all terminal sites are occupied. This is what is called *population matching. Error correction* refers to the fact that initial projections in the brain are often to inappropriate targets. The mechanism by which appropriate and inappropriate targets are segregated is not clear, although the fact that patterned activity seems to be necessary for neurons to segregate their connections appropriately could mean that aberrant neurons that lack correlation in their firings with the rest of the pattern could be detected as errors. In normal circumstances the majority of inappropriate connections do not survive. *Sculpting* refers to the fact that there is often a spatial pattern to neuronal loss. The central retina has a greater cell density than does the periphery in the adult. During normal development, neuronal loss is greater in the periphery than in the center, leading to the eventual adult pattern (Sengelaub and Finlay 1981).

Since competition for terminal sites is a key element in reducing the neuronal population and the number of axonal branches, it follows that destructive events that reduce the neuron population in one brain area may leave available target sites, leading to increased survival of neurons from another area. Because initial projections are more diffuse and often in error, such projections would survive as a consequence of early brain injury.

As pointed out by Janowsky and Finlay (1986), some likely candidates for such increased survival are the early diffuse callosal connections and ipsilateral corticospinal tracts, although the latter, which are known to be present after unilateral damage to the motor cortex, may be more a result of the sprouting of axonal branches from the contralateral tract. Cortical or thalamic damage could lead to decreased competition and increased survival of inappropriate connections. Damage to other subcortical nuclei or early germinal matrix cell loss leading to decreased cortical population in some areas might also lead to the survival of aberrant connections, although whether such a phenomenon is usual or not is unknown.

Of unknown but presumably considerable importance in determining the pattern of surviving axonal projections and synaptic connections is the role of early experience. This was amply demonstrated by Hubel and Wiesel in the visual systems of the cat (1963, 1965, 1970) and the monkey (Hubel, Wiesel, and LeVay 1977). During an early critical period between about four weeks and three months after birth, the closure of one eye in the kitten leads to a failure of ocular dominance columns to segregate normally in the striate cortex. Many more of the initial projections from the nondeprived eye survive than do those from the deprived eye, and the columns activated by the deprived eye are narrower than usual, whereas those from the nondeprived eye are wider. This alteration in pattern does not occur if eye closure is performed on the adult cat.

Since patterned neural activity seems to be crucial in determining the survival or loss of early neural connections, it is likely that both brain damage factors affecting cell loss and survival and early experience must interact to produce the eventual pattern of connectivity. How or what experiences are crucial and which parts of the brain are most susceptible to such influences are not known. However, it is typically found that variables related to social and environmental factors are often stronger determinants of outcome in prematurely born infants than are variables related to neurological factors.

Axonal Sprouting

Although much recent attention and speculation has focused on alterations in cell loss and axon retraction as consequences of early brain damage, there is considerable evidence that sprouting of new axonal connections may be of equal or greater importance. The extent and degree of axonal sprouting were shown to be related to age in several studies (Cotman and Lynch 1976; Fujito et al. 1984). Fujito et al. (1984) reported the results of several studies involving the placing of lesions in the sensory-motor area of the cortex in cats and the measurement of neural connections in the red nucleus. After damage to the ipsilateral cortex, there was evidence of sprouting from the contralateral cortex to replace the lost innervation. The likelihood of such sprouting was much greater in younger kittens and was almost nonexistent in adult cats.

Villablanca, Burgess, and Sonnier (1984) reported similar results after hemispherectomy in cats. In addition to less severe behavioral effects of early versus late lesions, they found that cortical frontal motor areas of the intact hemisphere sent axonal projections to the contralateral red nucleus and thalamus. Although they did not compare their results to those seen in lesioned adult cats, they did compare them to results in intact animals. In the intact cats, only ipsilateral projections were found. Most striking was the finding that the pattern of terminals for the abnormal contralateral projections was similar to that seen from ipsilateral projections in intact animals, indicating a reorganization process that mimicked the normal pattern. The authors hypothesized that their observations were due to the sprouting of new projections but admittedly were not able to rule out as an alternative explanation the survival of normal early projections that normally retract.

Although axonal sprouting may be extremely important in explaining recovery and plasticity after early brain damage, the extent to which it mimics normal connections should not be overestimated. Schneider (1973, 1979) demonstrated the development of abnormal neural connections in the hamster due to both dendritic and axonal sprouting, which in turn led to abnormal behavior patterns, causing him to question the adaptability of compensatory reactions to early brain injury.

Myelinization

Neural transmission is enhanced by the presence of myelin, which insulates the neural axon and increases the speed of depolarization down the axon. Myelin originates from glial cells, which show a rapid increase in number (*myelin gliosis*) immediately before the onset of myelogenesis. The nuclei of the glial cells enlarge, and premyelin lipids form in the cytoplasm of the cells. Finally, myelin sheaths, composed of lipids and proteins, are deposited around the axons of those neurons that must traverse any distance.

Yakovlev and Lecours (1967) extended the earlier work of Fleschig (1920) identifying the dates of myelinization of various regions of the human brain. Subsequent studies by Gilles, Shankle, and Dooling (1983) generally agreed with earlier findings, except that earlier ages of onset of myelinization were found in several tracts, especially the corpus callosum and anterior commissure. The most striking finding of Gilles, Shankle, and Dooling was the wide individual variation in the age of onset in different brains. Both they and Yakovlev and Lecours found wide variation between brain areas in the cycles of myelinization between onset and completion. Although the spinal cord begins myelinization somewhat earlier, the data of both Yakovlev and Lecours (1967) and Gilles, Shankle, and Dooling (1983) are in agreement that, with this exception, myelinization in the central nervous system generally does not begin until at least twenty weeks of gestation.

Some of the fiber systems myelinate quite early, particularly those of the brainstem related to the vestibular and cochlear systems, presumably for functional reasons related to primitive reflexes. In fact, Gilles, Shankle, and Dooling (1983) found an age of onset of less than twenty weeks for the medial longitudinal bundle in the brainstem.

Specific thalamocortical projections to the calcarine area and the pre- and postcentral somesthetic and propriokinesthetic areas myelinate early (in the first year of life), although the geniculotemporal projections to the auditory area take much longer to myelinate. Cortical projections subserving simple motor and sensory functions myelinate shortly thereafter and essentially in a similar time frame (Yakovlev and Lecours 1967).

Nonspecific thalamocortical projections myelinate later and do not complete the cycle of myelinization until well into childhood. The fiber tracts that myelinate latest, especially in terms of the completion of myelinization, are those of the reticular formation and the intracortical association fibers of the frontal, parietal, and temporal lobes. These latter fibers may continue to accumulate myelin well into adulthood. The cerebral commissure are intermediate between these extremes and continue myelinization nearly to adolescence (Yakovlev and Lecours 1967). The delayed onset and protracted cycle of myelinization of association cortex, particularly frontal areas and reticular projections, have figured into several explanations of attention problems, impulsive behavior, and poor problem solving in young children.

Leviton, Gilles, and Dooling (1983) were able to identify instances and sources of delayed myelinization in fetal and infant brains. Low birth weight or short gestational age, neonatal infections, siblings with seizures, and maternal anemia, third-trimester bleeding, and cigarette smoking (more than one pack per day) were all related to delayed onset of myelinization. Dobbing and Sands (1973) speculated as to the role of postnatal malnutrition in disorders of myelinization. More recently, Chiappelli et al. (1990) found that prenatal exposure to alcohol interfered with postnatal myelogenesis in rats.

The Development of the Cerebral Vascular System

In discussing the development of the cerebral vascular system, Pape and Wigglesworth (1979) emphasized the distinction between the embryonic and fetal periods of prenatal growth. Most authors agree with Streeter's (1951) distinction that the fetal stage begins with the formation of marrow in the humerus, which Lemire et al. (1975) estimated to occur usually around fifty-two gestational days. The distinction is important with regard to cerebrovascular development primarily because the stages of vascularization have been described in much greater detail in the embryo than during the fetal period (e.g., Duckett 1971; Padgett 1948). The distinction is somewhat arbitrary with regard to the actual development of the cerebral vascular system, since the development of some of the main venous architecture of the brain transcends the two stages. Other than with regard to the occurrence of arteriovenous malformations, the fetal period is of greater immediate importance so far as early brain injury is concerned.

Embryonic Stages

The development of the arterial system in the brain proceeds at earlier stages than does that of the venous system. According to the initial work by Padgett (1948) and later studies summarized by McLone and Naidich (1989), the basic arterial system largely develops between four and nine weeks of gestation. The initial stages include the emergence of the internal carotid arteries from the aortic arch and the development of longitudinal neural arteries that later become the basilar artery. As the external carotid and the basilar arteries begin to form, the internal carotid develops connections with the longitudinal neural artery to form the posterior communicating artery. By about five to six weeks gestational age, the vertebral, anterior cerebral, and superior cerebellar arteries begin to form, and by six weeks the internal carotid has formed divisions into the choroidal, middle cerebral, and anterior cerebral arteries. The middle cerebral artery develops several branches, which spread over the embryonic cerebral hemispheres, and the posterior cerebral artery begins to develop before the ninth gestational week.

The initial stages of vascularization of the cerebral hemispheres begin about the seventh week of gestation with the development of the *vascular tunic* (McLone and Naidich 1989). This tunic spreads over the neural epithelium through the developing subarachnoid space and goes through four embryonic stages (Duckett 1971). Initially, stem vessels from the vascular tunic penetrate the cortical anlage to the underlying intermediate zones. In the following two weeks they divide, sending out capillary-sized branches parallel to the cortical and ventricular surfaces. Within another three weeks, two more stages occur. A second wave of stem vessels arising from the pial vasculature either send out more parallel vessels or connect with vessels of the mantle layer and send off branches to the germinal layer.

The venous system of the brain develops later than the arterial system, with some venous patterns not being fully evident until term or even after birth (Padgett 1956). The cerebral cortex remains essentially avascular until term, at which time it rapidly acquires a venous drainage system, whereas the deep cerebral structures are vascularized some time before term (Towbin 1978).

The beginning of the venous drainage system dates from the formation of the primary head-sinus at about five weeks gestational age. This is the major early venous drainage from the brain and later feeds into the internal jugular vein as the latter develops. Around six to seven weeks, the subarachnoid space and meningeal layers are developing. As the hemispheres increase in size, the venous channels in the dural and pial layers become more separated and larger veins develop to traverse the subarachnoid space to reach the dural sinuses. At this stage, the veins and arteries cross each other, usually at right angles, but with vulnerability to arteriovenous malformations, in which there is influx of arterial flow into a vein (McLone and Naidich 1989).

In the next stages the primary head-sinus withers and is replaced by more definitive sinus development, such as the sigmoid sinus, marginal sinus, and, later, superior sagittal sinus. Around nine weeks gestational age, the great cerebral veins begin to form, including the vein of Galen and, at about twelve weeks, the basal cerebral vein. Further venous drainage patterns develop slowly as the cerebral hemispheres develop.

The Fetal Period

At the end of the embryonic period, the peripheral vascular system is sending branches inward and the cerebral arteries have developed, although the basal branches of the middle and anterior cerebral arteries are much larger, relative to other arteries supplying the cerebral hemispheres, than they will be at later stages of development. As the cerebral hemispheres develop, the cortical branches of the cerebral arteries become increasingly complex and tortuous (Kier 1974).

Pape and Wigglesworth (1979) described the development of the finer arterial branches and the capillary beds in the cerebral hemispheres in some detail. In the preterm fetus the major structural feature of the basal ganglia is the subependymal germinal matrix, which is situated mainly over the head and body of the caudate nucleus. The major blood supply to this area is from the recurrent artery of Heubner and the choroidal artery and lateral striate artery branches.

The source of more than 80 percent of intraventricular hemorrhages in newborns is the vascular bed of the germinal matrix (Pape and Wigglesworth 1979). A large capillary bed under the ependyma, over the whole caudate region, is most developed in the superficial and deep layers of the germinal matrix. The central mass of matrix tissue is relatively avascular (Pape and Wigglesworth 1979).

The arterial system in the developing fetal cortex shows extensive interconnections between adjacent stems of the same artery and between adjacent stems of different arteries. As pointed out by Pape and Wigglesworth (1979), this reflects the fact that the arteries only recently were part of a single vascular plexus and it is why the typical boundary zone infarcts observed in adult brains do not occur in the fetal brain. At term, when there is some regression of this rich interconnectedness, the classic patterns of infarcts are more likely to occur.

Between twenty-four weeks of gestation and term there is a marked increase in the blood supply to the cerebral cortex. At twenty-four weeks gestation the cortical vessels are primarily long spiral vessels that branch off of the peripheral vessels and run at right angles to the cortical surface, nearly to the ventricle wall, where they divide into the capillary bed. About twenty-eight weeks, increasing numbers of short cortical arteries have developed between the longer perforating arteries. As the cortical cells continue to develop in terms of the elaboration of their dendritic processes and the cortical gyri develop, there is a parallel increase in the development of short cortical arteries to supply the metabolic needs of the cortical cell structure. At the same time, the perforating arteries increase primarily in size and in the development of branches into the future white matter area (Pape and Wigglesworth 1979).

By thirty-two weeks gestation the germinal matrix has all but disappeared. Those vessels that supplied the matrix tissue are superseded in size by the other cerebral arteries. Heubner's artery and the choroidal arteries remain as the chief supply of blood to the medial aspects of the head of the caudate nucleus and the body and tail of the caudate, respectively (Pape and Wigglesworth 1979). At the same time, there is a gradual shift in the major targets for the cerebral blood supply from the brainstem and basal ganglia to the cerebral cortex.

The Midbrain and Cerebellum

The pattern of arterial development to the midbrain and cerebellum is similar to that of the cerebrum. The major difference is that the cerebellum is still immature enough at term that the major development of short vessels has not occurred (Pape and Wigglesworth 1979). Otherwise, there is a similar pattern of long perforating vessels and a rich surface capillary bed developing from the vascular plexus in the leptomeninges. In addition, separate arteries supplying the deep cerebellar nuclei enter via the cerebellar peduncles.

In the cerebellum the fetal pattern of blood supply, which consists of dense capillary beds in the core of the folium and on the surface, with a relatively avascular layer in between, is paralleled by the venous system. These patterns seem to be responsible for the primary sites of cerebellar hemorrhage in the newborn being in the cortical area just below the pial capillary network or related to venous infarct in the core of the folium (Pape and Wigglesworth 1979).

Venous Drainage

The deep venous system drains the blood supply from the basal ganglia, white matter, and germinal matrix in the fetus. Drainage is by way of the thalamostriate veins and septal and basal veins to the vein of Galen. Although there is a cortical venous system, which drains most of the cortical and superficial white matter areas that are supplied by the short cortical arteries, many of these arteries drain instead into branches of the thalamostriate system (Pape and Wigglesworth 1979). As gestation increases, there is increasing drainage from intermediate white matter areas related to more extensive development of branches from the perforating arteries into capillary beds at that level. At the same time, the network of cortical veins increases as the short cortical arteries continue to proliferate.

The germinal matrix tissue has a poorly defined capillary-venous system that drains into either fine branches of the thalamostriate vein or directly into the thalamostriate or branches of the internal cerebral vein. As the germinal matrix thins out from thirty weeks gestation onward, the basal ganglia drain primarily into striate veins that terminate in the basal vein.

Implications for Brain Damage

The pattern of development of the vascular system in the brain has a direct bearing on the most likely location of damage at different stages of fetal development. Most authors agree that one of the major causes of brain damage in the fetus or prematurely born neonate is hypoxia-induced hemorrhage (Schulte 1988; Towbin 1978; Wigglesworth and Pape 1978). Under normal circumstances, cerebral blood flow in the adult brain does not respond directly or passively to changes in systemic blood pressure within the physiological range (Lassen 1959). Autoregulation mechanisms that contract or dilate the cerebral vessels are triggered by changes in the extravascular tissue in response to increases or decreases in the levels of oxygen or carbon dioxide (Lassen 1974). These mechanisms maintain a constant cerebral blood flow in the face of changes in systemic pressure within the physiological range. Wider fluctuations in the systemic blood pressure can cause a failure of the autoregulation mechanism (Oleson 1973).

In the newborn and especially in the prematurely born newborn, the autoregulation mechanism is easily overridden (Pape and Wigglesworth 1979). In newborn infants, including prematurely born infants with respiratory distress, cerebral blood flow is more closely related to systemic pressure than to any other factor, including tissue pH, oxygen, or carbon dioxide (Lou, Lassen, and Friis-Hansen 1977).

Lou, Lasson, and Friis-Hansen (1979) demonstrated that a state of hypoxia in the distressed newborn could lead to hypotension. Then, because of immaturely developed mechanisms of autoregulation of blood pressure, this hypotension could result in subsequent hypertension in an attempt to restore blood pressure and a consequent breakdown of the capillary bed, primarily in the subependymal germinal matrix. Lou, Griesen, and Tweed (1988) formally outlined the sequence of events beginning with hypoxia-related impairment of autoregulation followed by hypotension-inducing hypoxic-ischemic infarction, which is followed by blood pressure increases leading to periventricular hemorrhage, which spreads into infarcted tissue and induces perihemorrhagic ischemia. The initial hypoxic insult in their scheme may be as minor as normal vaginal delivery if the delivery is premature, since studies of autoregulation of blood pressure in fetal lambs have shown it to be very fragile and sensitive to minor fluctuations in arterial oxygen concentration. As Towbin (1978) pointed out, various factors that may occur before birth may also result in hypoxia. Naeye and Peters (1988) included severe maternal anemia, third-trimester hypo- or hypertension, and multiple births as causative factors leading to antenatal hypoxia.

Towbin (1978) and Pape and Wigglesworth (1979) gave similar and elegant descriptions of the relationships between fetal age and the site of intracranial hemorrhage. The development of a more elaborate vascular system in the subcortex basal ganglia area than in the cortex is ample justification for the site of hemorrhage to be predominantly subcortical with decreasing gestational age. Data from autopsy of fetuses and infants of various gestational ages, presented by Dooling and Gilles (1983), indicate a peak in germinal matrix hemorrhage around twenty-four to twenty-seven weeks. Deep white matter hemorrhages increase in prevalence up to full term. Cortical hemorrhages, in their series, remain a small and fairly constant percentage from twenty weeks of gestation to term.

Intraventricular hemorrhage arises most often from hemorrhage in the germinal matrix and occurs primarily in preterm infants of less than thirty-two gestational weeks, and most often of less than thirty weeks (Pape and Wigglesworth 1979). The most frequent site of germinal matrix hemorrhage is over the head of the caudate nucleus opposite the foramen of Monro. Eighty-five percent of germinal matrix hemorrhages occur in this region (Leech and Kohnen 1974). The state of maturity of the germinal matrix vascular bed influences the site of hemorrhage. Hambleton and Wigglesworth (1976) reported that, in infants of twenty-eight weeks gestation or less, the hemorrhage is more likely to occur over the body of the caudate. There is an equal frequency of germinal matrix hemorrhage in either hemisphere, and bilateral hemorrhage is present in about 50 percent of cases (Leech and Kohnen 1974).

The rupturing of blood into the lateral ventricles can lead to post-hemorrhage hydrocephalus. Clotted blood occurs at the site of rupture as well as around the choroid plexus and may spread throughout the ventricular system. One or both ventricles may become dilated, depending on whether the clot moves through or occludes the foramen of Monro. When the whole ventricular system is filled, the blood often extends into the subarachnoid space, preventing normal drainage and resorption of cerebrospinal fluid (Wigglesworth 1988).

Towbin (1978) and Pape and Wigglesworth (1979) disagreed sharply regarding the vascular site of germinal matrix hemorrhage. Towbin (1978) regarded venous infarction as the most common hemorrhagic occurrence, whereas Pape and Wigglesworth (1979) cited rupture of the fine capillary bed as the usual source of hemorrhage and venous infarction as a secondary phenomenon. Wigglesworth (1988) reported that both types of hemorrhage could occur and pointed out the differing pathological appearance of each. Hemorrhages due to venous infarction tend to remain acutely localized around the thalamostriate vein or its branches and are often unilateral. Small capillary bleeds are more often bilateral and often spread into associated white matter areas because of a preexisting region of periventricular leucomalacia. The typical site is the optic radiation at the trigone of the lateral ventricles or the deep white matter near the foramen of Monro, especially at the juncture of the internal capsule and the corpus callosum (Shuman and Selednik 1980). Wigglesworth (1988) speculated that the latter type of hemorrhage may be the source of a relatively high incidence of spastic diplegia associated with intraventricular hemorrhage.

Intraventricular hemorrhage typically develops postnatally in the premature infant. Most frequently, hemorrhage occurs two to three days after delivery (Dyer et al. 1973). With increasing gestational age, there is a stronger association between intraventricular hemorrhage and respiratory distress syndrome associated with hyaline membrane disease (Wigglesworth et al. 1977). Pape and Wigglesworth (1979) offered the hypothesis that, in the more immature infant, postnatal circulation may itself be so fragile as to initiate the events leading to intraventricular hemorrhage. As gestational age increases, additional precipitating events are required to cause intraventricular hemorrhage. Apnea of prematurity is known to be associated with intraventricular hemorrhage, and other stressors, such as asphyxia, hypothermia, or infection, may also lead to the syndrome (Pape and Wigglesworth 1979).

In addition to intraventricular hemorrhage, primary hemorrhage may occur at other sites in the brain of the newborn. These will be discussed in considerably less detail because either they occur much less often or their consequences are more benign than those of intraventricular hemorrhage.

Subarachnoid hemorrhage is a relatively common finding on autopsy of infants who died shortly after birth or were stillborn. Dooling and Gilles (1983) reported leptomeningeal hemorrhage as the most common site of hemorrhage in their series. As mentioned previously, intraventricular hemorrhage may involve a spread of blood from the ventricular system into the subarachnoid space, usually involving posthemorrhagic hydrocephalus. Bleeding from the fine vessels of the leptomeningeal plexus also occurs and is usually a result of an anoxic episode (Larroche 1977) but may result from hemostatic failure (Courville 1971). Pape and Wigglesworth (1979) indicated that this is rarely a cause of death and usually does not lead to any particular handicap. Subarachnoid hemorrhage is more often seen in the preterm infant but may occur at term also (Amiel-Tison 1973). A related lesion involving subarachnoid hemorrhage over only the convexity of the brain may have more serious consequences. The typical finding is a firm clot of blood, usually over the occipital or temporal lobe, with two-thirds reported over the temporal lobes and usually on the left side (Larroche 1977). Compression effects of the clot may be thought to cause more severe consequences than generalized subarachnoid hemorrhages (Pape and Wigglesworth 1979).

Cerebellar hemorrhages occur in approximately 10 percent of infants with very low birth weight (Pape, Armstrong, and Fitzhardinge 1977). As mentioned earlier, the most usual site is the cerebellar cortex, which is heavily vascularized. Occasionally, hemorrhage occurs in the subependymal layer of the roof of the fourth ventricle (Pape and Wigglesworth 1979). The functional significance of cerebellar hemorrhage is uncertain, although coordination or balance difficulties would be expected to ensue, given the normal role of the cerebellum in these activities.

Cortical hemorrhage is seen most often in term infants but is relatively uncommon even then (Dooling and Gilles 1983). It is most often associated with severe asphyxia, which may involve arterial infarcts (Friede 1975). Primary white matter hemorrhages usually occur in preterm infants and are associated with severe birth asphyxia (Pape and Wigglesworth 1979).

Nonhemorrhagic ischemic lesions are fairly common in the newborn and have been increasingly implicated in functional handicaps during later development. They may occur in either the preterm or the term infant but are more prevalent in the preterm (Smith, Reynolds, and Taghizadeh 1974).

The most common ischemic lesion in the preterm infant is periventricular leucomalacia, a condition named for the characteristic "white spots" of necrotic tissue in the periventricular white matter. Periventricular leucomalacia is thought to represent a process of necrosis of tissue due to lack of oxygenation related to episodes of hypotension (Sinha et al. 1985). It begins at the boundary zones between the medullary artery branches entering the white matter from the cortex and the branches of the thalamostriate artery, which supplies the ependyma and adjacent periventricular white matter (DeReuck, Chattha, and Richardson 1972; Takashima and Tanaka 1978). Pathologically, large areas of periventricular leucomalacia become liquefied and then cystic, with the cysts gradually disappearing but impairment in myelination and glial scars remaining (Dubowitz, Bydder, and Mushin 1985).

Since the typical lesion in periventricular leucomalacia includes the white matter areas through which the corticospinal tracts pass, it is considered to be the lesion chiefly responsible for spastic diplegia (Pape and Wigglesworth 1979). Lateral extension of the lesion affects the arms as well as the legs and may extend into association and commissural fiber tracts. More posterior lesions in the optic radiation would be expected to interfere with vision, and auditory pathways may also become involved. Pape and Wigglesworth (1979) discussed the likelihood of severe motor and mental handicap and sensory impairment caused by extensive white matter destruction of fiber pathways as a result of periventricular leucomalacia, even without cortical lesions.

Some of the biochemical changes that lead to cell death after hypoxia or ischemia are well known. Others, such as alterations in neurotransmitters, are only in initial stages of investigation (Novotny 1989).

Changes in ion gradients include an increase in extracellular potassium and a decrease in sodium, chloride, and calcium ions. The increase in intracellular calcium has been implicated as a cause of cell death (Siesjo 1981).

One of the earliest cellular changes in response to hypoxia or ischemia is increased glycolysis and glycogenolysis leading to an increase in the level of lactic acid and a decrease in the levels of brain glucose and glycogen (Vanucci and Duffy 1977). In the newborn, the subcortical gray matter has a higher rate of glucose utilization than does the cortex, an observation that has been cited as another explanation for a higher incidence of subcortical disease in the asphyxiated newborn (Novotny 1989). Decreases in the level of phosphocreatinine and increases in the level of inorganic phosphate are also correlated with glucose utilization and lactate production and have been cited as good prognostic indicators for outcome in newborns (Hope et al. 1984).

Hemorrhage or hypoxia-ischemia in the premature infant may cause damage to the developing brain in a variety of ways. The mechanisms may not be as simple as they might appear, although substantial cell degeneration in a large area can lead to functional loss. As such lesions become chronic, the initial devitalized tissue and blood are replaced by scarring and cavitation. Large chronic lesions of this sort are found at autopsy in children with cerebral palsy and mental retardation (Towbin 1978).

Interactions between the Timing of Injury and the Age of Assessment

Although the research of Kennard (1936, 1938, 1942) is most often cited because of her finding that earlier brain damage results in greater sparing of function (the "Kennard principle"), her other finding, of equal importance, was that the extent of the impairment varied depending on the age at which the animal was tested. Some behavioral deficits may not be apparent until the animal reaches the age at which the damaged structures would normally be involved in mediating the behavior. This finding has most often been cited with regard to the so-called silent or delayed effects of damage to prefrontal cortex (Goldman 1976).

Nonneman et al. (1984) examined issues related to the development of prefrontal cortex, the head of the caudate nucleus, and the mediodorsal thalamus in monkeys. As indicated earlier, these connections are good candidates for damage related to premature birth because of the proximity of germinal matrix hemorrhage to the caudate. Lesions of either the dorsolateral frontal cortex or the orbital frontal cortex in adult monkeys produced deficits on a spatial delayed response task. However, when two-month-old monkeys were lesioned and tested, dorsolateral frontal lesions had no effect on performance, whereas orbital lesions produced a deficit. When early-lesioned animals were tested at later ages, the opposite effect was seen: dorsolateral lesions produced a deficit, whereas orbital lesions did not (Goldman 1971, 1972). Early lesions of the caudate and mediodorsal thalamus produced deficits at both younger and older ages (Goldman 1974; Tucker and Kling 1967).

Although Nonneman et al. (1984) cited the above studies as evidence that the caudate, mediodorsolateral thalamus, and orbital frontal areas mature early, while the dorsolateral frontal cortex matures later, it is not clear what this really means. Synaptogenesis, or the formation of synaptic contacts, is, presumably, a crucial factor in establishing the readiness of a cortical area to mediate behavior. Goldman-Rakic (1987) showed that measures of synaptic density indicate that all cortical areas mature concurrently in this respect. Synaptogenesis matures earlier in subcortical areas such as the caudate nucleus and superior colliculus than in the cortex.

In both cortical and subcortical areas, the synaptic density reaches a peak in early development that is well above that found in adulthood. Thereafter, there is progressive elimination of synapses until the adult level is reached. It is not clear, from the available data, that synapse elimination progresses at similar rates across all cortical areas.

If synaptogenesis is concurrent in different cortical areas, then the formation of synapses cannot account for differential mediation of behaviors by different cortical areas. This is not to say that synaptogenesis is not necessary for various behaviors, since a variety of behaviors in the rhesus monkey seem to emerge at the time of the peak formation of synapses. This includes the ability to perform the spatial delayed response task by unoperated monkeys (Goldman-Rakic 1987). Fischer (1987), in a response to Goldman-Rakic (1987), pointed out that the peak period of synaptogenesis in rhesus monkeys at two to four months postnatally corresponds to seven to twelve months postnatally in the human. This is the time of several major developmental accomplishments in sensorimotor development.

If synaptogenesis cannot account for the differential role of various cortical areas in mediating behavior at different ages, then there are other candidates, such as the progression of myelination, which is quite different for different areas and extends well into later development in the prefrontal cortex. Also, synapse elimination may progress at different rates for different cortical areas.

A reasonable general hypothesis, implied by both Goldman-Rakic and Fischer, is that cortical maturation is a necessary condition for the accomplishment of some tasks at some ages but that the maturation of cognitive abilities is also a process that builds upon itself and is not simply a matter of the development of brain structures. Assuming this to be the case, the solution of any particular cognitive task could involve different areas of the brain, depending on the use of different cognitive abilities at different ages. This is Luria's (1980) concept of functional reorganization.

If different areas of the brain are involved in similar behaviors at different ages, then brain damage could lead to results similar to those observed by Goldman (1972) in lesioned monkeys. Some tasks might show no effect of damage to a cortical or subcortical site at early ages but might show impaired performance at a later age, when the abilities mediated by the damaged site would normally be used to perform the task. It is also possible that damage could lead to early impairment but not later impairment if the performance of a task were able to be organized using other brain areas at later ages. Still, some tasks might be sensitive to brain damage at all ages if the same abilities were always used to solve the task or if certain crucial skills could not develop to serve as a basis for later cognitive development.

2

Genetic Disorders

A Brief Overview of Genetics

There is hardly a field in which progress has been so rapid as genetics. Chiefly, this has had to do with molecular genetics, although population genetics has had a substantial influence on the theorizing regarding inherited behavior and the transmission of biological and behavioral disorders.

At the heart of current genetic theory is the structure of deoxyribonucleic acid (DNA), as first described by Watson and Crick (1953). Genes are made up of stretches of DNA, which are helix-shaped double coils of ring-shaped carbon-nitrogen molecules of one of the four nucleotide bases: adenine, guanine, thymine, or cytosine. The spiral structure of DNA has been described as like a ladder or staircase, the "rungs" or "steps" of which are composed of pairs of opposing nucleotide bases. The base pairs are always formed by bonds of either adenine and thymine or, alternatively, guanine and cytosine. Genes are located on chromosomes, and chromosomes are located in the nuclei of our cells. Humans have 46 chromosomes, around 100,000 genes, and 3–3.5 billion base pairs of nucleotides.

DNA is involved in two functions that are extremely important for an understanding of genetic effects. The first is the translation of DNA structure to ribonucleic acid (RNA) so the DNA information may pass from the nucleus to the cytoplasm of a cell and be used as a code for making proteins. In DNA translation the DNA double spiral splits apart and one side is transcribed into a new molecule of RNA, which is similar to the original DNA except that uridine is substituted for thymine as a base. The RNA molecule travels outside the nucleus to ribosomes situated in the cytoplasm, where the base sequences, in sets of three, are translated into amino acids. The amino acids in turn form proteins or specialized proteins used in chemical reactions, called *enzymes*. In this way, the genetic code contained in the DNA controls all of the chemical processes in the body.

The other function of DNA is to transmit genetic information from one generation to the next. In doing this, the DNA splits and each side of the spiral duplicates the other, yielding two identical DNA molecules where once there was only one. In the process of meiosis, specialized cells, called *gametes,* are formed as either sperm or egg cells, each containing only one member of each pair of chromosomes. During fertilization, the sperm and egg combine to yield zygotes with all twenty-three pairs of chromosomes, half from each parent.

Genes are located on the chromosomes. Each chromosome has a long arm (denoted q) and a short arm (denoted p) that come together at a centromere. Chromosomes represent long sequences of genes. Each gene is composed of segments of DNA that code for amino acids, and thus each gene codes for a specific enzyme or protein. Genes are not as regularly arranged within the DNA as this account would imply, since they are broken into segments, some (exons) that code for the protein and some (introns) that seem to act as spacers. When the gene is read into RNA, there is a two-step process in which the RNA corresponding to the introns is deleted.

Inheritance refers to the transmission of genes from one generation to another. The basic laws of inheritance were worked out by Mendel in 1866. The crucial assumption is that, since any pair of chromosomes represents genetic material from both parents, there are duplicate genes, or alleles (which are, in fact, alternate forms of the same gene), on the two chromosomes. The location of either allele on the chromosome is called its *locus*. As Mendel demonstrated, two alleles do not yield a compromise, but rather each allele is either dominant or recessive. A dominant allele produces its effects whether the other allele is dominant or recessive. A recessive allele produces its effects only if the other allele is also recessive. Even though a recessive allele is not expressed in a particular individual, it may be passed on to the next generation, in which case the parent with the recessive gene is called a carrier.

Genes that reside on any of the chromosomes other than the X or Y sex chromosomes are referred to as having autosomal inheritance, since these twenty-two pairs of chromosomes are called autosomes. Autosomal inheritance may be dominant or recessive. Just because a gene is inherited as a dominant allele does not ensure that it will be expressed in the phenotype. In fact, simple rules of dominant or recessive inheritance apply to only some genetic traits. Dominance may be incomplete, leading to some compromise or blending between traits. Codominance also occurs, as in human blood types, where both alleles contribute to the phenotype. Many traits are also controlled by several alleles (polygenic inheritance). The expression of a gene may be variable for these and other reasons. The likelihood that a gene will be expressed is referred to as its *penetrance*.

Genes that are carried on a sex chromosome have a different mode of inheritance depending on whether the recipient is male or female. Since females have two X chromosomes, an allele may be recessive in the mother but be expressed in her son, since he has only one X chromosome. This is referred to as X-*linked recessive inheritance*. Recessive inheritance can also be passed to a daughter who inherits the dominant allele from the father, in which case she is heterozygous for the gene and is a carrier.

Mendel's principle of the independent assortment of genes often does not hold up in reality. Although the chromosomes display independent assortment, genes on the same chromosome are inherited together, a phenomenon referred to as *gene linkage*. Even gene linkage, however, has relatively routine exceptions because, during meiosis, when homologous chromosomes pair to form tetrads, material is exchanged between the homologues. This process is called *crossing over* or *genetic recombination*. Since genes near each other tend to remain linked even during recombination, the resulting inheritance patterns can be used to determine gene locations.

Genetic disorders may be due to single autosomal genes, be sex-linked, be polygenic, or be due to chromosomal abnormalities. Chromosomal abnormalities most often involve the duplication of a chromosome as a result of nondisjunction during meiosis. Down syndrome, for instance, is a result of an extra twenty-first chromosome. Duplications of the X and Y chromosomes are not uncommon, nor is deletion of the Y chromosome (Turner syndrome). Partial duplication may result from the translocation of a portion of a chromosome so it is attached to another while two normal chromosomes are already present. Partial deletions or inversions of a portion of a chromosome with respect to the rest of the chromosome may also occur.

Single-Gene Disorders

Phenylketonuria

Phenylketonuria (PKU) is a well-recognized recessive single-gene disorder that affects 1:10,000–20,000 live births (Benson and Fensom 1985). The nonfunctional gene codes for the enzyme phenylalanine hydroxylase, which is involved in the hydroxylation of phenylalanine (Phe) to tyrosine (Choo et al. 1979). Affected individuals cannot convert phenylalanine to tyrosine, resulting in inadequate levels of tyrosine in the brain, which affects the levels of dopamine, norepinephrine, and serotonin in the central nervous system (Butler et al. 1981).

Since the 1950s it has been known that the restriction of dietary Phe can avert the mental retardation associated with PKU (Bickel, Gerrard, and Hickmans 1954; Williamson et al. 1981). Questions have arisen, however, as to the effects of delayed or early terminated dietary treatment, as well as whether the elimination of gross retardation also eliminates mild cognitive and learning problems.

Untreated individuals with PKU are usually severely retarded and exhibit a variety of behaviors that might be loosely defined as disinhibited (Paine 1957). Delayed dietary treatment results in less severe forms of the disorder (McKean 1971). With treatment begun in infancy, IQ levels are usually in the normal range but often below matched or sibling controls (Koch et al. 1984).

More recently, the age at which dietary restriction can be relaxed has been moved upward to eight to ten years or even adolescence (Fishler et al. 1989). Fishler et al. (1989) found that reading, spelling, and IQ suffered if children were taken off the restricted diet between ages six and ten. However, even those maintained on the diet showed declining scores on measures of arithmetic, language, and perceptual skills equivalent to those children who went off the diet at age six. Visual and visuomotor abilities were deficient in both groups of children with PKU, compared to unaffected siblings. Michel, Schmidt, and Ratzler (1990) also found impairment of Performance IQ, visual perception, and mathematics in early-treated children with PKU at age five. Mathematical problems remained at age six, and high levels of plasma Phe were related to lowered Performance IQ. Interestingly, speech and language measures have not proven to be impaired in early-treated children with PKU, nor have they been related to concurrent dietary control of Phe intake (Ozanna, Krimmer, and Murdoch 1990).

Welsh et al. (1990) undertook a detailed study of cognitive functioning in early-treated four- to five-year-old children with PKU to test a specific hypothesis regarding the cognitive deficit found in spite of early dietary treatment. Briefly stated, their hypothesis was that, even with dietary treatment, there is insufficient conversion of Phe to tyrosine, resulting in lowered levels of tyrosine in the brain. This leads to lowered levels of dopamine, epinephrine, and serotonin, but specifically the depletion of dopamine affects cognition. The depletion of dopamine is hypothesized to impair executive function through its effect on synaptic transmission in the prefrontal cortex. Welsh et al. defined executive function as "the ability to maintain an appropriate problem solving set for attainment of future goals." From the maintenance of such a problem-solving set comes impulse control, organized search, planning, and flexibility of behavior. Operationally, such a set can be defined as age-appropriate performance on measures of visual search, verbal fluency, motor planning, and complex strategic problem solving in the absence of distraction from the task strategy or perseveration on old response sets.

Welsh et al. compared eleven early-treated children with PKU to a control group matched on IQ, age, and ethnicity. Both groups were mostly female, and socioeconomic status was slightly higher in the control group. Performance on the various cognitive measures within the PKU group was also examined in relation to concurrent Phe blood level, the mean of all past Phe levels since birth, and the highest Phe level during infancy, before dietary treatment.

Both the children with PKU and the controls were given a battery of cognitive measures which included a visual search task, a measure of verbal fluency, a rapid motor sequencing task, and a planning task (Tower of Hanoi). Performance across all four tasks was also averaged to yield an executive function composite score. In addition, a picture recognition task, measuring short-term memory, was administered as a control task on the assumption that it did not involve executive function.

The results of the study were quite clear-cut. While not differing on Verbal, Performance, or Full-Scale IQ or on the control task of picture recognition, the children with PKU performed significantly worse than the controls on the executive function composite score and on each individual task. Both the concurrent Phe level and the mean lifetime Phe level were negatively correlated with the executive function composite score at significant levels.

The results of the study by Welsh et al. (1990) provide evidence that, even in patients with early-treated PKU, the incomplete control of Phe by dietary methods has a negative effect on cognitive function. Furthermore, the significant correlation between the concurrent Phe level and cognitive function indicates that the effect of Phe is ongoing and, presumably, amenable to further treatment. With regard to the mechanism and pathway for producing Phe effects, the confirmation of their hypothesis that executive functions are primarily what are impaired supported the model of frontal lobe dopamine deficiency developed by Welsh et al. The model needs further exploration but is useful for conceptualizing a number of other disorders, most obviously attention deficit hyperactivity disorder and, possibly, Tourette syndrome (Comings 1990).

Neurofibromatosis (Von Recklinghausen Disease)

Neurofibromatosis is one of the least studied inherited disorders, in terms of its cognitive characteristics. It is inherited as a single-gene autosomal dominant disorder and is characterized by multiple fibrous tumors on peripheral, spinal, and cranial nerve roots. Early reports generally concluded that mental retardation was common in this disorder, but more recent studies suggest a less clear cognitive picture. Carey, Lamb, and Hall (1979) reported that just under 10 percent of 131 patients were mentally retarded. Samuelsson and Riccardi (1989) reported that 45 percent of 71 patients in a total population sample were in the borderline to mild range of mental retardation and 2 patients were moderately retarded. Wadshy, Lindehammer, and Feg-Olofsson (1989) found that 11 percent of children with neurofibromatosis were mentally deficient, whereas Stine and Adams (1989) found lower than average IQs but no cases of obvious mental retardation in their survey. They also reported that IQ levels showed an increase with age. Carey, Lamb, and Hall (1979) reported an association between macrocephaly and retardation in their sample.

Shprintzen and Goldberg (1986) pointed out that learning disabilities characterized a fairly large proportion of the cases they saw and that earlier reports of a high incidence of mental retardation may have confused intellectual retardation and learning disabilities. Carey, Lamb, and Hall (1979) found learning problems in 11 percent of their patients. Stine and Adams (1989) reported a 37 percent greater incidence of learning disabilities in patients with neurofibromatosis than in their siblings. Learning problems occurred in visual perception, spelling, and arithmetic. Wadshy, Lindehammer, and Feg-Olofsson (1989) found difficulties in reading and spelling in 41 percent of their sample and behavior problems in 28 percent.

The specific type of cognitive disability related to academic learning has not been identified thus far in persons with neurofibromatosis, nor has the pathological mechanism for producing cognitive deficits been isolated. Shprintzen and Goldberg (1986) suggested that the chief problems may be related to attention and distractibility, which, in combination with low average or borderline IQ, impairs academic learning in a nonspecific way. Whatever the difficulty, Samuelsson and Riccardi (1989) found that, even with normal intelligence, individuals with neurofibromatosis typically attained lower levels of academic and vocational achievement than did their unaffected relatives.

Duchenne Muscular Dystrophy

Although primarily thought of as a neuromuscular disease, Duchenne muscular dystrophy (DMD) has long been known to be associated with some cognitive impairment. Recent advances in identifying the gene locus for DMD on the p21 segment of the X chromosome and in identifying a gene product, dystrophin, promise eventual understanding of the mental as well as physical aspects of the disorder.

How to characterize the cognitive picture in DMD had been a topic of much research and some controversy. The questions have revolved around two issues: whether the deficit is global or selective and whether it is static or progressive. The global deficit hypothesis has gone out of favor with increasing evidence that language is more impaired than visual-perceptual ability, usually apparent as a Verbal-Performance discrepancy on the Weschler Intelligence Scale for Children-Revised (WISC-R) (Karagan 1979; Karagan and Zellweger 1978; Marsh and Munsat 1974). The presence of a verbal deficit has not been unanimously accepted, as some authors have pointed to psychodynamic or experiential factors as interfering with verbal expression in DMD (e.g., Mearig 1979). However, this is a minority point of view and the evidence in favor of diminished verbal abilities is almost overwhelming.

It is quite clear that neither overall intelligence nor verbal abilities decline with age in DMD. The reverse (i.e., that the deficit does not diminish with age) is not so clearly true. Intellectual and particularly verbal impairment have been shown to be present from early ages (Kaplan, Osborne, and Elias 1986; Smith, Sibert, and Harper 1990). Smith, Sibert, and Harper (1990) studied the early cognitive, language, and locomotor development of thirty-three boys with DMD who were six years old or younger (mean age, 3.4 years). Both the children with DMD and a control group of unaffected boys were assessed three times over a one-year period. In addition to assessing both differences and change in cognition, language, and locomotor scores, the investigators related the results to assessments of the quality of the home environment, maternal intelligence, and the presence of behavior problems.

Smith, Sibert, and Harper (1990) found that, even at such young ages, the youngsters with DMD were deficient, compared to controls, in overall cognitive development and especially in locomotion and speech. Both the children with DMD and the control subjects remained static in terms of quotients derived from the cognitive and language measures over the one-year period, while the subjects with DMD decreased in locomotor scores. Interestingly, maternal intelligence and the quality of the home environment were both positively correlated with cognitive and language measures in the control group but *not* for the subjects with DMD. Conversely, behavior problems were negatively correlated with cognitive and language scores in the group with DMD but *not* in the control subjects. Locomotor scores were not related to behavior problems in either group.

Besides confirming early cognitive and language impairment in DMD, the results of Smith, Sibert, and Harper (1990) suggest two other hypotheses. First, verbal and cognitive deficits are more likely to be biologically related to the disease than to experiential or reactive factors. The quality of the home environment was *less* related to cognitive development in children with DMD than in the control subjects, suggesting a weaker effect of experience. Second, the fact that behavior problems were correlated with cognitive and language scores but not with locomotor scores suggests that behavior problems themselves may be secondary to cognitive deficits rather than reactive to the loss of motor ability.

Despite the evidence that cognitive and verbal deficits are present at early ages in DMD, there is also some evidence that they may diminish with age. Sollee et al. (1985) found that younger subjects with DMD were impaired in language and attentional-organizational abilities but not visuomotor abilities. Older subjects with DMD were impaired only on timed motor tasks. Sollee et al. suggested that the language and attentional-organizational impairment characteristic of younger children with DMD might disappear with increasing age.

One of the authors set out to test this hypothesis using a cross-sectional design with DMD boys younger and older than ten (Dorman, Hurley, and d'Avignon 1988). Our own sample of twenty-five older DMD cases was pooled with those of Marsh and Munsat (1974; $n = 34$) and Liebowitz and Dubowitz (1981; $n = 42$). Full-scale, Verbal, and Performance IQ data had been reported for each subject in these earlier reports.

There were no significant differences between the age groups on any of the variables. However, the younger group (n = 48) had a significant 7.94-point difference between Verbal and Performance IQ, whereas the 3.48-point superiority of Performance over Verbal IQ in the older group (n = 53) was not significant. Although this seemed to support the suggestion of Sollee et al. (1985), it was noted that the distribution of Verbal IQ scores in the older subjects was bimodal. Nearly the same percentage of older as younger subjects had Verbal IQ scores less than 75; however, 40 percent of the older subjects had Verbal IQ scores greater than 95, compared to 25 percent of the younger group. We suggested that some, but not all, of the younger children with DMD might "outgrow" their verbal disability, pushing the mean Verbal IQ higher but leaving a significant number with continuing impairment. Only longitudinal research would confirm or deny this hypothesis.

The nature of the cognitive disability was examined by Whelan (1987) and in a second study by Dorman, Hurley, and d'Avignon (1988). In the latter study we assessed each of fifteen older male subjects with DMD with a battery of nineteen psychological tests measuring aspects of simultaneous spatial information processing, auditory sequential information processing, auditory perception and analysis, expressive speech, receptive speech, Verbal IQ, reading, and spelling. Nearly one-half (seven) of our subjects with DMD were cognitively impaired, as defined by having more than three cognitive scores more than one standard deviation below the normative mean for their ages. As a group, subjects with DMD were most impaired on measures of auditory sequential information processing and phonemic awareness and on a test of judgment of the spatial orientation of lines.

The seven cognitively impaired boys were remarkably similar in their areas of impairment. These included auditory sequential information processing, auditory analysis, expressive and receptive speech, Verbal IQ, and reading. Even the errors that they made on various tests were often similar: an inability to isolate a designated phoneme or reassemble a word without it on a sound deletion test, phonological and circumlocutory errors in naming, and errors based on nonphonetic strategies in reading. All seven were classified as dyslexic on the Boder Test of Reading-Spelling Patterns.

It was our impression that the cognitive deficit, when it was present, in older boys with DMD was an auditory-language deficit similar to that reported in many dyslexic readers (e.g., Bradley and Bryant 1978). Whelan (1987) added the additional factor of deficits in immediate verbal and nonverbal memory in a study that compared subjects with DMD to those with spinal muscular atrophy. Verbal fluency was also impaired in Whelan's study, although no overall verbal deficit was found.

It is not clear why any cognitive abilities should be impaired in DMD, much less a specific subset related to verbal abilities, auditory processing, memory, and reading. Dystrophin, the gene product that is deficient in DMD, has been found in the brain as well as at the neuromuscular junction (Nudel et al. 1989). However, its role in the brain is not known. Kakulas (1992) speculated that it may be implicated in the maintenance of normal neuronal migration and cited his own earlier findings of migratory errors in the brain of mentally impaired subjects with DMD (Rosman and Kakulas 1966). More recently, Jagadha and Becker (1988) also found heterotopic cells in the brain of subjects with DMD. More striking, however, was the attenuation of dendritic length and arborization found in visual cortex pyramidal cells. Al-Qudah et al. (1990) found no abnormalities using magnetic resonance imaging to look for structural brain changes in patients with DMD.

The neuropathological basis for the cognitive deficit in DMD remains obscure. Because of its known link to a genetic cause and because of the similarity of the deficit to other poorly understood disorders, such as dyslexia and more general learning disabilities, it continues to hold promise for providing substantial insight into brain-behavior relationships.

Fragile X Syndrome

Fragile X syndrome has been cited as the leading known cause of mental retardation (Hagerman 1992). Its incidence is approximately 1 in 1,000 births (Sherman 1991). The actual genetic abnormality in fragile X has received extensive study and has been described in increasingly greater detail during the last several years. The genetic defect itself seems to be located at the Xq27.3 site and has been characterized as an unstable repetitive CGG sequence of abnormal length (Oberle et al. 1991; Yu et al. 1991). The length of the repetitive CGG sequence has been related to the expression of the clinical syndrome (Rousseau et al. 1991). Recently, the mode of inheritance, either from the mother or from the father, has been implicated as important in determining whether a female child is affected. Hinton et al. (1992) examined both cognitive and molecular genetic expression of fragile X related to the parent from whom it was transmitted. They found that heterozygote girls who inherited the fragile X from their fathers were similar to normal subjects on cognitive measures and had repeat DNA sequences longer than normal but shorter than those of heterozygotes whose inheritance was from the mother. The latter group were also significantly more impaired on the measure of freedom from distractibility from the Weschler Adult Intelligence Scale-Revised (WAIS-R) and on visual memory as measured by the Benton Visual Retention Test.

Verkerk et al. (1991) identified a candidate gene, labeled FMR-1, which seems to fail to produce protein in the presence of an expanded CGG sequence. The current work on the molecular genetics of fragile X is moving forward very rapidly, and a review is beyond the aim of the present chapter. Of some interest, however, is the finding that the CGG repeat sequence expands when passed through a female carrier. The CGG sequence will enlarge in about 80 percent of the male subjects who receive the fragile X gene from an unaffected female carrier. However, if the sequence has already enlarged and the mother is affected, all of her sons who receive the gene (50 percent of her sons) will be affected and show the full syndrome.

Moderate to profound mental retardation is common in persons with fragile X syndrome, although the proportion who show various levels of retardation is currently impossible to estimate, given that most cases are identified as retarded first and as having fragile X second. We are seeing increasing numbers of studies of mildly affected individuals with normal IQ and learning disabilities. Some of these studies will be reviewed later.

The topic that has received the greatest attention in the behavioral and psychological literature has been the association between fragile X syndrome and autism. Brown et al. (1982) first reported an association between the two disorders. The percentage of fragile X male subjects in autistic samples has ranged from 0 (Venter et al. 1984) to 20 (Blomquist et al. 1985; Brown et al. 1986). Hagerman (1992) concluded that the overall rate of fragile X males among autistic males is about 7 percent. More rarely, fragile X females have also been reported (Edwards et al. 1988).

Einfield, Molony, and Hall (1989) pointed out that the likelihood of autism is generally higher in the developmentally disabled population and compared fragile X males and females to a similarly developmentally disabled control group. The two groups did not differ in the percentage of cases fitting a diagnosis of autism, leading Einfield et al.

to conclude that there was no association between the two disorders. This conclusion was echoed by Fisch (1992), who performed a meta-analysis of nineteen studies of autistic males and twenty-one studies of retarded males, each of which ascertained the percentage of cytogenetically positive fragile X cases. The percentage of fragile X cases in the samples of mentally retarded subjects was 5.5 and in the samples of autistic subjects was 5.4. From these results, Fisch concluded that the attributable risk for autism (i.e., the proportionate excess risk of autism associated with exposure to fragile X) was 0.

Reiss and Freund (1992) took an approach somewhat different from that of either Einfield, Molony, and Hall (1989) or Fisch (1992). Rather than asking whether or not fragile X posed an increased risk for a diagnosis of autism, they asked whether any of the individual behaviors associated with autism occurred at a higher rate in fragile X males. Their control group was age-matched non–fragile X males who were also matched on IQ. In fact, the subjects with fragile X were significantly more impaired than their developmentally disabled counterparts on six of the sixteen diagnostic criteria for autism from the *Diagnostic and Statistical Manual of Mental Disorders,* second edition, revised (DSM-II-R), and differences on two more criteria were nearly significant. Significant differences, favoring more impairment for the fragile X subjects, were found in social play (more isolation), nonverbal communication (gaze aversion and gesturing), verbal communication (abnormalities of rate and volume and perseveration), and repetitive behaviors (hand flapping and rocking).

Hagerman (1992) pointed out that, whether or not individuals with fragile X contribute an excess number who fit the diagnostic label of autism, the *majority* display a number of symptoms associated with autism. These include gaze avoidance, hand flapping, and vocal perseveration, as well as problems with attention and impulsivity. Some of these symptoms, such as gaze avoidance, which has been claimed to occur in 90 percent of cases (Hagerman 1992), are extremely interesting because they raise the question of whether a genetic condition can produce a specific behavioral manifestation (i.e., a "released" behavior, as is found in the innate behavior patterns studied by ethologists).

Cognitive Studies

A number of studies have examined the question of whether fragile X syndrome is associated with a characteristic cognitive profile. The question is probably easier to answer with regard to higher functioning individuals, in whom it might be expected that intraindividual variation in cognitive abilities would be more evident. The question is complicated, however, by findings that indicate that milder cases may have a different genetic mutation from more severe cases, by the possibility of subtypes related to cognitive patterns (Fisch et al. 1992), and by the presence of cognitive deficits in heterozygous female carriers that may be different from those found in positive males (Mazzocco, Hagerman, and Pennington 1992; Steyaert et al. 1992). Since the expression of physical and behavioral characteristics seems to be directly related to the length of the CGG sequence, which in turn varies according to gender and the mode of inheritance, it is reasonable to begin with an assumption that differences in cognitive expression represent differences in degree on a continuum, unless the evidence demands a more complex explanation.

Hagerman (1992) summarized the findings with regard to cognitive deficits in high-functioning males. IQ values are reported to range from borderline to normal, and it seems that learning disabilities are routinely present. These are reported to be in the areas of mathematics, visuomotor coordination, abstract reasoning, pragmatics, and attention. Conversely, strengths include single-word vocabulary, visual matching, reading, and spelling.

In a study that, at least, had the potential to explore some of these issues regarding cognition, gender, and the mode of inheritance, Cianchetti et al. (1992) examined cognitive profiles in forty-eight members of a large family, all of whom could trace their fragile X status back to a single woman heterozygous for fragile X. The members ranged in age from five to eighty-four, although nearly all were adults. All of the male subjects positive for fragile X had IQ scores below 50. Because of their low IQs, they were all given the Weschler Preschool and Primary Scale of Intelligence (WPPSI), rather than the WAIS, but all were adults. Their worst scores were on the Similarities and Block Design subtests, and their best were on Vocabulary.

Only one other subject, a fragile X–positive female, had an IQ below 70 (42). The one other fragile X–positive female had an IQ of 93. All other subjects, who included fifteen fragile X–negative males, eight negative females who were the daughters of normal transmitting males or the mothers of positive males, and fourteen negative females who were unclassifiable but who could have been heterozygous for fragile X or homozygous for the normal allele, were indistinguishable from one another based on their position in the pedigree. Their IQ scores on the WAIS, as well as their scores on the Bender Gestalt and Wechsler Memory Scale, were normally distributed, and they ranged in IQ from 70 to 125. No pattern of Verbal-Performance discrepancies was noted. The fuller expression of fragile X, with low IQ, was found primarily in the later generation male subjects. The authors took this to support a hypothesis of a stepwise mechanism of sequential mistaken recombinations.

Although language, and particularly vocabulary, has generally been found to be a strength, relative to other cognitive skills, in fragile X males, it has been a characteristic finding that some language, speech, and voice problems are often found in such subjects (Paul et al. 1984). Sudhalter and colleagues conducted a series of studies aimed at identifying just what the language disability (or disabilities) is (or are). Sudhalter et al. (1990) found that, compared to persons with either Down syndrome or autism, fragile X males showed more perseverative language, which they defined as either phrase repetition, sentence repetition, or repetition of talk about the same topic. To explain perseveration, Sudhalter, Scarborough, and Cohen (1991) examined expressive syntactic ability by testing a hypothesis that impaired syntactic competence led to perseverations in situations where more sophisticated syntactic constructions were called for. They found no evidence that syntactic competence was any more delayed than overall language ability or that syntactic ability in fragile X males correlated with perseverative language behavior.

A more positive finding emerged from the study by Sudhalter, Marianon, and Brooks (1992). Their subjects included eleven fragile X males ranging in age from six to forty-one years. They were matched to eleven normally developing four year olds (seven boys and four girls). Subjects were asked to respond to sentences of four types: contextually constrained sentences that required completion by supplying items of factual knowledge or experiential knowledge and contextually unconstrained sentences that required either factual or experiential knowledge.

The fragile X subjects were less able than the controls to supply either contextually constrained or unconstrained information. However, they had a disproportionate degree of difficulty with completing contextually unconstrained sentences (e.g., Grown-ups think about . . .). These findings fit a hypothesis that the perseverative speech found in fragile X males is a function of their decreased ability to produce appropriate words when contextual constraints fail to narrow the possible candidates.

Sudhalter, Marianon, and Brooks (1992) provided an attractive hypothesis but one that must be treated very tentatively. Other studies have found relative strengths in vocabulary, for instance, whether measured as a receptive skill (Kemper, Hagerman, and Altshul-Stark 1988) or as an expressive skill, as in the study of Cianchetti et al. (1992)

mentioned earlier. Furthermore, it is possible that both perseverative responding and difficulty generating appropriate words to finish contextually unconstrained sentences represent a more basic defect in generating novel response alternatives that may not even be confined to language.

The progression of the cognitive deficit in fragile X males was studied by Fisch et al. (1992). Previous studies by Lachiewicz et al. (1987) and Hagerman et al. (1989) indicated that IQ generally declines with age in fragile X males. Fisch et al. (1991) had found inconsistencies in such declines, with some subjects showing declines, some increases, and some remaining stable. In their most recent study, Fisch et al. used cluster analytic methods to determine whether they could identify two groups based on different patterns of IQ changes with age.

Indeed, two groups were found, one in which IQ remained stable over an approximately three- to fourteen-year test-retest interval and another group who averaged a decline of nearly four times the standard error of the test (Stanford-Binet) over the same interval. Various statistical procedures eliminated such potentially confounding biases as that one group was simply older at pretest and had already undergone a decline in IQ. The authors noted that the decline seems most dramatic during puberty and may be related to characteristics of the test requirements, failure to develop more abstract reasoning skills, or neurobiological progression of some sort, although the last has not been demonstrated. They speculated that the existence of two subtypes may represent different mutations, an interesting possibility, given the variability in the underlying molecular genetic disorder related to the history of inheritance.

Studies of Heterozygous Females

Hagerman (1992) expressed the hope that the study of heterozygous females, particularly those with normal IQ, will lead to an understanding of the mildest effects of the fragile X gene and thereby clarify some of the issues regarding subtle learning disabilities and emotional-behavioral problems. Other researchers seem to share this perspective, since the number of cognitive and psychological studies of heterozygotes has kept pace with, and perhaps even recently surpassed, those of positive males.

The available findings regarding cognitive functioning in heterozygous female subjects are by no means consistent. This probably stems from several sources, not the least of which are small sample sizes, the inclusion of females with different degrees of expression of the fragile X gene in different researchers' samples, and differences in the mode of inheritance (father versus mother) between samples. There is no doubt that any genuine conclusions regarding the cognitive functioning of heterozygotes should be constrained by the latter two variables.

The areas that have received the greatest attention have been IQ, memory, and problem solving. There is a consensus that IQ levels are related to the degree of expression of the fragile X gene in terms of the degree of fragility shown as the percentage of defective cells in cytogenetic studies. Kemper et al. (1986) and Cronister et al. (1991) found lower IQs in women with greater than 2 percent fragility than in those with less. Heterozygotes with comparable expression to that of positive males are most often retarded. Various percentages for the proportion of retarded versus normal IQ heterozygotes have been reported, with the percentage of normal IQ women ranging from 50 (Hagerman 1992) to 66 (Mazzocco, Hagerman, and Pennington 1992). Most studies that have found intellectual impairment have found that freedom from distractibility (Digit Span and Arithmetic subtests) from the WAIS is most affected (Hinton et al. 1992; Steyaert et al. 1992), but scores on some Performance subtests, usually either Block Design or Object Assembly, are also low (Kemper et al. 1986; Steyaert et al. 1992).

In the study by Hinton et al. (1992), fragile X–positive heterozygotes who inherited the gene from their mothers showed deficits in visual memory on the Benton Visual Retention Test, as had the subjects of Miezejeski et al. (1986). However, Mazzocco et al. (1992) found no differences and even some relative strengths in positive female subjects performing long-term memory tasks that did not require the processing of complex information.

Grigsby, Kemper, and Hagerman (1992) used a variety of verbal learning and memory tasks to compare fragile X–expressing heterozygotes to two control groups. One control group was composed of fragile X–negative carriers and siblings of the index group. The other, a "neurological control" group, was composed of females with either a history of mild head injury or learning disabilities. The fragile X females took significantly more trials to learn a list of ten unrelated words but performed no worse than either control group on delayed recall of the list thirty minutes later. Neither were there differences between any of the groups on a verbal-visual paired associate learning task or on the verbal paired associate memory task from the Wechsler Memory Scale. In addition, no differences were observed on a version of the Brown-Peterson interference recall task. The only other significant difference was found in the impaired performance, relative to both of the control groups, of the fragile X–positive female subjects on the Digit Span subtest of the WAIS-R.

As the authors pointed out, this study was perhaps most remarkable because of the difficulty in showing any impairment at all in the fragile X–expressing subjects. It is all the more remarkable in that the fragile X subjects averaged sixteen and eleven points lower on Verbal IQ than the fragile X and neurological controls, respectively. Grigsby, Kemper, and Hagerman (1992) interpreted the limited deficits that were found as being possibly related to frontal lobe impairment, although this does not seem like a hypothesis that immediately comes to mind in reviewing their results. They cited a previous study that found such frontal lobe deficits when analyzing neuropsychological data from single case reports (Grigsby and Myers 1987).

The hypothesis of frontal lobe deficits in fragile X females was explored in more depth by Mazzocco, Hagerman, and Pennington (1992). Their subjects were ten fragile X women, each of whom had at least 2 percent cytogenetic expression of the fragile X gene, and a control group of mothers of non–fragile X developmentally disabled children. The tasks presented to the subjects in the study required complex problem solving, the following of rules in the face of stimulus cues to behave differently, and the giving up of one response strategy for another or alternation between two response strategies based on stimulus cues. Fragile X subjects were generally not impaired relative to controls, except on those aspects of the problems that required them to consider a large number of features of the problem to generate a response strategy. Measures of perseveration related to changing response strategies did not produce differences between the groups. In one sense, the results were counter to what would have been predicted from a frontal lobe impairment hypothesis, although they imply a limitation in the awareness needed to generate complex strategies in fragile X women, which might also reflect frontal lobe impairment. Previously, Mazzocco et al. (1992) had found problems with perseveration among fragile X women on the Wisconsin Card Sorting Test, a traditional measure of frontal lobe functioning.

Although the frontal lobe deficit hypothesis seems to have only limited evidence behind it, it offers an attractive explanation for some of the psychiatric findings in fragile X females. Hagerman (1992) martialed a fair amount of factual and circumstantial evidence in favor of the idea that some of the emotional problems found in fragile X females may be linked to frontal lobe deficits. She pointed out that the problems with topic maintenance and disorganization in cognitive processing, particularly with affective stimulation, may be related to schizotypal features, social anxiety and withdrawal, and a tendency to be easily overwhelmed by multiple stimuli. Interestingly, depression may not be explainable in the same terms. Depression seems to be related to low or even no expression of the fragile X gene (Reiss et al. 1989; Sobesky 1991) and to the presence of learning disabilities. Hagerman speculated that the depression may be reactive to the presence of learning disabilities.

Fragile X syndrome is an interesting disorder for a number of reasons. In our opinion, the various manifestations of cognitive problems in various groups can most parsimoniously be placed on a continuum of severity, with different types of learning, memory, and problem solving skills appearing to be impaired depending on the severity of the general cognitive deficit. This may not turn out to be the case, but a more complex formulation would be only a back-up position, so to speak, if the simpler one would be found wanting.

Fragile X shares with other genetic disorders the advantage of rapid progress in molecular genetics, which holds the promise of leading to fairly precise biobehavioral connections. The behavioral manifestations of the disorder may turn out to be as important as or more important than the cognitive ones in this regard. Most likely, as Hagerman (1992) suggested, the cognitive and behavioral symptoms are related to one another in most instances. However, certain behavioral symptoms, such as gaze aversion, may turn out to be relatively "pure" manifestations of the genetic abnormality. The best evidence for this would be some documentation that the behavior was responsive to the same environmental cues and that its structure was very similar across subjects. Current research strategies, involving primarily frequency counts or categorical classification of the presence or absence of such behaviors, do not lend themselves to this type of analysis.

Tourette Syndrome

Tourette syndrome has come into prominence in recent years for two chief reasons. First, the incidence and prevalence of the disorder have become recognized as much higher than had previously been thought. Current estimates of prevalence have ranged from 1:1,000–1.400 (Burd et al. 1986; Caine et al. 1988) to as high as 1:100 (Comings 1990). Second, Tourette syndrome is now generally recognized to be genetically related to several other behavioral disorders, most notably attention deficit hyperactivity disorder (Comings and Comings 1987) and obsessive-compulsive disorder (Comings and Comings 1987;

Frankel et al. 1986). Comings (1990) suggested that Tourette syndrome may be genetically related to as wide an array of disorders as conduct problems, sexual exhibitionism, phobias and panic attacks, manic-depressive disorder, some forms of autism, and perhaps a number of other disorders sharing the characteristics of lack of behavioral inhibition or obsessive-compulsive types of thinking or behavior.

The evidence in favor of a common pattern of cognitive deficits in Tourette syndrome cases is not very strong. There is no positive evidence of anything other than a normal IQ distribution in Tourette cases (Bornstein, King, and Carroll 1983; Hagin 1982). On the other hand, learning disabilities have been reported in a number of studies (Burd, Kauffman, and Kerbeshian 1992; Cohen, Leckman, and Shaywitz 1983; Hagin et al. 1982; Sutherland et al. 1982). Comings (1990) suggested that there may be a genetic relationship between Tourette syndrome and dyslexia, principally on the basis of his own findings of a high association between the two disorders on the basis of self-reports (Comings and Comings 1987). He also suggested that Tourette syndrome may involve dysfunction in frontal lobe dopaminergic systems and that Tourette subjects should do poorly on measures related to frontal lobe functioning (Comings 1990).

Twenty-three patients with Tourette syndrome were examined neuropsychologically by one of the authors (C.D.) in association with Dr. B. Comings. All patients were referred because of a combination of Tourette syndrome and either attention deficit hyperactivity disorder or learning disabilities, or both. Twenty-one clients were male. Their ages ranged from six to forty years old, although only two were over twenty-one. Because of the age range and because they were not all referred for the same problem, no standard battery of neuropsychological tests was given to all of them. However, the same areas of functioning were assessed with different instruments in most cases, and several measures had been given to approximately three-fourths of the clients. The mean Full-Scale IQ of the group, based on either the WISC-R ($n = 21$) or the WAIS-R ($n = 2$), was 101.3; the mean Verbal IQ was 100.3 and the mean Performance IQ was 102.9. Subtest scaled scores were quite similar, with the lowest being Comprehension (9.3) and the highest being Picture Completion (11.5). Academic achievement was, as expected because of the referral bias, below IQ levels. On the Wide Range Achievement Test-Revised (WRAT-R), the mean Reading score was 92.4, the mean Spelling score 90.3, and the mean Arithmetic score 91.0.

In the group as a whole, there were no obvious weaknesses in language functioning in the areas of auditory discrimination, receptive speech, or expressive speech. The one consistent weakness was in short-term auditory memory. Nineteen of the subjects received the Spreen-Benton Sentence Repetition Test and obtained a mean standard score of 83.1. Only five subjects had scores within the average range on this test. In contrast, scores on motor and visuoperceptual functioning were unimpaired. Finger tapping speed averaged a standard score of 114.9 with the dominant hand and 115 with the nondominant hand. Three individuals were left handed. On Benton's Judgment of Line Orientation Test, twenty-one clients averaged a standard score of 100.7. Thirteen clients receiving the Hooper Visual Organization Test (a measure of visual closure) obtained a mean score of 104.1.

The ability to follow a behavioral plan in the face of distraction was assessed with the Fruit Distraction Test for the younger subjects and the Stoop Color-Word Test for the older subjects (some subjects received both). On the Fruit Distraction Test, the extra time to name the color of the stimuli when they were incorrectly colored yielded a mean standard score of 93.2 and the increase in errors due to the incorrect colors yielded a standard score of 95.8. Subjects performed below their IQ levels, but not outside the average range. The eight older subjects who were given the Stroop obtained an average standard score of 88.8. Fifteen clients were old enough to receive the Wisconsin Card Sorting Test. Nine performed at average levels or above, whereas four (27 percent) showed some degree of perseverative responding.

The above data do not really prove very much except in a sort of negative way. Given that the clients were all referred because of attention deficit hyperactivity disorder or learning disabilities as well as Tourette syndrome, the results are not unexpected. Academic problems, short-term verbal memory problems, and difficulty resisting distraction or, occasionally, with switching set are not uncommon in such a sample, with or without Tourette syndrome. No unique pattern of test scores was evident, and the group actually appeared relatively unimpaired for a learning-disabled sample. This might be because they also demonstrated histories of behavioral problems, often quite severe. In fact, two of the subjects had been diagnosed as autistic at one time in their lives. Nearly all were being medicated, and the majority continued to show some evidence of motor and vocal tics.

One remarkable finding was the good scores on the majority of the motor and visual-perceptual measures. This was remarkable because a few clients had absolutely terrible handwriting. In fact, a behavior that was evident in a small subset of clients was one that the authors have rarely seen in other clients, very messy handwriting with a tendency to impulsively write the wrong letter or number and then scribble out the effort in such a way that it was sometimes hard to see the eventual product. This was interpreted as disinhibited motor behavior that might be another manifestation of the underlying problem causing the motor tics.

Disorders of Chromosome Number

Sex Chromosome Abnormalities

Sex chromosome abnormalities include some well-known disorders. Turner syndrome (45,X) and Klinefelter syndrome (47,XXY) are just two of these. One reason for discussing them together is that they form almost a continuum of variations on the theme of XY combination. Bender et al. (1986), for instance, described a series of studies of sex chromosome abnormalities in which they looked for variation in common effects through a range of disorders that included 45,X, mosaic conditions of 45,X/46,XX, 45,X/47,XXX, 46,XX/47,XXX, partial monosomies of 45,X/46,XXq− and 46,XXq−, and the "extra" chromosome disorders 47,XXY, 47,XXX, and 47,XYY.

In a survey of school-age cognitive functioning in their sample of forty-six children representing different numbers of each of the variations of sex chromosome abnormalities, Benders et al. found only two subjects who were clearly retarded intellectually. Unfortunately, this finding cannot be translated into the straightforward generalization that sex chromosome abnormalities do not affect intelligence. The mean IQ of the group with sex chromosome abnormalities was fourteen points below that of a control sample. Some conditions were represented by only one or two subjects, and in others, most notably 45,X and 47,XXX, the mean IQ levels were below average, although still within the normal range. Subjects with mosaic conditions were generally more intelligent and indistinguishable from controls.

Sizable Verbal-Performance IQ differences were not unusual in any of the groups with sex chromosome abnormalities, except the subjects with mosaic conditions. Such differences favored Performance IQ, except in the group with Turner syndrome, who showed the reverse pattern of lower Performance than Verbal IQ. Nevertheless, all groups, including 45,X girls but not mosaics, showed some evidence of speech or language and auditory memory impairment. Spatial deficits were present in the 45,X and 47,XXX girls but not in the 47,XXY or 47,XYY boys nor the mosaic subjects. Motor skill impairment was present in all of the groups with sex chromosome abnormalities except those with mosaic conditions.

By looking at the spectrum of sex chromosome abnormalities, one might be able to generate some hypotheses regarding the effects of sex chromosomes on cognitive development that could not be generated by studying specific groups with sex chromosome abnormalities. An obvious hypothesis is that the duplication of a sex chromosome has less deleterious effects on cognition than does the duplication of an autosome. In fact, the same may be true of some sex chromosome abnormalities and survival. Klinefelter syndrome (47,XXY), for instance, has a substantial incidence of 1:500–800 male births and is not found in much greater proportion in spontaneous or medical abortions, although Turner syndrome is (Carr and Gedeon 1977). With regard to intellect, disorders of sex chromosome number represented only 3 of 274 (1.09 percent) institutionalized males with moderate mental retardation in a recent survey. In contrast, nine patients (3.25 percent) had Down syndrome (Volcke et al. 1990). Nielsen and Wohlert (1990) found no children with mental retardation among the 78 with sex chromosome abnormalities surviving from a total population of nearly 35,000 live births over a thirteen-year period.

Attempts have been made to link the effects of extra or missing chromosomes to differences in language and visuospatial abilities via the concept of influences on lateralized cerebral development, usually with the underlying assumption that sex chromosome abnormalities may represent exaggerations of normal sex-related differences in both physiological and cognitive development (Hier, Atkins, and Perlo 1980; Netley and Rovet 1982). Netley and Rovet (1982, 1983) presented the most specific hypothesis. Citing evidence that the length of the cycle of mitosis is affected by the presence or absence of extra or the typical number of chromosomes (Barlow 1973; Polani 1977), Netley and Rovet hypothesized that the absence of an X chromosome, as in Turner syndrome, would increase brain growth rate by shortening the cell cycle, allowing inadequate time for right hemisphere development. Conversely, the presence of an extra X chromosome, as in 47,XXX or 47,XXY, would slow brain growth rate and result in a delay in the maturation of the left hemisphere.

The hypothesis proposed by Netley and Rovet is bold, if simplistic. There have been other suggestions that the right hemisphere matures more slowly than the left, and this has been invoked as an explanation for the ability of the right hemisphere to "take over" language functions after early left hemisphere injury (Witelson 1987). As Bender et al. (1986) pointed out, the hypothesis runs into some difficulties simply in accounting for the findings regarding verbal and spatial abilities in the various groups with sex chromosome abnormalities. As mentioned previously, 47,XXX girls seem to have a spatial deficit that is more severe than that found in 47,XYY boys, which is opposite to the prediction. On the other hand, verbal abilities are more impaired than spatial abilities in 47,XXX girls, and their overall greater impairment of cognitive skills typically results in *all* of their abilities being lower than those of other groups with sex chromosome abnormalities. The 47,XYY male subjects also present a problem for the Netley and Rovet hypothesis, since they are decidedly unimpaired in spatial abilities but are impaired in language (Bender et al. 1984b; Graham et al. 1988). Of course, 47,XYY males are not "missing" an X chromosome, at least compared to normal males. This may reduce the contradictory status of their lack of spatial deficits, but it does little to explain why they would have language problems, for they do not have an "extra" X chromosome either. By ignoring the sex of the chromosome and counting only their number, the hypothesis fits a little better, since it would predict spatial deficits in 45,X and language deficits in 47,XXX, 47,XXY, and 47,XYY, but the spatial deficit in 47,XXX would still be unexplained.

The presence of verbal or spatial deficits may be more closely related to the degree to which individuals with sex chromosome abnormalities are phenotypically male or female than to the actual number of X chromosomes. If this were the case, then we might look to hormonal influences as a source of hypotheses regarding the development of cognitive strengths or weaknesses. Such hypotheses have been proposed by Money (1973; Money and Erhardt 1972), Reinisch (1976; Reinisch, Gandelman, and Spiegel 1979), and Hier, Atkins, and Perlo (1980). Geschwind theorized regarding embryological hormonal influences, lateralized cerebral development, handedness, and reading problems (Geschwind and Behan 1982; Geschwind and Galaburda 1985). Interestingly, Netley and Rovet (1982) found an excess of left handedness in 47,XXY males, although they dismissed hormonal theories because of the supposed greater influence of hormones at puberty than in early development (Netley 1988). Recently, Netley (1992) found that testosterone levels at puberty were related to lowered Verbal IQ in 47,XXY males.

A hormonal hypothesis is attractive, since it has also been used to explain normal female-male differences in verbal and, particularly, spatial abilities and has, interestingly, been tied to maturation rates (Waber 1977). Hormonal influences need not be confined to a specific developmental period when used as an explanatory variable. In some instances the influence may be early in prenatal development and in others at puberty, depending on the chromosomal abnormality and on what is being explained. There are problems with this hypothesis too, since Bender et al. (1986) pointed out that 47,XXY and 47,XYY boys have similar cognitive profiles but different hormonal effects, with Klinefelter males having hypogonadism while 47,XYY males do not. Netley (1992) found that testosterone levels in 47,XXY males were related to early onset of puberty, which, in turn, was related to higher Verbal IQ. Simple increased dosage effects, except by creating permanent changes in neuroendocrine function, probably do not apply to such theories, since the inactivation of the extra X chromosome should occur very early in development, similar to the situation in normal females (Lyon 1962). Even here, however, Zang (1984) proposed a scenario in which gene dosage effects could occur in a minority of cases. The whole area is certainly not simple, and the intricacies necessary for sensible theorizing are largely out of our league. Although a broad spectrum approach to sex chromosome abnormality may offer one approach to the characterization of cognitive deficits in such disorders, more detailed examination of some of the more common disorders is also useful.

47,XXY (Klinefelter Syndrome)
A vast number of psychological studies of males with the 47,XXY karyotype have yielded a generally consistent picture of the cognitive characteristics associated with this syndrome. First, intelligence is usually normal; mean scores are often between 90 and 100, and IQs can be in the superior range (Bender et al. 1986; Nielsen and Sorensen 1984; Ratcliffe 1984). Verbal IQ is often lower than Performance IQ (Graham et al. 1988; Netley and Rovet 1982; Pennington et al. 1982). However, a minority of studies failed to find such a pattern (Ratcliffe 1984; Ratcliffe et al. 1982). Although clumsiness and delays in motor development have also been reported (Bender et al. 1986; Nielsen and Sorensen 1984), visuomotor deficits have not (Bender et al. 1986). School achievement is greatly affected, relative to what might be expected on the basis of IQ results. Ratcliffe (1984) found 50 percent of subjects in special education, and Bender et al. (1986) and Graham et al. (1988) reported impaired reading and spelling, even in subjects who were not placed in special education.

The language deficit in 47,XXY individuals has received the most attention. Difficulties with short-term auditory memory and more problems with expressive than receptive language were reported in several studies (Graham et al. 1988; Walzer et al. 1978).

Graham et al. (1988) compared fourteen XXY and fifteen control subjects, ten of whom were karyotypically normal and five of whom had a familial autosomal translocation. Ages ranged from five to twelve years. Each child was assessed with the WISC-R and a battery of twenty-one language, memory, reading, and spelling tests.

On the WISC-R the 47,XXY subjects had lower Verbal and Full-Scale but not Performance IQ scores than the control subjects. On the various language measures, the 47,XXY subjects were primarily deficient, relative to both the controls and the normative data, on the measures of expressive speech, processing of rapid auditory material, and auditory memory and were much less so on receptive language measures. Within the expressive speech area, deficits were apparent in word-finding, syntactic production, and narrative formulation, but not in articulation. Both oral and silent reading measures of accuracy, speed, and comprehension were deficient in the 47,XXY group, as was a measure of the ability to decode words phonetically. Spelling was also deficient.

The above findings support the claim by Bender et al. (1986) that 47,XXY males are often dyslexic and that, among groups with sex chromosome abnormality, they come closest to having a "pure" learning disability. Indeed, the pattern of deficits shown by 47,XXY males is typical of many dyslexics and seems to be a cognitive phenotype very similar to that which we have found in Duchenne muscular dystrophy (Dorman, Hurley, and d'Avignon 1988). This is no doubt a similarity that is considerably removed from the direct genetic effects of the two conditions but may reflect a dysfunction of the left cerebral hemisphere in both cases, the similarity probably being more functional than physiological.

Klinefelter syndrome has also engendered a great deal of research on noncognitive psychological functioning. It is unclear whether 47,XXY males are overrepresented in either criminal or psychiatric populations. Although most efforts to control for confounding factors in determining these issues have focused on lowered IQ, it seems even more reasonable to control for reading disability, which is known to predispose boys toward both behavioral and delinquent problems. Of equal interest, and a more consistent finding, has been the indication that 47,XXY males may show a characteristic personality profile of low energy, social timidity, and passivity (Netley 1988; Nielsen and Sorensen 1984). Nielsen and Sorensen (1984) reported that testosterone treatment at puberty improved the energy level and ability to concentrate in their sample of 47,XXY subjects. Most interesting, in their study Nielsen and Sorensen found greater psychological problems in adult 47,XXY men even when they were compared to karyotypically normal but hypogonadal controls. Any attempt to isolate a causal mechanism is made even more complicated by Netley's (1992) finding that unaltered testosterone levels were related to the level of Verbal IQ and age of onset of puberty in 47,XXY boys. The untangling of all of these issues may provide us with considerable insight into the relationships between sex chromosome, brain development, reading, and behavior.

47,XYY Syndrome
47,XYY ought to provide a mirror-image disorder to 47,XXY, but of course it does not, nor does it even come close. In fact, the few studies of 47,XYY males that have examined their cognitive abilities in any detail have found them quite similar to 47,XXY persons (Bender et al. 1984b). Bender et al. (1986) speculated that, given their similarities in cognitive abilities, including reading disability and good visuospatial skills, the brain organization of 47,XXY and 47,XYY may be quite similar. This would create problems for a theory of lateralized brain development that utilized the number of extra X chromosomes as a crucial variable.

45,X (Turner Syndrome)
Turner syndrome has generated more research on cognitive abilities than has any other sex chromosome abnormality. In one of the earliest studies on cognitive functioning in a sex chromosome abnormality, Alexander, Walker, and Money (1964) identified a deficit in direction sense in 45,X females, which has continued as a consistent, albeit not the sole, finding regarding the cognitive abilities of 45,X girls.

The original finding of a specific spatial deficit in 45,X syndrome and its subsequent replications were particularly exciting because it represented one of the very first pieces of evidence that a specific cognitive deficit could result from a chromosomal abnormality (Money 1973; Money and Alexander 1966). Subsequent studies have broadened the definition of the deficit to include copying shapes (Silbert, Wolff, and Lilienthal 1977), difficulties with spatial rotation (Rovet and Netley 1982), and problems with handwriting and mathematical disability (Pennington et al. 1982).

Although spatial deficits are, in fact, a consistent finding in 45,X subjects, several studies have found additional deficits outside of the visual-perceptual domain. Waber (1979), for instance, found as much evidence of a verbal deficiency as a visual-spatial deficit in her sample of eleven 45,X subjects. Pennington et al. (1985) found that Turner syndrome patients performed more like women with diffuse brain injury than like women with right lateralized injury, as had been suggested by Money (1973) and Silbert, Wolff, and Lilienthal (1977). Bender et al. (1986) mentioned the tendency toward increased ear infections in 45,X subjects as possibly responsible for language deficits, and attention and hyperactivity as contributing to generally decreased performance, no matter what the test. Williams, Richman, and Yarbrough (1991) found that girls with Turner syndrome were similar to boys and girls who fit a nonverbal learning disability subtype. Both the subjects with Turner syndrome and the subjects with nonverbal learning disability were below average on a measure of short-term verbal memory. In addition, while the subjects with Turner syndrome were no worse than the subjects with nonverbal learning disability on measures of attention and impulsivity, there were wide variations on the latter measure in the Turner syndrome group, and their mean scores were more than one standard deviation below the normative mean for the test instrument.

The presence of some difficulties with short-term verbal memory in individuals with Turner syndrome has been reported by others (e.g., Bender, Linden, and Robinson 1989). However, studies utilizing the Wechsler tests continue to find little impairment of Verbal IQ and significant impairment of Performance IQ and, as a consequence, Full-scale IQ (Downey et al. 1991). Even the study by Williams, Richman, and Yarbrough (1991) failed to find impairment on the WISC-R Digit Span test when the Rey Auditory-Verbal Learning test (another measure of short-term verbal memory) was impaired.

It is still not clear just how far the cognitive impairment in Turner syndrome extends. Bender et al. (1986) found some Turner subjects impaired in verbal abilities and auditory memory, even though they were most impaired in spatial ability. Academic difficulties, in their sample, were never confined to just mathematics and usually extended to all school subjects. Of the 2 cases of mental retardation in their sample of 38 children with nonmosaic sex chromosome abnormalities, one was a case of Turner syndrome. Kleczkowska et al. (1990) found that below average IQ was present in 23 percent of 218 children with Turner syndrome seen at their center in Belgium. On the other hand, Nielsen and Wohlert (1990) found no cases of mental retardation in the individuals with Turner syndrome identified in a population incidence study in Denmark. Certainly, the picture remains unclear.

47,XXX Syndrome

The females with a 47,XXX karyotype were the most impaired of the groups with sex chromosome abnormality studied by Bender et al. (1986). Nearly all were impaired in language, though not so often in short-term auditory memory. Spatial abilities and neuromotor skills were also often impaired. Nine of the eleven were receiving special education.

The cognitive profile of 47,XXX girls has been noted to be similar to that observed in 47,XXY males and has led to the hypothesis that the number of extra X chromosomes has a crucial and similar effect on cognitive functioning (Walzer 1985). Language deficits and lower Verbal than Performance IQ have been consistent findings in both syndromes (Nielsen et al. 1982; Ratcliffe et al. 1982; Rovet and Netley 1983). What has not been reported so often is that a spatial deficit may also be present and that this may distinguish the 47,XXX and 47,XXY syndromes from each other. Bender et al. (1986) found that nearly one-half of their 47,XXX group were impaired in spatial abilities, whereas such impairment was rare in 47,XXY males. What was most clear for the 47,XXX individuals was that their cognitive abilities were often impaired across a number of areas, with corresponding difficulties in many areas of academic achievement.

Down Syndrome

Down syndrome is the leading known cause of mental retardation. The incidence is about 1:1,000 live births in the United States (Adams et al. 1981). With prenatal diagnosis (targeted toward women over age thirty-five, who are at greater risk), there has come a downward shift in maternal age, so 80 percent of Down syndrome births now occur to women under age thirty-five (Lott 1986).

Down syndrome is inevitably tied to an extra copy or a partial copy of chromosome 21, resulting from a failure of the chromosomes to separate during meiosis (nondisjunction) or, less frequently, from a translocation when a fragment of chromosome 21 attaches itself to another chromosome, leading to partial trisomy. Possibly the survival of trisomic individuals with Down syndrome is related to the fact that chromosome 21 is nearly the smallest human chromosome, containing only about 45 million base pairs of DNA, or 1.5 percent of the total genetic material. The resulting extra copy of chromosome 21 leads to 1.5 times the normal level of gene products coded by that gene.

Neuropathology

How the trisomic condition translates into neurological abnormalities has been the subject of intensive research. The research has pursued so many different directions that it is not possible to present even a summary of the findings. Two of the most intriguing hypotheses, though, are related to synaptogenesis and synaptic transmission.

With regard to synaptogenesis, Wisniewski et al. (1986) examined postnatal brain development of Down syndrome and control subjects in terms of neuronal density in the occipital, temporal, and prefrontal cortices and in terms of synaptic density and synaptic morphological findings in the visual cortex. Both of these issues were studied in relation to age. Neuronal density in area 17 (visual cortex) was less in subjects with Down syndrome at nearly all ages. In area 10 (prefrontal cortex), neuronal density was less up to one year of age but was similar thereafter. In the parahippocampal gyrus (area 28), the opposite pattern was found, with significantly less neuronal density only at ages eleven to fourteen (the upper age limits of the study). In both areas 17 and 28, the decreased neuronal density in patients with Down syndrome was most evident in granular layers II and IV. Synaptic density was reduced in the visual cortex of Down syndrome cases at birth and again at eighteen years of age but not between eight months and nine years. Synaptic density was highest in both groups at age eight months and then decreased thereafter to adult values at nine years for controls and, apparently at a somewhat later age, for subjects with Down syndrome. Presynaptic length and average surface area per synaptic contact were less in subjects with Down syndrome at all ages. Both measures of synaptic structure showed increases in control subjects up to nine years and in subjects with Down syndrome up to eighteen years.

Wisniewski et al. also found that overall brain weight and cortical thickness in areas 10 and 28 showed no differences between subjects with Down syndrome and control subjects at early ages, but differences emerged after age four in terms of weight and by age fourteen years in terms of neuronal density. This confirmed others' findings of postnatal brain growth arrest in Down syndrome.

The authors speculated that, because (with the exception of area 28) mean differences in neuronal density between subjects with Down syndrome and control subjects were present from birth, the bulk of the disturbance in neuronal development probably occurred prenatally. Similarly, with regard to synaptogenesis in area 17, differences at one day of age pointed to prenatal influences, and they hypothesized that a prenatal arrest 'of neurogenesis was the cause of both neuronal and synaptic density differences.

Nadel (1986) suggested that postnatal differences in the development of the granular cells in the hippocampal and parahippocampal regions might be related to arrested neuronal development during a second migratory-proliferative stage. He speculated on the role of the hippocampus in indexing the informational contents of the neocortex and in spatial integration of information and how deficiencies in these aspects of cognition might be similar in subjects with Down syndrome and Alzheimer disease.

The link between cognitive deficits in Down syndrome and those in Alzheimer disease has provided a framework for another line of research. One promising link has to do with neurotransmitter re-uptake. Superoxidase dismutase 1 (SOD1) is an enzyme that is coded by a gene on chromosome 21 and that, when overproduced, results in lipid peroxidation, which in turn affects neurotransmitter re-uptake and efficiency. The neuronal effect, in mice, is coupled with other effects similar to those of aging, which may give a clue to the cognitive impairment in both Down syndrome and aging.

Unfortunately, the SOD1 gene may not be overproduced in Alzheimer patients. Delabar et al. (1987) looked for gene duplications common to both Alzheimer disease and Down syndrome. Although the duplication of the SOD1 gene was found in subjects with Down syndrome, it was not found in Alzheimer patients. Instead, the beta-amyloid protein–encoding AD-AP gene was found in both disorders. This gene, as well as the oncogene ets-2, is located in a small subsection of chromosome 21, and both are found in patients with Alzheimer disease and Down syndrome. This suggests a common genetic basis for the Alzheimer-like changes in Down syndrome and true Alzheimer dementia.

The relationship between Alzheimer disease and Down syndrome is only one of the factors that makes this all-too-common disorder psychologically interesting. As the previously cited genetic studies indicate, the link with Alzheimer disease is not just by analogy. There is good reason to think that older persons with Down syndrome develop true Alzheimer disease at relatively young ages. In fact, the evidence in favor of similar neuropathological conditions in Alzheimer patients and in aging Down syndrome subjects is somewhat greater than that for similar clinical presentations. This is probably because of the gross premorbid differences in cognitive functioning between the two types of disorders.

Virtually 100 percent of patients with Down syndrome who are over forty years of age have neuropathological changes characteristic of Alzheimer disease (Lott 1986). Studies using light or electron microscopic analysis have confirmed a very high association between the two disorders. Pathological changes seen in individuals with Down syndrome, sometimes younger than thirty years and routinely over forty years, include neuronal loss, senile plaques, and neurofibrillary tangles.

Ball, Schapiro, and Rapoport (1986) summarized much of their own and others' research through the mid-1980s. Ball and Nuttall (1980) compared the brains of five Down syndrome patients, twenty-one to sixty-two years old, to the brains of normal controls and Alzheimer patients. Neuronal density in the hippocampus was similar between the Down syndrome and Alzheimer cases, and both densities were below that of normal controls. Similarly, both patients with Down syndrome and those with Alzheimer disease showed similar numbers of neurofibrillary tangles in the hippocampi and, again, more than the normal controls. Moreover, examination of the location of neurofibrillary tangles in the hippocampus revealed similar areas of vulnerability for normal subjects and patients with Down syndrome or Alzheimer disease.

Aside from the deficits noted previously in neuron and synapse density (in particular the absence of granular cells), in impaired synaptic transmission, and in the presence of pathological changes associated with aging, no specific neurological abnormality has been associated with Down syndrome. Gross abnormalities in brain weight, shortened frontal-occipital diameter, steep occipital ascent, and opercular or superior temporal gyrus hypoplasia have generally been found. Lott (1986, 20) concluded, however, "Where focal neurological deficits are noted, further investigation usually uncovers a coexisting disorder unrelated to [Down syndrome] or a secondary complication of the syndrome." Nadel (1986) proposed that granular cell hippocampal abnormalities may, in fact, be a focal deficit with wide-ranging effects. He also proposed that a more "modular" view of cognitive development, in which impairment is more specific to those cognitive functions based on late-maturing neural systems, rather than a "general purpose" view of impairment has a better fit with the neurobiological data. We will now see how such considerations fare in the light of the data on cognition.

Cognitive Development

The most complete data available on cognitive development in persons with Down syndrome are provided by Carr, both from her own longitudinal study (Carr 1988) and from her extensive review (Carr 1985). Three clear-cut findings emerge from both sources: (1) there is a rapid decline in IQ in children with Down syndrome after the first years of life, and the decline becomes progressively less steep with increasing age; (2) females have higher IQs than males; and (3) children raised at home have higher IQs than those raised in institutions or foster homes.

With regard to the decline in IQ with age, the usual IQ figures reported for children with Down syndrome at six months or one year are surprisingly high, given the level to which they sink by about age four. Dameron (1963), Ramsay and Piper (1980), and Carr and Hewett (1982) all reported IQs in the 70 to 94 range at six months and one year in samples with IQs of 46 to 51 at two to three years. Carr (1988) reported mean IQs of 80 at six months, 45 at four years, 37 at eleven years, and 41.9 at twenty-one years. As Carr (1985) pointed out, the decline in IQ begins before much language or abstract reasoning is required by the infant tests that have been given. This is less clear in the case of language, since some language begins to be required by even infant tests at their upper ages of fifteen to twenty-four months. Carr (1988) reported that language scores on the Reynell Language Scales lagged behind IQ scores at age eleven in her sample of forty-nine children with Down syndrome.

Wishart (1991) reported the results of her ongoing studies of learning abilities in infants with Down syndrome. One set of studies involved assessment of the development of an object concept. Surprisingly, the infants with Down syndrome who were between the ages of four months and two years nine months were very close to the normal infants in making transitions to higher levels of object concept development. However, the infants with Down syndrome showed some difficulties related to their low-level engagement in tasks that had already been passed and marked avoidance of tasks that were more than one step beyond their current developmental status. In fact, Wishart found that failure on previously mastered tasks seemed to reflect a genuine loss of competence.

Several operant learning tasks were also studied. Infants with Down syndrome were found to rely on reinforcement generated by others, even when they could generate greater rewards themselves. Furthermore, an enhanced early success rate led to greater reliance on self-generated reinforcement and better consolidation of early learning. Finally, serial IQ testing indicated that it was not uncommon for infants to fail tasks that had been passed only a week earlier, usually because of deficient task engagement.

Wishart's conclusion from the above studies was that infants with Down syndrome demonstrate a counterproductive learning style, characterized by a failure to engage fully in easy tasks, avoidance of difficult tasks, and reliance on others when it is not necessary. She did not identify such deficits as due to poor motivation, although such a conclusion might be a matter of definition. As she pointed out, clinicians need to take into account the learning style that she identified when attempting early intervention to improve the cognitive development of infants with Down syndrome.

Early intervention has a substantial history in children with Down syndrome and has achieved mixed results. Gibson and Harris (1988) conducted a meta-analysis of the results from twenty-one early intervention studies with Down syndrome infants. Results were analyzed in terms of six developmental categories representing general motor growth, socialization status, eye-hand/fine-motor coordination, speech and language, cognitive-academic skills, and intelligence. Short-term gains were most consistently found in the categories of eye-hand/fine-motor coordination, socialization, and intelligence, with less consistent evidence of an effect on general motor growth, speech, and language or cognitive-academic skills. Long-term effects were confined essentially to socialization skills.

Gibson and Harris argued that most early intervention programs focused on fine-motor coordination and self-help skills, the latter being heavily sampled by measures of socialization. Short-term IQ gains in infancy may reflect the preponderance of fine-motor items on developmental tests, and later declines in IQ to the levels of nonintervention subjects may reflect the greater importance of language and cognitive items at older ages.

Early intervention is surely fighting an uphill battle in the case of Down syndrome. Children with Down syndrome seem most promising at their earliest ages. If early IQ scores from the first year were simply maintained, they would double the eventual IQ of most children with Down syndrome. However, as Wishart (1991) pointed out, even when small differences on quantitative assessments between infants with Down syndrome and control subjects are shown, the infants with Down syndrome give evidence of a deficient learning style. Substantial differences between home-reared and institutionalized or foster home-raised Down syndrome children on IQ measures suggest that differences in learning style may be responsive to environmental variables. Still, home-raised infants and even infants involved in early intervention do decline substantially in cognitive abilities as they get older.

Although meager long-term gains from early intervention may not justify enthusiasm regarding the attainment of normal levels of cognition in children with Down syndrome, neither do they justify complete despair. Socialization gains, in particular, may allow greater participation in normal activities that has a substantial influence on the quality of life. Meanwhile, continued biological and learning studies may reveal new avenues for improving cognitive development.

Academic Skills

One of the most fascinating findings in persons with Down syndrome is their relatively advanced reading ability relative to their other cognitive skills. Carr (1988) confirmed this finding in her own research. At age twenty-one reading recognition scores averaged two years above vocabulary age scores, while reading comprehension was fourteen months above vocabulary. Arithmetic showed no such acceleration and was compatible with vocabulary scores. Several individuals with Down syndrome were reported to read on their own, for pleasure.

Buckley (1985) reported similar, if not more dramatic results. She cited evidence from a behavioral intervention project at McQuarrie University in Australia, which showed that eight students obtained reading levels nearly equal to their chronological ages, despite IQs ranging from 48 to 67. Reading comprehension was more impaired but still above IQ-based expectations. Reading skills were also higher than receptive or expressive language skills and, in some cases, substantially so. Buckley suggested that reading ability may be used to promote the development of language in children with Down syndrome and cited in support of this idea the extensive anecdotal report of Duffen (1976) regarding his daughter.

Buckley also suggested that a greater facility with visual as opposed to auditory stimulus input may be responsible for the advanced reading skills of individuals with Down syndrome. This is a novel idea, for it contradicts most current theorizing regarding reading acquisition, which places auditory processing skills and language development at the core of reading. Her suggestion is not without support, however. Several studies demonstrated greater difficulty with auditory than visual memory (Marcell and Armstrong 1982; McDade and Adler 1980). Opposite to normal subjects, individuals with Down syndrome are typically better on visual than auditory short-term memory. Marcell and Weeks (1988) attempted to determine whether this relative deficit in auditory short-term memory was a true memory phenomenon or might be secondary to verbal expressive deficits that interfered with responding. They utilized auditory and visual memory tasks in which responding was either oral or manual. Subjects with Down syndrome were compared to both nonretarded subjects and retarded, non–Down syndrome subjects. The mode of response had no effect on performance, and the Down syndrome subjects had the greatest difficulty in auditory memory tasks. Not only were they deficient compared to the other groups, but also only the Down syndrome subjects failed to show a superiority of auditory over visual memory.

If children with Down syndrome read at an accelerated rate but have deficient auditory memory and rely more on visual processing skills, are they learning to read in a different way from most children? Buckley thinks so. She presented a provocative analysis of Down syndrome reading which ought to have incited a great deal of further research, although we are not aware that it has. She cited several cases of the development of reading at quite young ages in children with Down syndrome, often below four or five years of age. According to her, children with Down syndrome do not learn to read phonetically. In fact, they learn whole words and access meaning directly from print, rather than recoding the words phonologically. As evidence for this, she cited their tendency to produce semantic errors consisting of the substitution of words with similar meaning rather than sound.

The obvious problem with Buckley's analysis is that it presents the dilemma of how the meaning of printed words would exist in the first place to be accessed. In adult cases of "deep dyslexia" (Coltheart 1980), the assumption is that the print lexicon is tied to a larger language system. Buckley suggested that, in Down syndrome, reading is equivalent to learning a "first language." That is, the meaning of printed words is established by experience with printed words themselves, this experience running ahead of auditory-verbal language skills. If this were so, then semantic errors should consist primarily of substitutions of other words learned through reading (reading vocabulary should exceed auditory-verbal vocabulary). Buckley suggested that auditory-verbal language may be built up from reading, a reversal of the usual process (though it may not be so unusual at more advanced reading levels).

Buckley went on to suggest that reading may be based primarily on right-hemisphere processing of visual language in Down syndrome. Given that her analysis of reading skill is accurate, which is based more on clinical observation than on research, the right-hemisphere hypothesis is still tenuous. Although there is some evidence that semantic errors may be produced after left visual hemifield presentation of words in fluent readers, this does not imply that the lexicon of

Down syndrome persons is organized similarly, since theirs is built up during the acquisition phase of reading and is not, apparently, part of a larger language system. What is more, there simply is no reason to think that the right hemisphere would assume such an importance for language in this condition.

A result related to some of the above issues was recently obtained by Cossu, Rossini, and Marshall (1993). They examined the question of whether phonemic awareness (the ability to produce responses based on explicit awareness of the phonemic structure of words) was present in children with Down syndrome who were relatively good readers. They matched ten Italian children with Down syndrome with a mean age of 11.4 years to a group of younger normal children with a mean age of 7.3 years. The respective IQs of the two groups were 44 and 111. There were no differences between the groups on accuracy of reading regular and irregular words (in Italian, *irregular* refers to the location of the stress within the word, since most words are phonetically regular).

Besides the obviously remarkable reading skill shown by such intellectually impaired children with Down syndrome, two other results, of even greater importance, were obtained. First, the children with Down syndrome also were equal to the normal subjects in reading nonwords, constructed by changing one letter in a real word that had also been read accurately. This result is counter to what would have been predicted from Buckley's (1985) analysis, since the children with Down syndrome would not have had experience reading the nonword. It would imply some phonological decoding skill (although words composed of nonsense syllables would be a better test).

In their second result, Cossu, Rossini, and Marshall (1993) found that the children with Down syndrome were grossly deficient on a number of phonemic awareness tasks, whereas the normal control subjects were not. Cossu et al. used this finding to argue that the "meta-linguistic" skill of phonemic awareness is not necessary for reading.

Aside from its implication for normal reading, the study by Cossu, Rossini, and Marshall (1993) is important in apparently demonstrating that children with Down syndrome possess some phonetic reading ability. Since that was not the main point of their study, their demonstration is not absolutely convincing, particularly with regard to whether reading skills are learned using phonetic analysis in children with Down syndrome. Certainly, phonetic reading could be a skill that emerges from whole-word reading, although not with awareness of the strategy for producing responses, since two of the tasks failed by the majority of the children with Down syndrome were oral spelling and "phonemic synthesis," the blending of a sequence of isolated letter-sounds into a word. Both of these tasks seem to require an awareness of letter-sound correspondences.

Further studies of reading in individuals with Down syndrome are needed. The intriguing questions seem to be related to the extent of phonetic reading ability such children really have, the verification of high rates of semantic errors, and the extent to which reading comprehension is functional, as well as whether it really does exceed auditory language comprehension. If the last finding were true, it would call for a reexamination of most current ideas about language, not just reading.

Generally the mathematical abilities of individuals with Down syndrome are not particularly advanced relative to their general intelligence and are considerably behind their reading skills. As early as 1942, Pototzky and Grigg observed that, among Down syndrome cases, 50 percent could perform simple additions, 35 percent knew multiplication tables, 30 percent could perform long additions of three-place numbers, and 30 percent could perform simple subtraction. Only 5 percent could do long multiplication and none could do subtraction of three-place numbers. Kostrzewski (1965) reported that only 2 percent of subjects with Down syndrome could perform simple addition.

Buckley (1985) again reported more encouraging data, although not on a par with the striking results in reading. As she pointed out, occasional case reports have indicated some spectacular skills, such as Duffen's (1976) report of his daughter's ability to add, subtract, and multiply multidigit numbers and to plot points on a graph. However, neither Nigel Hunt, who wrote his own biography (1966), nor W. W. Smith's daughter Judith (Smith 1976), both of whom were high achievers, could do much arithmetic compared to their reading skill.

From the McQuarrie University project, Thorley and Wood (1979) reported substantial development of counting and numeral identification skills in ten preschool age children with Down syndrome taught by a highly structured sequential arithmetic program. One five year old had developed simple addition skills.

An interesting account of a twenty-six-year-old woman with Down syndrome was given by Kennan (1984). Helen O., the subject, had an IQ of 49 on the WAIS-R. Although her arithmetic skills were quite elementary (WRAT grade level of 1.7), she had developed her own strategies for adding numbers. By writing the numerals 1 to 9 and placing a dot under each, she could add any two single-digit numbers by counting the dots up to one of the numbers and then, beginning again at the first dot but continuing her count from the last number of the previous count, counting up to the next number. She was able to perform similar additions using her fingers, rather than dots.

An interesting characteristic of Helen O. was that she was relatively obsessed with birthdays. She recorded the birthdays of all friends and even acquaintances in her calendar and reminded each as the birthday approached. She recorded dates of birth and calculated ages, even at times when the person had died several years earlier. Helen's perception of time segments and time differences was keen, but not precise. She was satisfied comparing ages by phrases such as "older than," "younger than," or "same" and differences in time until birthdays as "ahead of" or "behind." A few months was "not too long," whereas weeks were designated by number. Her own birthday, which was the central date in her life, was always either "coming up" or had "already" happened.

Helen O. is interesting because she used a system for temporal orientation that was, in terms of arithmetic precision, vague but nevertheless, for her, sufficiently structured to provide quite adequate orientation in time. She did not develop spectacular calculation abilities, as are found in autistic savants or even in some nonretarded but brain-damaged individuals (e.g., Dorman 1991a), as well as, of course, in some highly intelligent true savants such as John von Neumann (Poundstone 1992). This contradicts Lindsley's (1966) conjecture that such spectacular abilities in retarded people are largely a result of motivational factors. What is equally fascinating, however, is that her temporal concepts, by being evocative, particularly of either succession or distance, rather than precise, bear some resemblance to semantic errors in reading. As described by Coltheart (1980) and others, such errors reflect concrete, imagic meaning networks rather than precise phonological matches to words that are read. To the extent that this similarity is more than superficial, the reading achievement of persons with Down syndrome may be a product of a general style of using language, rather than being related to auditory versus visual skills per se.

One way to look at the reading of children with Down syndrome and Helen O.'s use of time concepts is to see them both as reflecting an arrest of language development at an early stage. For instance, the telegraphic style of speech that has been reported in children with Down syndrome is reminiscent of what Brown (1973) called "stage 1" development of grammar. Also, the use of limited descriptors for very broad classes of events or objects, a phenomenon referred to as "overextension" (Bee 1989), is characteristic of the beginning speech of two year olds (Clark 1973). Overextension may be an apt description for both Helen O.'s time concepts and typical semantic reading errors.

To say that the language development of individuals with Down syndrome is arrested at an early stage is not news. In fact, much of their cognitive development seems to be arrested. What both Helen O. and those children with Down syndrome who read well add to this picture is the evidence that strategies for reading and temporal orientation, and perhaps much more, can be more highly developed, though they must make do with limited language facility. This would suggest that teaching strategies pay more attention to non–linguistically based meta-cognitive development and less to traditional language-based cognitive expansion. We tend to think of meta-cognition as the use of language-based knowledge, rules, and strategies. However, a little thought about skill development in, say, sports activities should make it clear that this is not always the case. Furthermore, work on mental rotation in both humans (Shepard and Metzler 1971) and, more recently, baboons (Vauclair, Fagot, and Hopkins 1993) indicates that nonverbal problem-solving strategies can be used on visual tasks. Perhaps the reported greater progress of Down syndrome children using signing as a tool for communication and socialization (Le Provost 1983) is an indication that moving away from dependence on auditory-vocal language has some advantage for persons with Down syndrome.

3

Congenital Malformation Syndromes

Because of the vagaries of nature, the number of malformation syndromes is almost unlimited. This chapter, however, focuses on only those syndromes that represent a substantial incidence, such as hydrocephalus and microcephaly, or that are of particular psychological interest, such as agenesis of the corpus callosum, Williams syndrome, and velocardiofacial syndrome. Although genetic disorders are covered in chapter 2, a clear-cut distinction between genetic and nongenetic disorders is difficult to maintain in the case of malformation syndromes. Velocardiofacial syndrome, for instance, is apparently genetically based, as are some proportion of the cases of microcephaly and, perhaps, even hydrocephalus. These disorders might be thought of as producing obvious physical abnormalities that are nonprogressive, but such a definition does not clearly fit hydrocephalus and applies equally well to disorders such as Down syndrome. The division between this chapter and chapter 2 is, therefore, somewhat arbitrary and primarily reflects conventional ways of thinking about each disorder.

Both the volume of literature and its focus differ widely across the syndromes discussed in this chapter. Some of these differences reflect differences between the syndromes themselves. Hydrocephalus, for instance, is relatively common; it is most often associated with spina bifida, and the clinical picture in different cases has some degree of uniformity. All of these things permit a fairly comprehensive review of the cognitive manifestations of the clinical syndrome itself.

Microcephaly and agenesis of the corpus callosum, on the other hand, occur much less often as isolated syndromes, and a description of the "typical" clinical picture of either would be difficult to put together and less useful, since the clinical findings often reflect the associated abnormalities. For each of these syndromes, however, certain questions have emerged regarding the relationship between the brain abnormality and behavior. With microcephaly, the principal question of interest has been the relationship between brain size and intelligence. With agenesis of the corpus callosum, questions have focused on interhemispheric communication and the role of the transfer of neural energy between hemispheres in normal development. Williams syndrome and velocardiofacial syndrome represent important clinical problems with fairly regular features but may be of interest because they represent some degree of dissociation between behaviors of one type or another. Although the relationship between such behavioral patterns and underlying brain structure is not clear in either of these syndromes, the dissociations themselves have been studied because of their importance in our understanding of how cognitive factors interact, with implications for our understanding of normal development.

Congenital Hydrocephalus

Hydrocephalus may arise for a variety of reasons. Brain malformations, including the Arnold-Chiari malformation and the Dandy-Walker syndrome, may occur secondary to or associated with spina bifida, or the latter may occur without a neural tube defect. Hydrocephalus secondary to intraventricular hemorrhage does not represent a malformation syndrome, since it is related to prematurity and hypoxia; it will not be discussed in this chapter. Hydrocephalus may also occur secondary to congenital infection (e.g., toxoplasmosis). Congenital brain tumors may also cause hydrocephalus. Our discussion is limited to hydrocephalus arising as a congenital malformation syndrome, secondary to neural tube defects.

The Mechanics of Obstruction of the Flow of Cerebral Spinal Fluid

Hydrocephalus may be either *communicating* or *noncommunicating*. In the latter, there is either partial (stenosis) or complete (occlusion) obstruction of the aqueduct of Sylvius, preventing the flow of cerebrospinal fluid from the lateral and third ventricles to the fourth. Estimates are that 20–66 percent of cases of congenital hydrocephalus are noncommunicating (Warkany, Lemire, and Cohen 1981). Communicating hydrocephalus includes the flow of cerebrospinal fluid from the third to the fourth ventricle, but access to outflow into the subarachnoid space is blocked at the level of the foramina of Magendie or Luschka or the foramen magnum.

The Arnold-Chiari malformation is a lengthening of the cerebellum such that it stretches into and partially occludes the foramen magnum or may even reach the upper cervical spinal cord. The fourth ventricle is elongated. This malformation occurs in conjunction with spina bifida (Mayr et al. 1986) and may or may not be associated with aqueductal stenosis; therefore, it may or may not be noncommunicating.

The Dandy-Walker syndrome involves the development of a cyst-like structure in the roof of the fourth ventricle. The cerebellum may show associated malformations, and the brainstem and cervical spinal cord may be flattened and displaced. The foramen of Magendie is closed, as may be the foramina of Luschka. Obstruction of the flow of cerebrospinal fluid results in dilatation of the lateral and third ventricles and of the aqueduct of Sylvius.

Incidence

The incidence of congenital hydrocephalus varies because of a number of factors related to cause, geography, and time. The overwhelming majority of cases are associated with neural tube defects. Lorber (1965) reported that, in a series of 588 patients with obstructive hydrocephalus obvious before three months of age, 84 percent were due to some type of neural tube defect and 8.7 percent were uncomplicated hydrocephalus. Tumors and hemorrhage accounted for the remainder of the cases. Sovik, Van der Hagen, and Loken (1977) reported a sex-linked recessive trait for aqueductal stenosis that may account for a very small proportion of cases of uncomplicated hydrocephalus. Hydrocephalus has also been reported to occur in conjunction with cytomegalic inclusion disease (Hanshaw 1970) and toxoplasmosis (Feldman 1958; Kaiser 1985).

The cause of neural tube defects is not known, although poor maternal nutrition has been implicated in increasing the risk (Laurence, Miller, and Campbell 1980) and decreased intake of folic acid, found in many green vegetables, has been suggested as the crucial dietary factor (Laurence et al. 1981, 1983; Smithells et al., 1983). The incidence of neural tube defects, including spina bifida and anencephaly, has declined steadily in the United States and Great Britain over the last twenty-five years (Laurence 1985; Lorber and Ward

1985). Lawrence (1985) linked this decline to both rising standards of living and prenatal diagnosis leading to therapeutic abortion. Shurtleff (1986) pointed out that prenatal diagnosis and aggressive treatment, even prenatally and including cesarean delivery, will continue to maintain a reduced but substantial prevalence, partly because of attitudinal factors regarding abortion.

Geographic variations in the incidence of neural tube defects have been noted for some time (Elwood and Elwood 1980; Lemire et al. 1975). The higher incidence reported in England, Wales, Scotland, and Ireland as well as among Irish Americans in Boston has been suggested as due to environmental and/or nutritional factors (Laurence 1985). Increases in neural tube defects in times of famine lend some support to this point of view (Rogers 1976; Wynn and Wynn 1979).

Intelligence

There seems to be unanimous agreement that hydrocephalus, even when treated, usually lowers intelligence. Table 3.1 lists studies in which the mean IQ for a sample was reported. Although the samples vary in age and the type of hydrocephalus (most being cases of spina bifida and hydrocephalus), it is clear that no one reported a mean IQ in the average range. In fact, most of the studies specifically excluded cases with severe mental retardation, so the IQ figures may be considered to overestimate intellectual levels to some unknown extent. Laurence (1969) reported the lowest mean IQ (69.7) in a sample that did not exclude any cases. When patients with IQ below 40 ($n = 17$) were removed from the sample, Laurence reported a mean IQ of 84 for the remaining sixty-four cases, which was similar to other reports.

It is also clear from Table 3.1 that average intelligence is not uncommon in hydrocephalus. Virtually every sample has a standard deviation that reaches the average range of intelligence when combined with that sample's mean. A number of other studies reported the percentage of subjects with an IQ in the average or normal range, even though the mean IQ for the whole sample was not reported. Some of these studies also reported the percentage of retarded subjects. Shurtleff, Foltz, and Loesser (1973) found that 86 percent of patients with congenital hydrocephalus without meningomyelocele ($n = 22$) had an IQ greater than 80. Sixty-two percent of those with hydrocephalus and meningomyelocele ($n = 37$) had an IQ greater than 80. These figures excluded cases of infected shunts ($n = 41$), in which the number with an IQ above 80 dropped to 23–30 percent.

Table 3.1 Mean Intelligence Quotients Reported in Different Studies

Study	Disability	n	Age (years)	IQ Mean	SD
Laurence (1969)	Congenital hydrocephalus with and without spina bifida	81		69.7	
Spain (1974)	Hydrocephalus and spina bifida	86	5.1	82.9	
Anderson and Spain (1977)	Hydrocephalus and spina bifida	29	7.8	88.3	15.0
Soare and Raimondi (1977)	Hydrocephalus and spina bifida	128	7	87	
Dennis et al. (1981)	Hydrocephalus and spina bifida	33	8.7	89	12.33
Hurley et al. (1983)	Hydrocephalus and spina bifida	30	17.5	77.6	12.4
Tew and Laurence (1983)	Hydrocephalus and spina bifida	51	5	81.3	24.2
			10	81.2	25.3
			16	75.6	24.5
Dennis (1985a)	Internal hydrocephalus	16		88.8	13.32
	Internal hydrocephalus with bilateral cortical thinning	26		85.7	13.51

The studies reported above primarily included only children whose hydrocephalus had been treated with shunting. The effect of un-treated hydrocephalus is more difficult to ascertain because intellec-tual prognosis is usually a factor in determining whether to treat a child (Shurtleff 1986). Cases may include those in which the hydro-cephalus is "spontaneously arrested" and in which a decision not to treat was made on the basis of a poor prognosis for survival or for intellectual and physical outcome. Nevertheless, some figures are available. Laurence (1958) reported on 182 patients who had not been treated. Fifty-seven percent had an IQ greater than 85. Hagberg and Sjogren (1966) reported on 62 spontaneously arrested cases. Thirty-seven percent had an IQ greater than 90, 38 percent were "educable but retarded," and 25 percent were severely retarded. Shurtleff, Foltz, and Loesser (1973) reported that 40–60 percent of patients with untreated hydrocephalus were retarded. These figures generally support a conclusion that untreated hydrocephalus has a poorer prognosis than does treated hydrocephalus and that the available figures concerning the effects of hydrocephalus on intelligence reflect both the condition and its treatment.

It might seem that the simplest way to determine the effects of hydrocephalus on intelligence, especially in the case of spina bifida, would be to compare the IQ scores of children who have spina bifida and either do or do not have an associated hydrocephalus. Some investigators have reported such figures. Spain (1974) found that 40 children with spina bifida and no hydrocephalus had a mean IQ of 99.9, compared to a mean IQ of 82.9 in 86 with hydrocephalus. Soare and Raimondi (1977) reported a mean IQ of 102 in 39 patients with meningomyelocele and no hydrocephalus, whereas 128 patients with associated hydrocephalus had a mean IQ of 87. The available evidence strongly suggests that, in spina bifida, the presence of an associated hydrocephalus lowers intelligence.

Factors That Lower Intelligence in Hydrocephalus
Factors that may or may not contribute to a lower IQ in hydrocephalic patients have been studied. Although several of the results are contradictory, some consistent findings have emerged.

The level of spinal lesions is related to intellectual outcome (Tew and Laurence 1979), with higher lesions having a poor prognosis. As a mechanism producing lower IQ, however, this is hardly an explanatory factor. The level of the lesion affects the likelihood of developing hydrocephalus, so some studies have produced results that may be redundant with those showing an effect of hydrocephalus on IQ. The degree of motor involvement is also related to the level of the spinal lesion and itself may affect intellectual outcome (Dennis et al. 1981; Lawrence 1964). In children with spina bifida and hydrocephalus, the correlation between the level of the lesion and IQ remains (Hunt and Holmes 1975; Shaffer et al. 1985). However, it seems most likely that this effect is mediated by other variables, such as the degree of motor impairment (Laurence 1969) and the site of the obstruction of cerebrospinal fluid (Dennis et al. 1981).

It seems reasonable to assume that a direct measure of the effects of hydrocephalus, such as the thickness of the cortical mantle, would be related to intellectual ability. This relationship has been difficult to establish. Shurtleff, Foltz, and Loesser (1973) found a relationship between the cerebral mantle width, defined as the frontal ventriculoskull distance, and IQ, but only if the cerebral mantle was less than 22 percent of the normal width for that age. A more linear relationship was found between a measure of estimated brain mass, taking into account both skull size and mantle width, and IQ. No patient with less than 60 percent of the normal brain mass for the age had a normal IQ.

Dennis et al. (1981) observed an even more complex relationship between cortical thinning and intelligence. The mean cortical width was not related to intelligence in their thirty-four cases. Neither was the cortical width in either the frontal or the occipital region when considered alone. Asymmetrical thinning of the cortex, with relatively greater thinning occipitally than frontally, was related to a lowered Performance IQ but not Verbal IQ. Furthermore, this result was found only in the children with intraventricular hydrocephalus and obstruction of the cerebrospinal fluid at the cerebral aqueduct or anterior third ventricle. There was no interaction between the effect of asymmetrical cortical thinning and the presence of ocular, motor, or seizure disorder, although all three of these factors had an independent influence on lowering Performance IQ.

The results with regard to cortical thinning are by no means clear. The findings by Shurtleff, Foltz, and Loesser (1973) and Dennis et al. (1981) seem to be contradictory, but Shurtleff et al. used a measure of brain mass, whereas Dennis et al. measured mantle width. The latter study demonstrated only an effect on Performance IQ; because a lowering of Performance IQ may also be reflected in the Full-Scale IQ, however, it is not clear whether the result of Shurtleff et al. pertains to global or selective intellectual impairment. The entire matter deserves further study. Both the method of measurement of brain volume (width versus mass) and the delineation of the type of hydrocephalus (communicating versus noncommunicating) and the site of the obstruction of cerebrospinal fluid seem to be pertinent independent variables. Similarly, dependent measures of cognitive ability must be sufficiently varied to assess whether the impairment is global or selective.

There is some theoretical significance to the answers to the questions regarding cortical thickness or mass, regional versus global thinning, and global versus selective impairment of cognition. Many cases of hydrocephalus represent an alteration in brain structure that begins prenatally. Defects in neural tube closure occur within the first month of gestation. The likelihood of reorganizing neural structures to compensate for tissue loss seems to be maximal in this type of disorder, although the continuation and even accentuation of the pathological process up to the point of treatment may affect neural plasticity. The findings by Dennis et al. are provocative in this regard because they seem to demonstrate a selective impairment of cognitive function based on diminished volume of a circumscribed cortical area relative to the cortex as a whole. This would imply limitations to cortical plasticity even when the damage occurs extremely early. Recent research using animal models has provided a suggestion that the occipital cortex may regenerate or develop alternative but functionally viable connections (e.g., Michejda 1984; Michejda and McCollough 1987); however, such alterations may be severely time limited (Bannister et al. 1987). The degree of reorganizational capacity of human cortex may be gauged in part by the outcome of children with congenital hydrocephalus. Although the results cited above imply a limit to this capacity, the unusual cases reported by Lorber (1983), in which high IQ was found in the presence of nearly absent cortical tissue, caution against any premature conclusions in this area.

Associated Influences on Intelligence
The level of the spinal lesion and the extent of cortical thinning are variables that are related to the structure of the nervous system and its influence on intelligence. Dennis (1985a, 1985b) used multivariate procedures (factor analysis and cluster analysis) to group biological and medical history variables that may be pertinent to cognitive functioning. With congenital hydrocephalus, subjects fell into two clusters: (1) those with internal (noncommunicating) hydrocephalus, aqueductal stenosis or anterior third ventricle (foramina of Monro) blockages, or spina bifida and Arnold-Chiari malformation and (2) similar subjects with known cortical thinning bilaterally. The former group had a slightly higher Full-Scale IQ (88) than did the latter (85), primarily because of a higher Verbal IQ.

Related to the pathological findings in these two groups were a number of medical variables concerning intellectual functioning. In addition to the presence of obstructive hydrocephalus and early signs of hydrocephalus, which were both related only to Performance IQ, spinal dysraphism, brain thinning, and the presence of a shunt were all related to both Performance IQ and Full-Scale IQ (but not Verbal IQ). Other factors, found across a number of conditions including hydrocephalus, such as eye signs, fine motor problems, and seizures, were also related to intelligence, although only seizures were related to Verbal IQ.

Dennis's study did not permit the identification of factors affecting IQ in hydrocephalus as opposed to other conditions (unless they occurred only in hydrocephalus). However, considerable research has examined medical variables such as shunt placement, infections of the central nervous system, and seizures in terms of their relationship to IQ in children with hydrocephalus.

Some studies equate the presence of a shunt with the presence of hydrocephalus (e.g., Anderson and Spain 1977), thus leading to an inverse relationship between shunt placement and IQ. In children with hydrocephalus, shunt placement as opposed to nontreatment is associated with improved intelligence. Since most children with congenital hydrocephalus undergo shunt placement, the question of whether the number of shunt "revisions" is related to intellectual outcome has been raised. Soare and Raimondi (1977) found no relationship between the number of shunt revisions and IQ in a sample of 167 children with spina bifida and hydrocephalus. Neither did Dennis et al. (1981) find any such relationship. Contrary to these findings, both Puri, Malone, and Guiney (1977) and Halliwell, Carr, and Pearson (1980) reported a negative relationship between the number of shunt revisions and IQ. Grant et al. (1986) raised an interesting question regarding the effects of shunting on hydrocephalic children. Citing some evidence that shunted children showed a greater Verbal-Performance split in IQ, favoring higher Verbal IQ, than did nonshunted children (e.g., Lonton 1979; Tew and Laurence 1975), they proposed that the tradition of inserting shunts through the right hemisphere might contribute to this discrepancy. In addition, they proposed that the left hemisphere might be more resilient with regard to the effects of such a procedure on language skill. Such a proposal actually has some support from evidence cited by Dennis (1985a, 1985b) regarding the paucity of effects on Verbal IQ as opposed to Performance IQ of a number of brain injury variables.

Although Grant et al. had only a limited number of cases available, they examined the effects of left-hemisphere shunting when it occurred (usually after complications with a previously placed right-hemisphere shunt). Additionally, they determined that several patients had "reversed laterality" on the basis of tasks presented to either the right or the left visual field. Their results indicated that shunting through the language area does not impair language to the extent that shunting through the right hemisphere impairs visual perceptual abilities. However, a selective deficit in reading skills was noted in the children shunted through the language area.

These results by Grant et al. should be evaluated with caution. Their sample size was extremely small, with only ten subjects in each group (right-hemisphere shunts versus right- and left-hemisphere shunts). The "reversed laterality" group contained only three subjects.

Their results were significant in only one analysis—poorer visuo-spatial skills in the right hemisphere–shunted group. All groups continued to show a superiority of verbal over visual skills. We describe the study in some detail because it represents an attempt to determine the effect of one aspect of hydrocephalus (i.e., shunting) on the pattern of cognitive skills seen in such children.

A more clear-cut relationship between intellect and one medical factor pertinent to hydrocephalus was demonstrated by those investigators who examined the influence of shunt-related infections on IQ. Shurtleff, Foltz, and Loesser (1973) found that 14 percent of children with hydrocephalus without myelomeningocele and 38 percent of children with myelomeningocele and hydrocephalus were retarded if no history of infection was present. The same two groups showed 70 percent and 77 percent retardation, respectively, when infection was present. McLone et al. (1982) found an equally dramatic effect of infections on the IQ of hydrocephalic children. Eighty-six children with myelomeningocele and hydrocephalus but no history of infection had a mean IQ of 95. Forty-two children with the same disorder but also a history of shunt infection had a mean IQ of 73. Although the result did not reach statistical significance, there was a suggestion that the earlier the infection occurred, the greater the degree of retardation.

Another medical variable that has been consistently related to intellectual outcome in hydrocephalus is the occurrence of seizures. Stellman, Bannister, and Hillier (1986) found the incidence of seizures to be 29.6–54.2 percent in children with congenital hydrocephalus. More than half of the children had had only an isolated seizure incident, often related to raised intracranial pressure or shunt infection. Children with seizures were more likely to have an IQ below normal than were those without. Similarly, frequent and persistent seizures were much more highly related to low IQ than were isolated seizure episodes. Generalized and focal seizures were approximately equally likely to occur.

Dennis et al. (1981) found seizures to be associated with lower Performance and Full-Scale IQs as well as with a larger discrepancy between Verbal IQ and Performance IQ. Neither the type nor the frequency of seizures was related to IQ in their study. However, the presence of a right-hemisphere seizure focus on electroencephalogram was related to diminished Performance IQ relative to Verbal IQ.

The above-mentioned medical variables that have been found to affect intelligence in hydrocephalus may be primarily related to treatment. Certainly, the side on which a shunt is placed or the presence of shunt infection is a treatment-related phenomenon. Seizures may also be related to shunt infections but occur with raised intracranial pressure or may simply be a consequence of the brain malformation. At any rate, such treatment-related medical variables serve to obscure the relationship between the anatomical abnormalities found in hydrocephalus and cognitive functioning.

Donders, Canady, and Rourke (1990) used multivariate procedures (stepwise discriminant analysis) to predict intellectual outcome in a sample of five- to eight-year-old children who had been shunted for hydrocephalus in the first year of life. The presence of additional medical problems in infancy and the presence of ocular defects at the time of testing were the best predictors of low IQ.

Language

It is a general finding that Verbal IQ is higher than Performance IQ in many children with hydrocephalus (Anderson and Spain 1977; Dennis et al. 1981; Hurley, Laatsch, and Dorman 1983). It is also generally thought that the higher Verbal IQ found in such children does not necessarily represent intact language abilities. As mentioned previously, Dennis et al. (1981) found relative cortical thinning occipitally, right focal seizures, motor problems, visual problems, and site of the blockage of cerebrospinal fluid flow all to be related to lowered Performance but not Verbal IQ. The majority of the children in their study had a Verbal IQ but not a Performance IQ in the average range. When both the Verbal and Performance IQs of a sample are below average, the same discrepancy is usually found, however (Hurley, Laatsch, and Dorman 1983; Tew and Lawrence 1983). Hurley, Laatsch, and Dorman (1983) demonstrated that the "split" in Verbal and Performance skills was not an artifact of lowered IQ itself. They matched thirty hydrocephalic patients with thirty nonhydrocephalic patients on the basis of age and Full-Scale Wechsler IQ. Both groups had mean IQs below the normal range (77 and 78). The hydrocephalic group's split between Verbal IQ and Performance IQ (7 points) was significantly greater than that found in the control group (1 point).

Despite evidence of relative strength in the verbal area, weaknesses have also been found. Hadenius et al. (1962) identified a "cocktail party syndrome" in children with hydrocephalus. This syndrome was characterized by "a peculiar contrast between a good ability to learn words and talk, and not knowing what they talk about." Several clinical descriptions of such behavior have been offered (Anderson and Spain

1977; Hagberg and Sjogren 1966; Ingram and Naughton 1962). It has been suggested that the syndrome should occur particularly in those children with larger differences between Verbal IQ and Performance IQ (Badell-Ribera, Shulman, and Paddock 1966).

Tew attempted a quantitative study of cocktail party syndrome in children with hydrocephalus and spina bifida (Tew 1979; Tew and Lawrence 1979). Cocktail party syndrome was judged to be present if four of the five following characteristics were observed: (1) perseverative speech, (2) excessive use of social phrases, (3) overly familiar manner, (4) a habit of introducing personal experience into the conversation in irrelevant and inappropriate contexts, and (5) fluent and well-articulated speech. Children ware assessed in terms of intellectual, language, visuomotor, and social skills at age five, on reading and arithmetic at age seven, and on intelligence at age ten.

Compared to children with spina bifida and hydrocephalus who did not exhibit cocktail party syndrome, those who did were more likely to be female, to have required a shunt for their hydrocephalus, to have a lesion higher on the spine, to be more physically disabled, and to attend a special school. Although both groups of hydrocephalic children were less intelligent than a group of normal controls, the IQ scores of the group with cocktail party syndrome were also significantly lower than those of other hydrocephalic children. Differences between Verbal IQ and Performance IQ were present in both hydrocephalic groups but reached significance only in those with cocktail party syndrome.

Virtually every cognitive and academic measure given to the subjects at either five or seven years of age revealed substantially worse skills in the group of subjects with cocktail party syndrome than in the other hydrocephalic children. These differences were interpreted as related to the difference in intellectual level between the two groups. Similar differences were present on the Reynall Developmental Language Scales. Surprisingly, the subjects with cocktail party syndrome scored higher on the language comprehension measure than on the expression measure and showed a greater relative superiority of comprehension skills over expression skills than did the other hydrocephalic children or the normal controls. Thus, the characterization of the subjects with cocktail party syndrome as better at speaking than at understanding language was not substantiated by formal tests. By age ten, approximately half of the subjects with cocktail party syndrome had "grown out of" the syndrome. Those who continued to be rated as having the syndrome were likely to be female and to have a lower IQ.

Hurley et al. (1990) examined some of the cognitive characteristics of children and young adults identified as having cocktail party syndrome. Using the criteria listed by Tew (1979), they obtained fairly high interrater agreement (76–82 percent) on the presence or absence of each component of the syndrome. Fifteen of fifty (30 percent) hydrocephalic subjects (all with spina bifida) met the criteria for cocktail party syndrome. These subjects differed from the others by having lower intelligence on Verbal, Performance, and Full-Scale measures. Achievement scores in reading, spelling, and arithmetic were also lower, as were scores on a measure of comprehension of metaphorical language. There were no differences between the groups on the number of perseverative errors on the Wisconsin Card Sorting Test, a problem-solving measure often thought to measure frontal lobe–based skills.

To assess the extent to which IQ levels accounted for the differences between the groups, fifteen of the subjects without cocktail party syndrome were matched for Full-Scale IQ to the subjects with cocktail party syndrome. Those with cocktail party syndrome remained poorer in spelling and arithmetic skills but not in metaphorical language comprehension. Interestingly, no differences between Verbal IQ and Performance IQ were noted between the groups, but an additional subgroup of subjects designated as dysfunctional in daily living skills, with or without cocktail party syndrome, showed a larger Verbal-Performance discrepancy in favor of higher Verbal IQ than did other subjects. These results tend to support Tew's (1979) conclusion that cocktail party syndrome is found in lower IQ hydrocephalic subjects and is not associated with any characteristic cognitive pattern except perhaps poor academic skills.

Dennis et al. (1987) questioned the usefulness of the designation of cocktail party syndrome in hydrocephalic children. These authors favored a more comprehensive assessment of language abilities in hydrocephalic children and an attempt to relate language variables to medical factors (e.g., the cause of the hydrocephalus) and age. Their study of seventy-five children and young adults with both congenital and birth or neonatal problem-related hydrocephalus revealed several significant findings. Spina bifida with hydrocephalus impaired verbal fluency (measured by automatized naming), which the authors hypothesized might share a common cause with the visuomotor difficulties observed in this disorder. Generally, intraventricular (noncommunicating) hydrocephalus had a more deleterious effect on language understanding (comprehension of grammar) and word finding, whereas extraventricular (communicating) hydrocephalus had a more deleterious effect on fluency but not understanding. This finding prompted the authors to hypothesize that verbal fluency may be more related to subtentorial brain regions and that more central language processes such as lexical access and grammatical comprehension may be more related to a blockage of the flow of cerebrospinal fluid within the ventricular system. Both types of hydrocephalus were related to poor sentence recall, suggesting that "verbal memory systems (perhaps especially those mediated by brain regions surrounding the third ventricle) are especially vulnerable to disturbances of intracranial pressure."

The approach by Dennis et al. (1987) to the question of language development in hydrocephalic children and their results are among the more comprehensive in terms of the breadth of assessment of both language and medical variables. Although they decried the focus on so-called syndromes, like cocktail party syndrome, because these represent an unusual abnormality and tell little about the normal course of development in a condition, such syndromes may deserve explanation. It is not clear what cocktail party syndrome represents. It is a phenomenon that is striking enough to provoke clinical description (e.g., Anderson and Spain 1977; Taylor 1961), but it is possible that it represents merely a surprising degree of language usage in otherwise retarded children. Tew (1979) offered a number of possible variables related to upbringing and environment that might account for precocious use of social language in otherwise severely impaired children. Thus far, there is no good evidence that this syndrome is related to a special pattern of cognitive abilities. Although it has not been reported to characterize any subset of generally retarded children without hydrocephalus, cocktail party syndrome has been reported in Williams syndrome, a congenital anomaly syndrome that includes cardiovascular abnormalities, mental retardation, distinctive facies, voice abnormalities, and hypersensitivity to acoustic stimuli. Bennett, La Veck, and Sells (1978) found visuomotor and motor deficits in preschool-age children with this syndrome. MacDonald and Roy (1988) replicated this finding in seven older children (six to eleven years) who were compared to a control group matched for age, sex, and receptive vocabulary scores. They observed specific deficits on academic achievement and visuomotor measures in the children with Williams syndrome. Because this profile bears considerable resemblance to that observed in hydrocephalic children, it keeps alive the issue of whether there might be a relationship between disparities in language versus visuomotor behavior and the presence of cocktail party syndrome.

Rourke postulated a relationship between impaired visuomotor performance and overly talkative, socially inappropriate behavior in learning-disabled children and speculated that it might reflect right-hemisphere neurological disorder (Rourke 1987; Rourke and Strang 1983). Recently, he extended his right-hemisphere dysfunction hypothesis to include hydrocephalic children with visuomotor problems. Donders, Canady, and Rourke (1990) administered a comprehensive battery of neuropsychological tests to thirty hydrocephalic children who were five to eight years old. Although the children performed normally on many of the tests, they were specifically impaired on measures of complex visuospatial functioning. The authors concluded that such findings supported a hypothesis of posterior right-hemisphere dysfunction.

Fletcher et al. (1992) arrived at a similar conclusion to that of Donders, Canady, and Rourke. Their sample consisted of ninety children who were five to seven years old. Thirty-three children had hydrocephalus secondary to spina bifida. Eight had hydrocephalus related to aqueductal stenosis but without spina bifida. Twenty children had been born prematurely and had hydrocephalus secondary to grade III or grade IV intraventricular hemorrhage. Twenty-nine children had no hydrocephalus; of these, sixteen had been born prematurely and thirteen had normal histories. All children were tested two times, one year apart. On the first occasion the McCarthy Scales of Children's Abilities and a battery of verbal, visuospatial, visuomotor, and memory tests were administered. On the second occasion the WISC-R was administered.

Fletcher et al. found that hydrocephalic children were deficient on performance measures on both the McCarthy scales and the WISC-R. There was no effect of the cause of the hydrocephalus. There were no verbal-nonverbal discrepancies on memory tasks for the hydrocephalic subjects, although the hydrocephalics did worse than the nonhydrocephalics on both verbal and nonverbal memory tests. In addition, visuospatial tasks were performed less well by the hydrocephalic children whether or not a motor component was involved. Magnetic resonance imaging of the brains of the children in the study revealed thinning of the corpus callosum in nearly all of those with hydrocephalus secondary to either spina bifida or aqueductal stenosis. The correlation between the thickness of the corpus callosum and nonverbal skills was greater than that between the thickness and verbal skills. The authors concluded that either impairment of white matter in the right hemisphere or deficient connectivity between the hemispheres might be the source of nonverbal deficits.

Visuomotor Abilities

The association between hydrocephalus and impaired Performance IQ relative to Verbal IQ has been documented (Badell-Ribera, Schulman, and Paddock 1966; Hurley, Laatsch, and Dorman 1983). Visuomotor abilities have also been the subject of many investigations. In a series of studies that have generated several efforts at replication, Miller and Sethi (1971a, 1971b) examined visual perception and tactile perception in a relatively small sample ($n = 16$) of hydrocephalic children. Their methods of testing visual perception attempted to eliminate the confounding variables of motor performance or verbal labeling of stimuli. Their tasks involved matching to sample problems using difficult-to-label stimuli (Hindi letters) and matrix patterns of different complexity which also varied the degree to which background information was irrelevant to the solution of the task. They found that hydrocephalic children were inferior to controls in matching visual stimuli and that the control subjects' difficulty ignoring irrelevant background was magnified in the hydrocephalic children's performance.

On tactile matching tasks, the hydrocephalic subjects were not different from the controls when the sample and the match were explored with the same hand. However, when matching required intermanual communication because both hands were used, the hydrocephalic children's performance was worse than that of the controls. This finding prompted Miller and Sethi (1971b) to suggest that hydrocephalic children might have a "partial callosal dysfunction" syndrome due to a stretching of callosal fibers with increasing hydrocephalus.

Zeiner and Prigatano (1982) devised several experiments to test the hypothesis of partial callosal dysfunction with regard to hydrocephalic subjects. Their tasks involved same and opposite visual field matching tasks, unimanual and bimanual tactile matching tasks, and dichotic listening tasks. Although hydrocephalic subjects performed more poorly than controls on all of the tasks, they did not have significantly greater difficulty when communication between the two hemispheres was required to solve the task. Zeiner and Prigatano conceded that their subjects were generally more cognitively intact than those of Miller and Sethi, probably because Zeiner and Prigatano excluded any case with complications secondary to hydrocephalus. However, they established that hydrocephalus per se does not seem to disrupt interhemispheric communication.

Although the results of Miller and Sethi with regard to visual perception seem to eliminate the confounding variables of motor performance and verbal labeling, they do not rule out the influence of cognitive impairment on performance. In fact, some studies found impairment on visuomotor tasks but failed to distinguish such deficits from more general cognitive impairment (Grimm 1976; Sand et al. 1973). Tew and Lawrence (1975) administered the WPPSI and the Frostig Test of Visual Perception to fifty-nine children with spina bifida, thirty-nine of whom had some degree of hydrocephalus. Although the distribution of scores on the Frostig test was below normal, it closely paralleled the distribution of IQ scores.

Visuomotor impairment may reflect low IQ, but differences between Verbal IQ and Performance IQ scores are presumably independent of the general cognitive level. This is not entirely true, however, since the equivalence between Verbal IQ and Performance IQ holds much more for the middle range of IQ than for the upper and lower extremes. With higher IQ levels the Verbal IQ is more likely to be above the Performance IQ, and with lower IQ levels the reverse is true.

Hurley, Laatsch, and Dorman (1983) matched thirty hydrocephalic subjects (with spina bifida) to thirty controls on the basis of age and IQ. The hydrocephalic subjects showed a significant difference between Verbal IQ and Performance IQ, in favor of Verbal IQ, whereas the controls did not. The mean IQ of the two groups was 77.5, so the discrepancy between Verbal and Performance abilities did not seem to be a function of intellectual level. Dennis (1985a, 1985b) found that several variables in children's medical histories predicted Performance IQ but not Verbal IQ. It seems that visuomotor abilities may be vulnerable to adverse developmental influences that are less likely to disturb language development.

Measures such as the Frostig Test of Visual Perception or the Performance section of the Wechsler scales do not separate visual perception from motor skill. Several studies bear upon the issue of whether the major deficit in hydrocephalus is visual, motor, or both. There is ample evidence that motor skill alone is impaired in children with spina bifida and hydrocephalus, as shown by their difficulty with such tasks as handwriting (Cambridge and Anderson 1979). Sand et al. (1973) found that the Eye-Hand Coordination subtest of the Frostig was the most impaired scale in hydrocephalic children but also in children with spina bifida but no hydrocephalus. Since spinal cord abnormalities can themselves cause motor impairment (such as spasticity in the tethered cord syndrome), it is not surprising that spina bifida alone can impair motor abilities. This further complicates the issue of whether hydrocephalus per se impairs motor performance.

Grimm (1976) studied hand function on a measure that seems to place much more stress on coordination and strength than on visual perception (Taylor, Sand, and Jebson 1973). Hydrocephalic children were more impaired than were nonhydrocephalic children with spina bifida, although the latter were slightly below the normal range. Higher spinal lesions were related to poorer hand functions but also to the likelihood of developing hydrocephalus, a consistent finding that complicates the issue in cases of hydrocephalus secondary to spina bifida. Interestingly, Grimm also found deficits in tactile perception in hydrocephalic subjects. However, tactile deficits and motor deficits were generally unrelated.

The syndrome of "normal pressure hydrocephalus" (Hakim and Adams 1965) was originally reported in adults with dementia who showed enlarged ventricles but normal cerebrospinal fluid pressures. A characteristic finding in this condition is an improvement in motor abilities after the placement of a shunt. Furthermore, motor disturbance is a prominent symptom of the condition before shunting and a predictor of likely improvement after shunting. In this condition it seems clear that motor disturbance is related to the presence of hydrocephalus because the symptoms improve with relief of the hydrocephalus. Hammock, Milhorat, and Baron (1976) reported a similar syndrome in children with spina bifida. As was experienced with adults, they found that motor performance (as measured by the Tactual Performance Test) improved in some subjects after the placement of a shunt.

Despite the large number of studies that have established visuomotor deficits in hydrocephalic children, the exact nature of such deficits remains unclear and their practical significance is not well established. Simms (1986, 1987) examined the relationship between performance on visual perceptual and memory tasks and automobile driving and route-finding ability in real-life situations. Hydrocephalic young adults were compared to nonhandicapped peers. Although the hydrocephalic subjects performed less well on perceptual and memory tests, such tests were not very predictive of real-life abilities. General reasoning skill and experience were more strongly related to route finding and driving in traffic than were measures of perception and memory.

An interesting finding with regard to motor abilities in hydrocephalic children is that the incidence of left and mixed handedness seems to be elevated. Lonton (1976) found that mixed handedness was more prevalent in hydrocephalic children with spina bifida than in normal children. Children with mixed handedness also had lower

Verbal and Full-Scale IQ levels, as well as lower reading levels, than those of both right- and left-handed children. No differences in cortical thickness were found between the mixed-handed children and others, but more mixed-handed children had severe grades of lacunar skull deformities and higher meningomyeloceles. The correlation of mixed handedness with lower IQ is also found outside the hydrocephalic population. Soper et al. (1987) found that 45 percent of severely and profoundly retarded residents of a school for retarded children were ambiguous in handedness. They hypothesized that brain injury could account for this finding. It is possible that hydrocephalus is one of the brain injury factors that increases mixed handedness.

Academic Achievement

Given that the distribution of intelligence level in hydrocephalus is skewed toward lower values, it might be expected that academic levels would also be impaired. In fact, this is the case (Tew and Laurence 1972, 1975).

In 1975 Tew and Laurence found that hydrocephalic children with spina bifida were considerably behind their age-matched peers in all academic subjects. Although children with spina bifida and no hydrocephalus were also behind their nonhandicapped peers, the gap was not so large as when hydrocephalus was present. IQ scores were also depressed in the hydrocephalic subjects, and both academic achievement and visuomotor skills were closely related to IQ. Interestingly, although reading, spelling, and arithmetic were all impaired in the hydrocephalic subjects, the degree of impairment was greatest in arithmetic.

In 1984 Tew and Laurence reported again on the same sample, who were now sixteen to eighteen years old. They found a similar result. Both reading and arithmetic scores were significantly poorer than in control subjects, with arithmetic being the weaker skill. In addition, as judged by the passage of national examinations, those students attending special schools were at lower levels of academic skill than were their similarly handicapped peers who attended ordinary schools. The latter is also a common finding. Both Anderson and Spain (1977) and Halliwell, Carr, and Pearson (1980) reported lower academic achievement scores in reading and arithmetic for children with spina bifida and hydrocephalus attending special as opposed to ordinary schools. Unfortunately, the children in these samples differed in terms of intelligence as well as school placement, confounding a clear-cut interpretation of the results. However, Carr, Halliwell, and Pearson (1984) carefully matched twenty-two pairs of children for Full-Scale, Verbal, and Performance IQ. One member of each pair attended ordinary school and one attended special school. Reading scores between the two groups did not differ, but the children in special school were, on the average, more than one year behind the children in ordinary school in arithmetic achievement. Dodd (1984) obtained similar results in a sample of thirty-eight pairs of children in which there was no significant difference in IQ between those attending special schools and those attending ordinary schools. Arithmetic scores from the WISC were lower in the children attending special schools, but reading scores were not.

Social class may interact with biological factors to produce a more severe hydrocephalus at birth in children of lower social class (Lonton 1979). At present, the mechanism that might account for such an interaction is obscure, although the possibility that maternal nutrition could reflect social class and affect brain development certainly deserves consideration because there is evidence of such a mechanism in determining small head size (Brandt 1981). An equally intriguing finding is that a social factor such as school placement seems to affect arithmetic achievement selectively, and arithmetic achievement, in turn, is generally the weakest academic skill in hydrocephalic children. One might conclude that arithmetic, either because it is the more vulnerable skill in hydrocephalus or because of the nature of the learning of arithmetic itself, requires greater environmental support for development than does reading.

Barnes and Dennis (1992) conducted an in-depth study of reading ability in hydrocephalic children. Their subjects were fifty children ages six through fifteen matched to normal controls on the basis of age and grade. Twenty-four of the children had hydrocephalus secondary to spina bifida; the others had intraventricular hemorrhage (9), congenital or idiopathic hydrocephalus (6), aqueductal stenosis (5), Dandy-Walker cyst (3), arachnoid cyst (2), or choroid plexus papilloma (1). Reading measures were taken from the Woodcock Reading Mastery Test-Revised and included measures of word recognition, word attack (nonsense-word reading), single-word comprehension, and passage comprehension.

Unfortunately, Barnes and Dennis had IQ scores for only the hydrocephalic sample, not the controls. Thus, intelligence could not be used as a covariate in their between-groups analyses. The hydrocephalic subjects did have low-average to average IQ scores, with lower Performance than Verbal scores. IQ was significantly related to reading on all of the reading measures. Reading scores were lower in the hydrocephalic group only on the measures of word and passage comprehension, not on the measures of word recognition or word attack. Follow-up analyses indicated that reading comprehension was poorer than reading recognition in the hydrocephalic group and that passage comprehension was significantly related to the subskills of reading recognition and word comprehension.

It is not clear from the Barnes and Dennis study to what extent reading is actually impaired in hydrocephalic children. One would surmise that vocabulary is a limiting factor in the comprehension of passages, since such comprehension is related to single-word comprehension, which is also impaired. However, comprehension is also related to recognition skills, which are not impaired. The authors pointed out that recognizing single words does not measure other aspects of recognition, such as speed or effort, which may impair comprehension. When those hydrocephalic subjects who had average or better intelligence were analyzed separately, their reading recognition scores were still better than their passage comprehension scores, but their recognition scores were also slightly (but not significantly) better than those of the controls. The differences between the average-IQ hydrocephalic children and the normal controls were reported and were about one-half of a standard deviation on passage comprehension, but were not analyzed for statistical significance. Differences between the two groups were not apparent on any of the other reading measures.

The Barnes and Dennis (1992) study implies that hydrocephalic children are relatively impaired in reading comprehension but not reading recognition, either when their abilities are analyzed ipsatively or when they are compared to normal children. The data are actually more supportive of the former conclusion. This is not, however, the same as saying that their reading levels are impaired *relative to what would be expected on the basis of their intellect*. For instance, a pattern of overachievement in reading recognition, relative to intelligence, and expected achievement in reading comprehension would yield the same results if the average IQ of the hydrocephalic subjects was somewhat lower than that of the control group.

Our own data collected from children attending a residential school for handicapped students have some bearing on this issue. Most of the children in the sample had attended the same school throughout their education. Therefore, there was an opportunity to compare children with spina bifida and hydrocephalus to equally severely physically handicapped children with other conditions, such as cerebral palsy or

Table 3.2   Means and Standard Deviations of Intellectual and Academic
Test Scores

	IQ			Academic Score		
Subjects	Full-Scale	Verbal	Performance	Reading	Spelling	Arithmetic
Hydrocephalic	75.51	80.46	75.00	86.09	81.63	74.09
	(13.55)	(13.51)	(14.33)	(20.56)	(17.37)	(15.56)
Neurologically impaired	82.03	87.23	78.63	85.29	83.29	72.17
	(16.40)	(19.07)	(17.58)	(21.79)	(16.18)	(10.61)

muscular dystrophy, while controlling for educational experience. Table 3.2 lists the intellectual and academic achievement scores for two groups of thirty-five children each, one composed of just those children with spina bifida and hydrocephalus and the other composed of children with other neurological disorders.

The most interesting finding is that academic achievement scores in the hydrocephalic sample, especially in reading and spelling, were somewhat better than would be predicted on the basis of the IQ scores. Arithmetic, on the other hand, was more compatible with IQ. Arithmetic was also the weakest area of academic achievement for the hydrocephalic subjects, but this applied also to the mixed impairment group. This would imply either that arithmetic skill is especially vulnerable to a variety of neurological disorders or that the special education environment in which all of these students were taught was poor at developing arithmetic skills. Whichever is the case (and they both may be), it is clear that having a greater deficit in arithmetic skills than in reading or spelling skills is not a unique consequence of having hydrocephalus. In addition to viewing these data in terms of mean skill levels in each academic area relative to IQ variables, the investigators also examined them to determine which intellectual abilities were most highly related to the measures of academic achievement.

Table 3.3 provides the correlation coefficients between each of the intellectual variables and the academic variables for both the hydrocephalic subjects and the mixed neurologically impaired subjects. It is quite clear that intellectual test scores are generally good predictors of academic achievement test scores for both groups of subjects. Verbal IQ is also generally a better predictor of academic scores than is Performance IQ or even Full-Scale IQ. The pattern and size of the correlations are quite similar for the two groups, with the only substantial difference being in regard to the correlation between Performance IQ and arithmetic. The correlation is substantial (.63) in the

Table 3.3   Correlations between Intellectual and Academic Measures

IQ Measure	Hydrocephalic			Neurologically Impaired		
	Reading	Spelling	Arithmetic	Reading	Spelling	Arithmetic
Full-Scale IQ	.65[b]	.60[b]	.77[b]	.64[b]	.68[b]	.66[a]
Verbal IQ	.72[b]	.67[b]	.76[b]	.73[b]	.78[b]	.80[b]
Performance IQ	.42[a]	.36[a]	.63[b]	.39[a]	.39[a]	.31

[a] $p < .05$.
[b] $p < .001$.

hydrocephalic group and higher than that between Performance IQ and either reading or spelling, although still lower than that between either Verbal IQ or Full-Scale IQ and arithmetic. In the mixed neurologically impaired group, the correlation between Performance IQ and arithmetic is quite low (.31) and is the only nonsignificant correlation found in either sample.

These results are compatible with the hypothesis that the visuospatial deficits found among hydrocephalic subjects are related to their difficulty in doing arithmetic. This is not surprising because studies of children who are specifically disabled in arithmetic skills have found similar deficits on visuospatial tasks (Rourke and Strang 1978; Strang and Rourke 1985). As we assert in chapter 8, however, this correlational relationship between visuospatial skills and arithmetic does not necessarily signal a causal relationship. It is probably more surprising that a similar relationship was not found among the mixed neurologically impaired group. It seems likely that members of this group, who often had upper extremity motor impairment, were sometimes impaired in Performance IQ for purely motoric reasons and that this fact obscured any relationship between visuospatial ability and arithmetic skill.

The finding that reading and spelling skills were better than would be expected on the basis of IQ scores was somewhat surprising, although several of the studies reported above found reading to be less impaired than arithmetic in hydrocephalic children. We followed up this initial finding by examining discrepancies between IQ and scores on reading recognition and reading comprehension in a sample of forty hydrocephalic children, eight to nineteen years old, which included about half of those in the initial study and an additional twenty-three students. Reading skills were below normal for the age level in many cases. In fact, fifteen (37.5 percent) of the subjects had reading recognition scores below a fifth-grade level, and nine of these

(22.5 percent) had scores below a fourth-grade level. However, IQ scores were also below normal in many of the subjects. In terms of discrepancies between reading level and IQ, only two students had reading comprehension scores more than ten points below the Full-Scale IQ and only one had a reading recognition score more than ten points below the Full-Scale IQ. This student was also the only one whose shunt was placed through the left hemisphere. Twelve students (30 percent) had reading comprehension scores ten or more points higher than the Full-Scale IQ, and sixteen (40 percent) had reading recognition scores ten or more points higher than the Full-Scale IQ. These findings substantiate a degree of overachievement in reading in hydrocephalic children relative to their intellectual abilities. Such overachievement extends to both the recognition and the comprehension of what is read.

The discrepancies between IQ and reading in the hydrocephalic subjects could be partially but not wholly accounted for by their selective intellectual deficits. In many cases there were substantial discrepancies between Verbal and Performance IQ levels of a subject, so the Full-Scale IQ was a compromise between the two disparate scores. When this was taken into account, only three subjects (7 percent) had reading comprehension scores ten or more points higher than *both* the Verbal IQ and the Performance IQ. Eight subjects (20 percent) had reading recognition scores ten or more points higher than both the Verbal IQ and the Performance IQ. Looking at underachievement in terms of reading scores ten or more points lower than *either* the Verbal IQ or the Performance IQ, we see that the number of underachievers in reading comprehension increased to six (15 percent) and in reading recognition increased to five (12.5 percent).

The above findings indicate that most children with hydrocephalus read at a level compatible with their intellectual abilities. Because such children may show selective intellectual deficits, usually in visuomotor skills and Performance IQ, they often appear to read better than one would expect on the basis of their overall intellect. In fact, this is true for some hydrocephalic children, especially in terms of their reading recognition but less so with reading comprehension. In many cases, however, such apparent overachievement is an artifact of the lowering of their global IQ by poor perceptual-motor scores and their reading remains compatible with their verbal intelligence.

Agenesis of the Corpus Callosum

The syndrome of agenesis of the corpus callosum represents an intriguing anomaly, primarily because of the opportunity to contrast such patients with adult commissurotomy patients reported by Sperry and others (Gazzaniga, Bogen, and Sperry 1962, 1965; Gazzaniga and Sperry 1967). The adult who has undergone surgical section of the cerebral commissures demonstrates striking symptoms generally referred to as a hemispheric disconnection syndrome. These include, among other symptoms, an inability to match or recognize pictures presented in opposite visual half-fields or objects palpated with opposite hands or to cross-match from one visual half-field to the opposite hand. Odors identified by one nostril are not recognized by the other. Such a patient is unable to name what is seen in the left visual field or felt by the left hand or smelled by the left nostril, although recognition can be confirmed by pointing or gesturing using the left hand (Sperry 1986).

Generally, the person with callosal agenesis does not show symptoms similar to those of the commissurotomized patient, or at least not nearly to the same degree. The identification of those deficits that are present, the specification of compensatory mechanisms that reduce such symptoms compared to the commissurotomized patient, and the use of these findings to support speculation regarding the role of the corpus callosum in normal brain and cognitive development provide an interesting puzzle that has not yet been solved.

Agenesis of the corpus callosum does not usually occur in isolation, although it has been reported as an inherited abnormality with occasionally few other associated symptoms (Lynn et al. 1980). It is sometimes a postmortem finding in persons who have otherwise been neurologically asymptomatic (Warkany, Lemire, and Cohen 1981). Until 1968, of 250 reported cases of agenesis of the corpus callosum, 25 were without neurological symptoms (Loesser and Alvord 1968). The vast majority of cases have come to light because of the presence of associated abnormalities that produce neurological symptoms. Hydrocephalus is the most common of these and has been present in the majority of cases that have received intensive psychological study. This fact alone limits some of the generalizations that can be made from such studies.

The cause of callosal agenesis remains obscure for most cases. Nevertheless, it always occurs as an early embryological defect, and the exact timing of the insult, whatever it might be, largely determines the extent of commissural agenesis (Lemire et al. 1975). Jeeves (1986) outlined a timetable in which, if the insult occurs before the tenth embryonic week, all forebrain commissures will be absent. The anterior commissure alone will develop if the insult occurs during the tenth or eleventh week. After the eleventh week, both the anterior and the hippocampal commissures will develop, but not the corpus callosum. Although callosal agenesis may occur in conjunction with a variety of other brain malformations, it is not associated with any single brain anomaly except the development of a band of intrahemispheric fibers stretching occipitofrontally and known as Probst's bundle (Lemire et al. 1975). The presence of these fibers has led to speculation that most cases represent not true agenesis but rather misdirected growth of fibers (Rakic and Yakovlev 1968).

Initial reports of psychological findings in single patients with callosal agenesis indicated that these patients had no difficulty successfully performing the interhemispheric integration tasks most often failed by commissurotomized patients (Saul and Sperry 1968). A recent report by Koeda and Takeshita (1993) found at least one of the classic disconnection symptoms in two subjects with callosal agenesis. Both subjects were female, one eight and the other fifteen years old. Both subjects had a complete inability to name objects placed in the left hand. Such tactile naming was unimpaired with the right hand, and even with the left hand both subjects were able to discriminate the quality or shape of objects or to identify palpated objects by pointing at them when they could later see them.

The report by Koeda and Takeshita is somewhat anomalous, since this symptom of disconnection has not ordinarily been found in other subjects. The authors speculated that alternate pathways that might have developed, such as through the anterior commissure (which was present in one of the cases) or through the use of ipsilateral afferent pathways for tactile information, or even bilateral language representation might not have developed in these subjects because they had additional brain damage that might have limited neural plasticity. The actual explanation for the deficit (or the lack of such a deficit in other subjects) remains obscure, but a wealth of earlier studies examined cognitive functions in acallosal subjects in great detail. These studies, using larger samples or more sophisticated assessment procedures, revealed a relatively consistent pattern of deficits in acallosal subjects.

Ettlinger et al. (1972, 1974) studied four subjects with total agenesis of the corpus callosum, four with partial callosal agenesis, and four controls. All of the totally and partially acallosal subjects also had some other neurological disorder (seizures, epilepsy, meningocele), as did the control subjects. A large number of procedures were used to assess cross-hemispheric transfer. In neither study were dramatic differences observed between subject groups on the majority of interhemispheric transfer tasks. Ear asymmetries were evident in the acallosal subjects on a dichotic listening task. Although the group with total agenesis showed more left ear superiority, opposite from the other subjects, the authors were unable to unconfound the results from handedness findings. More subjects with total agenesis were also left handed, which might account for such asymmetries through reversed or bilateral speech representation. Since Witelson (1986) found that the size of the corpus callosum is increased in non–right-handed persons, it might seem that efficient callosal transmission is related to whether handedness is firmly lateralized to the left hemisphere and that the findings of Ettlinger et al. were not artifactual. However, the majority of their subjects with total agenesis were hemiparetic on the right side, which may account for left handedness on the basis of cortical damage unrelated to the corpus callosum.

In the subjects studied by Ettlinger et al., neither total nor partial agenesis groups were inferior to controls in reaction time tasks that presented visual stimuli to either the same or the opposite side of the required manual response. Acallosal subjects also were able to detect apparent movement errors in both vertical and horizontal planes, indicating interhemispheric integration of visual information across the midline. They were also unimpaired in stereoscopic depth judgments, thus able to integrate binocular information across the midline, and showed no difficulty localizing finger position on bimanual matching.

The only tasks in which the subjects with total agenesis were inferior to controls were those requiring tachistoscopic visual pattern matching of dot patterns presented to each visual field and cross-localization of tactile stimulation (Ettlinger et al. 1972, 1974). Despite a majority of negative results, both visual matching of perceptually complex stimuli and tactile localization have surfaced as fairly robust deficits observed in other acallosal subjects (Dennis 1976; Gott and Saul 1978).

Dennis (1976) reported on tactile discrimination and localization and manual coordination in two subjects with callosal agenesis: a twenty-one-year-old woman with total callosal agenesis and hydrocephalus and a fourteen-year-old boy with partial agenesis. Control subjects were hydrocephalic patients matched for age, sex, and IQ (all subjects had average IQ). Although there were no differences between the acallosal subjects and controls on either two-point tactile discrimination or inter- or intramanual identification of touched objects, acallosal subjects were deficient in identifying the number of fingers in between two that had been touched and in identifying which finger had been touched and the exact location of the stimulus. The first task (the number of fingers between those that had been touched) was entirely unimanual, but the most difficulty on the latter tasks was observed in the intermanual condition. Dennis considered both sets of positive findings to be indications of difficulty with tactile topographic localization, not necessarily related to interhemispheric transfer.

To confirm poor topographic localization of tactile stimuli in callosal agenesis, Dennis deprived one of the acallosal subjects of sensory input to a circumscribed area of the forearm for one week. In normal subjects this causes hypersensitivity, as indicated by a reduced threshold for sensory discrimination, in a homologous area of the opposite body side. Dennis found the acallosal subject to be hypersensitive to extended areas of both arms. Her interpretation of this result was that topographic skin stimulation is more diffusely represented in the acallosal brain. The rationale for this finding was that information regarding tactile location is primarily carried by ipsilateral fibers in the acallosal brain. Normal callosal transmission inhibits such ipsilateral input, which is less specific than contralateral input. In the acallosal brain the more diffuse ipsilateral input is dominant.

Dennis also reasoned that the same lack of callosal inhibition should lead to lack of suppression of diffuse ipsilateral motor innervation on either hand. Because of this, acallosal subjects should show more associated finger movements, both intra- and intermanually. In fact, this was the case with her subjects, although the subject with total agenesis showed more associated movements intramanually and the subject with partial agenesis showed more intermanually. This finding led Dennis to speculate that, in the case of partial agenesis, the preserved areas of the corpus callosum might allow the ipsilateral tracts a bimanual expression. In this case, partial agenesis could be more disruptive than total agenesis.

Some support for the hypothesis of callosal inhibition of ipsilateral input can be derived from a study by Lassonde et al. (1988). Comparing acallosal, callosotomized, and normal subjects on tactile matching tasks, they found that acallosal subjects took more time to match stimuli when both hands were used simultaneously than when one hand had explored the two stimuli sequentially. This was opposite to the results found in normal subjects or even callosotomized subjects. As Lassonde et al. pointed out, the lack of somatosensory connections through the anterior commissure (Pandya and Seltzer 1986) strongly suggests that bimanual matching is carried out using within-hemispheric integration of ipsilateral and contralateral tactile input. Thus, the acallosal subjects may rely on a functional but inefficient intrahemispheric system that is ordinarily suppressed in normal subjects. If this is true, however, the inefficiency of this compensatory mechanism should not be exaggerated. The acallosal subjects did not differ from normal controls in response accuracy on the tactile matching tasks and their unimanual response times were not different from those of IQ-matched controls. Their lack of response facilitation by the use of two hands was their most striking deficit, pointing to the deleterious effect of not being able to integrate input from two hemispheres more than to an inherent weakness in the mechanisms available to each hemisphere.

Lassonde (1986) placed a different emphasis on the significance of relative impairment on intrahemispheric tasks. Citing her own evidence of slower response times on intrahemispheric visual matching tasks in acallosal subjects (e.g., Lassonde et al. 1988), she speculated that, rather than intrahemispheric processes needing to be suppressed because of their inherent deficiencies, the role of the corpus callosum may be to activate each hemisphere, thus enhancing the hemisphere-specific processes that are ordinarily integrated on interhemispheric tasks. Lack of such facilatory activation in acallosal subjects could explain the less efficient intrahemispheric performance sometimes seen in such patients.

In support of her position, Lassonde (1986) reported two sets of results using visual presentations of stimuli to acallosal, callosotomized (total or partial), and IQ-matched and normal control subjects. One set of results indicated that both acallosal and posterior callosotomized subjects failed to make accurate binocular depth judgments even when the stimuli were located so as to project to the same hemisphere. The second study found that similar acallosal and posterior callosotomized subjects were inaccurate in pointing to the location of visual stimuli whether the visual field and hand were contralateral or ipsilateral. In the first study, a replication indicated that the results were apparent only under conditions of very brief presentation. In the second study, either prolonged practice or foveal presentation of the stimulus reduced the observed deficit. Lassonde interpreted her results as being compatible with a lack of hemispheric activation affecting intrahemispheric processing in both acallosal and callosotomized subjects.

At first glance it seems as though the two hypothesized roles of callosal transmission, either inhibitory or excitatory, cannot be distinguished on the basis of the results of behavioral tests. As these positions have been most clearly stated by Dennis (1976, 1981) and Lassonde (1986), however, they do allow the evidence to be weighed for or against each. Dennis's hypothesis is explicitly developmental. Lack of callosal inhibition and the reliance on uncrossed input and output pathways are assumed to reflect a failure to obtain a normal developmental outcome. Acallosal subjects have continued to utilize those ipsilateral connections that gradually lose behavioral significance in normal persons. Within such a developmental framework, it would probably not be predicted that subjects with intact corpora callosa during development that later were sectioned would show the same intrahemispheric deficits as acallosal subjects. In fact, it is not clear why callosotomized subjects would show any deficits at all on tasks that did not require the integration of information from the two hemispheres. That they do raises a serious objection to the developmental aspects of the inhibitory hypothesis, although not necessarily to the role of ongoing inhibition in suppressing ipsilateral processes from interfering with contralateral processes.

The developmental aspect of the inhibitory hypothesis can, perhaps, be evaluated from another angle. If ipsilateral suppression develops only over time and with age, then it might be expected that younger callosotomized subjects would show even more dramatic intrahemispheric deficits than older subjects. This would be predicted because the suppression of ipsilateral processes would be less established in younger subjects. Indeed, some of the behavioral deficits found by Dennis (1976) in her acallosal subjects, such as associated movements and poor tactile localization, are known to occur as normal developmental phenomena in younger children (Abercrombie, Lindon, and Tyson 1964; Kinsbourne and Warrington 1963). Lassonde et al. (1988), however, found better intrahemispheric performance in a younger callosotomized subject than in older children who had undergone callosotomy. Interhemispheric performance was also less impaired in the younger subject, as was the case with the callosotomized children reported by Geoffroy et al. (1983). Although these findings suggest less reliance on callosal functioning in younger children, they do not support the hypothesis that less reliance on callosal transmission is associated with greater ipsilateral control of behavior in younger children, unless one concedes that ipsilateral control may not be inferior to contralateral control. Data from normal children are equivocal with regard to this point, since some tasks, such as manual cross-retrieval of texture discrimination, show an increase with age, indicating improved callosal functioning (Galin et al. 1979), and other tasks, such as dichotic listening, show a steady increase in ear asymmetry with age (Bryden and Allard 1978), indicating greater separation between the hemispheres (Zaidel 1986).

Quite clearly, the developmental hypothesis of an inhibitory role of the corpus callosum can withstand any of the above results. It is not at all incompatible to predict fewer effects of callosotomy with decreasing age, greater interhemispheric transfer with increasing age, and greater separation of the specialized functioning of two hemispheres with increasing age, all from the same premise. The premise gets quite complicated, however, if one of its corollaries is that inherently diffuse ipsilateral processes develop as dominant modes of sensory and motor control in the absence of the corpus callosum. A more parsimonious hypothesis might be that ongoing inhibitory and excitatory callosal influences achieve greater control over sensory and motor functions with age. Both their congenital absence and their removal by callosotomy have the similar effect of decreasing the selection of the appropriate ipsilateral or contralateral pathway, depending on whether one hemisphere is more specialized to process the particular type of stimulus. This hypothesis predicts similar effects of callosal agenesis and callosotomy, since the callosal role is assumed to be ongoing rather than developmental. It also predicts an interaction between the type of task (specialized to be processed by one or the other hemisphere or not) and age (in normal subjects). Thus, tasks that are better performed by one hemisphere than the other will show an increasing separation with age in terms of which hemisphere receives the input or organizes the output. Agenesis or callosotomy will increase the degree of asymmetry in such tasks but not impair performance when input/output laterality and hemisphericity coincide. Whether callosal influences are primarily inhibitory or excitatory, or both, remains unclear and, perhaps, cannot be decided on the basis of behavioral data alone.

Evidence for the above hypothesis, other than that already cited, is meager. One finding in accordance with the task × hemisphere × corpus callosum status portion of the hypothesis was reported by Lassonde (1986). In the task in which subjects pointed to visual locations, normal subjects showed a handedness × visual field effect in that they performed better when the hand and visual field were homologous. The effect was less pronounced in the left field/left hand condition. Callosal agenesis and callosotomized subjects showed a dramatic right-hand advantage when the stimulus was in the right visual field. In fact, the acallosal and totally callosotomized subjects were similar to normal subjects in this condition. Assuming a specialization of the left hemisphere for manual control of pointing, these data indicate that lack of callosal function does not impair performance when the hemisphere receiving the input and controlling the output is the one that is specialized to perform the task. By way of contrast, both the left and right hands were inferior to those of the controls when the stimulus was presented in the left visual field. Differences in handedness were also less dramatic. This would indicate that failure to modulate the activity of the hemisphere that is poorly suited to perform the task (whether modulation is inhibitory or excitatory) results in impaired performance by that hemisphere. However, a similar lack of callosal modulation in the hemisphere that is better suited to perform the task does not impair performance, although interhemispheric transfer to motor output from the opposite hemisphere is, naturally, impaired, producing the large handedness × visual field effect.

The role of inhibitory influences of the corpus callosum has not been discussed solely in terms of the suppression of ipsilateral neural processes. Another role that has achieved some attention is that of the suppression of bilateral development of cerebral specialization. In other words, cerebral lateralization of function has been hypothesized to depend on intact function of the corpus callosum.

The clearest statement of the hypothesis that the corpus callosum suppresses the bilateral development of otherwise hemisphere-specific abilities was by Ferris and Dorsen (1975). They studied four subjects, two with total callosal agenesis and two with partial acallosal syndromes due to lipomas of the corpus callosum. Interhemispheric transfer deficits were found primarily on more complex tactile-motor tasks and were demonstrated by a lack of transfer of training from one hand to the other. More elementary functions involving the integration of information regarding tactile recognition from both sides of the body were unimpaired. However, there was some difficulty with cross-responding when verbal information was presented to one visual field and the response was made with the opposite hand. This was in contrast to better performance when the visual field and hand were on the same side. There were no absolute differences between sides when the visual field and hand were on the same side, nor were there deficits in word recognition in either visual field. This latter finding prompted Ferris and Dorsen to invoke bilateral language representation as an explanation, since there was evidence of impaired interhemispheric transfer but no left field deficit, as might be found in a commissurotomized subject who had only left-hemisphere language representation.

The results reported by Ferris and Dorsen are not entirely convincing, since the argument for bilateral representation rests on the assumption of a lack of interhemispheric transfer. Similar interhemispheric deficits either were not found by other investigators (Gott and Saul 1978; Saul and Sperry 1968) or were found primarily in terms of increased response latencies, which implicate less efficient compensatory mechanisms for the integration of the two hemispheres rather than disconnection (Lassonde et al. 1988). As Jeeves (1986) pointed out, the evidence that the two hemispheres are equally good at language tasks in acallosal subjects also was not supported by dichotic listening studies (Jeeves 1979). Moreover, motor control, as demonstrated by handedness, is usually lateralized, and most often to the right hand, in acallosal subjects (Chiarello 1980).

Gott and Saul (1978) reported a case in which bilateral language representation was confirmed using amobarbitol injection. Their subject was left handed, and whether or not the failure to lateralize language was related to callosal agenesis cannot be decided because left-handed people are known to have a greater incidence of bilateral language representation than normal. Neither that subject nor their other, right-handed acallosal subject showed any difficulty naming objects flashed to either visual field, but also neither showed any difficulty with manual identification of objects when the visual field and hand were opposite.

Jeeves (1986) reported that acallosal subjects generally show a right visual field advantage for reading words or letters that is similar to but sometimes smaller than that found in normal subjects. Donoso and Santander (1982) reported a case in which right visual field reading was absent and speculated that there was also an absence of the anterior commissure, thus approximating a commissural disconnection. Their case argues against a role of the corpus callosum in preventing bilateral language representation, since reading was clearly lateralized, albeit in reversed fashion, in their subject.

Ferris and Dorsen (1975) also pointed to the generally below-average abilities of their subjects on both language and perceptuomotor tasks as consistent with bilateral development of cortical areas specialized for both types of skill. Their argument was similar to that put forth to explain a lack of development of higher level language or perceptuomotor skills after early hemispherectomy (Kohn and Dennis 1974). Since only a limited amount of cortical area is available to support cognitive activities, the lack of specialization of cortical function results in a compromised development in which the more basic language and perceptuomotor skills can be supported by the available cortical area but higher level functions, such as those that develop later, have no room for growth. In acallosal subjects, this could happen in both hemispheres, almost as if they developed as "double hemidecorticates."

Dennis (1981) reported language deficits in an acallosal subject that were quite similar to those she reported in subjects who had undergone hemispherectomy (Dennis 1980; Dennis and Whitaker 1976). Although her subject had average verbal intelligence (though the Verbal IQ was 23 points below the Performance IQ), deficits were apparent on tasks requiring naming by rhyme cues, syntactic comprehension, sentence repetition, production of complex sentences, and meta-linguistic and pragmatic comprehension of language. The subject was also poor at an auditory selective attention task and in identifying CV syllables on a dichotic listening task.

Two recent reports confirmed the deficits in syntactic comprehension and naming by rhyme cues in acallosal subjects. Sanders (1989) found deficient sentence comprehension, particularly on passive constructions, in a six-year-old girl with callosal agenesis. Temple, Jeeves, and Villaroya (1989) found deficits in both recognition and production of rhyme in two children with callosal agenesis, a ten-year-old girl and a fourteen-year-old boy.

Although her subject's deficit in syntactic comprehension, pragmatic use, and understanding of language and meta-linguistic knowledge were similar to those found in left-hemidecorticated subjects, Dennis hesitated to conclude that this was due to bilateral speech or perceptuomotor representation. Her main argument was that too many other explanations could account for her findings and that bilateral representation could be neither ruled in nor ruled out on the basis of her data.

With regard to her subject's deficits in the selective attention and identification of CV syllables presented dichotically, Dennis was more willing to suggest an explanation: in this case, the ability to suppress competing speech sounds with spectral-temporal overlap required the inhibition of ipsilateral auditory input, which was absent because of a lack of callosal transmission. Dennis's explanation is in keeping with her earlier hypothesis regarding deficient suppression of ipsilateral input for tactile processing. Since similar attentional deficits have not been reported in other acallosal subjects, the question remains open as to whether the phenomena that Dennis observed require an explanation that invokes the absence of the corpus callosum.

The relative lack of interhemispheric transfer abnormalities in acallosal subjects has prompted a search for compensatory mechanisms to explain such apparently normal functioning. Both bilateral cognitive representation and increased use of ipsilateral processes are potential compensatory mechanisms. The other major candidate has been the use of preserved interhemispheric commissures, especially the anterior commissure, to maintain communication between the two hemispheres. Those deficits in interhemispheric transfer that have been found most often have involved either slow response times or deficits in accuracy with more complex stimuli.

Lassonde et al. (1988) found that response time on tasks that required interhemispheric integration of either visual or tactile information was slower in acallosal subjects than in IQ-matched or normal controls. Although this difference was also apparent on intrahemispheric tasks, the acallosal subjects did not increase their speed on tactile exploration when using two hands simultaneously, as did the control subjects. These results are not entirely clear; Lassonde et al. raised the possibility that a lack of callosal activation of either hemisphere could produce the same result, especially since intra- as well as interhemispheric deficits were noted. However, the lack of bilateral response time facilitation on the tactile tasks is relatively convincing evidence of slow interhemispheric transfer. This would imply that information is being communicated between hemispheres but that the noncallosal pathways that carry such communication are less efficient than is normal callosal transmission.

Gott and Saul (1978) found that cross–visual field matching of simple stimuli (objects, shapes, words, or numbers) was unimpaired in two subjects with callosal agenesis. However, when the stimuli were perceptually complex (i.e., Chinese ideograms or two-digit number pairs), a marked cross-field matching deficit was noted. Somewhat similarly, simple tactile matching between hands was unimpaired but transfer of tactile-motor learning on Halstead's Tactual Performance Test was quite deficient. Ferris and Dorsen (1975) had found similar difficulties with intermanual transfer of learning on the same task in their three acallosal subjects. Ettlinger et al. (1972, 1974) had earlier found that, although simple visual stimuli provided no difficulty on cross–visual field matching tasks, more complex dot patterns revealed a deficit in their acallosal subjects.

Taken all together, the above series of results provide fairly consistent evidence of limits to interhemispheric transfer in acallosal subjects based on the complexity of the stimulus or task requirements. Most of the authors who found such results took them to indicate an upper limit to the efficiency of compensatory interhemispheric communications, probably via the anterior commissure. It is not really clear, however, that the anterior commissure can be relied on to perform even this inefficient role. If it does, this would seem to be an added function requiring interhemispheric connections that do not ordinarily exist. Pandya and Seltzer (1986) summarized a great deal of the accumulated evidence regarding the commissural location of fibers connecting different areas of the two hemispheres in rhesus monkeys. Anterior commissural connections are generally limited to the orbitofrontal cortex, the superior temporal region, portions of the inferotemporal area, and lateral and medial portions of the parahippocampal gyrus. Somatosensory and visual connections do not traverse the anterior commissure, but neither are primary visual cortex connections found in the corpus callosum in rhesus monkeys.

The anatomical evidence places a great deal of weight on the development of abnormal interhemispheric connections via the anterior commissure, perhaps more so than increased use of those pathways that already exist. This would seem to favor alternative compensatory pathways and mechanisms such as subcortical connections (yet to be fully delineated) or increased reliance on ipsilateral connections. At this stage in solving the anatomical puzzle regarding interhemispheric connections, it is not possible to rule out any possibilities. Since it is known that many more interhemispheric fibers exist early in development than are retained (Innocenti 1986), it remains possible that compensatory mechanisms in cases of callosal agenesis rely on an increased survival of such noncallosal commissural fibers, creating a situation genuinely anatomically different from but functionally similar to the normal brain.

Anatomical studies have generally yielded results that have been more reliable and specific yet have generated more conservative speculation than have behavioral studies. The results of anatomical studies may be applicable to the inhibitory-excitatory debate that has been generated by the behavioral data, although at least one group of anatomically oriented researchers rejected the whole debate as "wild interpretation" (Berlucchi, Tassinari, and Antonini 1986). The bulk of evidence from both anatomical and physiological studies has continued to support a hypothesis of a major role of callosal fibers in providing continuity of representational fields across the midline, especially for points near the vertical meridian (Antonini, Berlucchi, and Lepore 1983; Lepore, Ptito, and Guillemot 1986). This is clearly the case with regard to vision (Antonini, Berlucchi, and Lepore 1983; Berlucchi, Tassinari, and Antonini 1986) but is also a reasonable interpretation of the data with regard to somatosensory connections, even if the concept is sometimes stretched to include a "functional midline" (Lepore, Ptito, and Guillemot, 1986).

In addition to the majority of homotopic interhemispheric callosal connections that provide such cross-midline continuity, however, some studies have identified callosal fibers that project to areas predominantly serviced by ipsilateral connections (Cusick and Kass 1986). The pertinence of such callosal connections is that they presumably augment intrahemispheric processing in some way and that their absence in acallosal subjects could explain intrahemispheric deficits simply on the basis of information deprivation. However, such information deprivation would be present only in the situation in which both hemispheres are normally activated (i.e., bilateral stimulation or cross-hemisphere tasks). With input and output restricted to the same hemisphere, no information would ordinarily be transferred from the opposite hemisphere. The fact that acallosal subjects do show deficits on such tasks strengthens the case for a nonspecific facilitatory or inhibitory role for some callosal connections. It is still not clear, however, that such a role is developmental rather than ongoing, nor that it applies equally to both hemispheres when one hemisphere is specialized to perform a task. It would be quite interesting if it proved that transmission through such callosal projections to areas that transmitted primarily intrahemispherically was asymmetrical, depending on whether the behavior function was lateralized or not. It is perhaps not too "wild" to speculate that normally one hemisphere inhibits the other from doing what it is not good at doing, even when experimenters try to bypass such normal roles by restricting information to a single hemisphere.

The study of cases of callosal agenesis has generated a good deal of speculation regarding the normal role of the corpus callosum in development. It has probably been wiser to focus on the effects of callosal agenesis on specific tasks known or hypothesized to depend on callosal function than to attempt to delineate a typical pattern of cognitive effects of callosal agenesis. As Bigler et al. (1988) pointed out, the majority of cognitive weaknesses found in acallosal subjects will be secondary to other types of abnormalities associated with but not necessarily related to the absence of a corpus callosum.

Williams Syndrome

Williams, Barratt-Boyes, and Lowe (1961) first identified Williams syndrome, which includes supravalvular aortic stenosis, a distinctive facial appearance, hypersensitivity to sound, occasional infantile hypercalcemia, and mild to moderate mental retardation. The basic defect in the disorder seems to be metabolic, and abnormal production of the hormone calcitonin has been identified as a marker for the syndrome (Culler, Jones, and Deftos 1985). Other abnormalities associated with the syndrome include oral and dental defects, large ears, and a hoarse voice. A genetic or even chromosomal basis for the disorder has not been ruled out.

Some authors reported cognitive impairment as a coexistent feature of Williams syndrome (Arnold and Yule 1985; Bennett, La Veck, and Sells 1978; Jones and Smith 1975b). Bennett, La Veck, and Sells first noted the marked discrepancy between the levels of language and visuospatial skills in children with this disorder. On the McCarthy Scales of Children's Abilities, the Perceptual and Motor scores were more impaired than the language scores. They also noted that retesting some of their subjects indicated no change in their cognitive level with age.

MacDonald and Roy (1988) replicated the findings of Bennett et al. in a sample of seven children with Williams syndrome, using a battery of tests of language, academic, visuomotor, and motor skills. Compared to age-, sex-, and vocabulary-matched controls, their subjects were deficient on visuomotor and academic tasks but not on language and motor tasks. In fact, the visuomotor deficit was so consistent and severe that Macdonald and Roy were prompted to suggest that it was an invariant feature of the syndrome.

Bellugi, Sabo, and Vaid (1988) reported an in-depth cognitive study of three children with Williams syndrome who were eleven, fifteen, and sixteen years old. Overall cognitive development of all three children was below normal, with Wechsler IQ scores ranging from 43 to 66. When IQ and mental age scores from repeated testing over intervals as long as five years were examined, it was found that mental age remained relatively constant, reaching an apparent plateau at about seven years.

Bellugi, Sabo, and Vaid found two quite striking dissociations in the abilities of their subjects with Williams syndrome. The first involved a higher level of language skill than would be predicted from the overall levels of cognitive ability. Expressively, their sentences were lengthy, ranging from 8.6 to 13.5 morphemes, and were grammatically well formed, with use of complex syntactical structures. Receptively, the subjects were able to comprehend syntactically complex sentences and to predict correct grammatical endings based on beginning sentence fragments. Despite substantial conceptual impairment, their ability to produce and process language was quite good.

The second dissociation found by Bellugi, Sabo, and Vaid was in the area of visual perception. The children with Williams syndrome were impaired across a variety of visuospatial tasks. These included drawing and block construction tasks as well as motor-free tasks that required judgment of the orientation of lines or spatial transformations of visual stimuli. The ability of the subjects to trace designs that they could not copy was taken as evidence that their impairment was not primarily motor. MacDonald and Roy (1988) also found that purely motor tasks were unimpaired in their subjects. Both drawing and construction of block designs revealed the subjects' inability to integrate the components of the tasks into a spatially intact gestalt, despite attention to each of the components as a separate entity. Bellugi, Sabo, and Vaid remarked on the similarity of this style of visuomotor performance to that reported in adults with right-hemisphere lesions.

In contrast to their defective performance on spatial tasks, the same subjects performed at average levels on tests of visual "closure" and facial recognition. Although both the spatial tasks and the closure and facial recognition tasks have been found to be sensitive to right-hemisphere lesions (Benton et al. 1983), their dissociation has been reported by other authors (Neville 1988) and may be related to the anterior-posterior dimension of the right hemisphere.

There are at least two reasons why the findings reported in Williams syndrome may have a significance well beyond the characterization of an unusual metabolic disorder. Behavioral dissociations that arise during development in neurologically impaired children allow us to frame hypotheses regarding the interaction between different psychological abilities. For instance, although a certain level of conceptual ability might be thought necessary to support complex syntactic comprehension and expression, such may not be the case. Certainly, the three subjects with Williams syndrome studied by Bellugi, Sabo, and Vaid showed such language skills well beyond those normally seen in children whose global cognitive development has not reached a level of concrete operations. Such a finding could be construed to support a more "modular" conception of syntactic processing (Fodor 1983).

The peculiar pattern of better language than visuomotor skills, even with low intelligence and hyperverbal, socially disinhibited behavior reported by several observers of children with Williams syndrome (Jones and Smith 1975b), prompted some authors to compare them to subjects with "cocktail party syndrome" as seen in hydrocephalus (MacDonald and Roy 1988). The descriptions of the two syndromes sound similar, but it is not clear to what extent the similarity is impressionistic or can really be documented. In neither disorder is there any obvious reason why a developmental dysfunction without a focal locus should produce such behavioral dissociations nor, in some respects, resemble focal right-hemisphere brain injury. Rourke described similar behavioral characteristics in other children and suggested that the right hemisphere really is damaged in such cases, although the evidence for such a cause is most often quite weak and, circularly, based on psychological test performance (Rourke 1987; Rourke and Strang 1983). Rourke argued convincingly that the behavioral pattern of verbosity and social disinhibition and the cognitive pattern of impaired visuospatial skills are probably associated. Appealing as this formulation may be, Hurley et al. (1990) could not find such an association in hydrocephalic children specifically noted for "cocktail party" behavior. Williams syndrome may offer an additional avenue for the study of this interesting issue.

Microcephaly

Incidence and Etiology

Microcephaly has been variously defined as a head circumference more than two standard deviations below the mean (Ross and Frias 1977) or more than three standard deviations below the mean (Book, Schut, and Reed 1953). The causes of microcephaly are also varied. Microcephaly is a symptom rather than a diagnostic entity and as such may stem from a wide variety of causes. The common circumstance that leads to a smaller cranium is a defect in brain development, since skull growth is determined by brain growth rather than vice versa. Cowie (1987) suggested that, regardless of whether the determinant is genetic or secondary to some other insult, the most likely period of disruption of brain development which might lead to microcephaly is the first half of the second trimester of pregnancy. Dobbing and Sands (1973) also suggested that the timing of the brain insult, rather than its cause, may be most important in producing a microcephalic brain. Others, however, such as Warkany, Lemire, and Cohen (1981), have claimed that the above considerations apply only to what they call "primary" microcephaly. In their terms, "secondary" microcephaly also occurs in cases where brain development is normal until it is affected by a disease process in later fetal life or even during the neonatal period. Occasionally, the disease process may occur even beyond the neonatal period, as in the "walnut brain" syndrome described by Laurence and Cavanaugh (1968).

Some of the material in this section was previously published in Dorman (1991b).

Most authors make a distinction between "true" microcephaly and other types of secondary microcephalic symptom. Warkany, Lemire, and Cohen (1981) regarded "true" microcephaly as that in which only the skull and brain and no other organ systems are affected. In their opinion, this limits true microcephaly to those cases of autosomal recessive inheritance in which associated abnormalities are not found (e.g., Kloepfer, Platou, and Hansche 1964). Estimates of the incidence of such genetically determined and unisymptomatic microcephaly have been in the 1/40,000 range for the general population (Book, Schut, and Reed 1953; Quazi and Reed 1975).

Cowie (1987) criticized the proposal that "true" microcephaly comprises a single condition. He pointed out that some clinical features that have been postulated as pathognomonic for this disorder have not been found in different samples. Several of these involve such behavioral characteristics as posture and temperament (Penrose 1963), as well as certain facial features (Baraitser 1985).

Microcephaly occurs as a symptom in a large number of genetic syndromes. Autosomal recessive inheritance has been reported (Hankenson, Ozonoff, and Cassidy 1989; Teebi, Al-Awadi, and White 1987), as has autosomal dominant or even X-linked inheritance (Bavinck et al. 1987; Kawashima and Tsuji 1987). Microcephaly also occurs as a result of environmental causes, including maternal and fetal malnutrition (Brandt 1981), and teratogens, such as maternal consumption of alcohol (Warkany, Lemire, and Cohen 1981). Microcephaly has been reported in congenital rubella syndrome (Streissguth, Van Derveer, and Shepard 1970), cytomegalic inclusion disease (Weller and Hanshaw 1962), and phenylketonuria (Denniston 1963). It is also a common symptom in Down syndrome (Warkany and Dignan 1973).

Intelligence

Given the myriad etiological factors that may lead to microcephaly, generalizations regarding its relationship to intelligence are difficult to make. Some studies have reported that virtually all persons with microcephaly are mentally retarded (O'Connell, Feldt, and Stickler 1965; Pryor and Thelander 1968). Unfortunately, it is not clear whether bias introduced from sampling clinical populations affects the conclusions of these studies. Sells (1977), using a criterion of head size more than two standard deviations below the mean for age, sampled 1,006 school-age children and found that 1.9 percent qualified as microcephalic. Those children thus classified were indistinguishable from their normocephalic peers on tests of intelligence.

Even within the clinic-referred population, the association between head size and intelligence may not be as dramatic as some reports have indicated. Sassaman and Zartler (1982) examined the charts of 990 children referred for developmental delay to a medical evaluation clinic. Data on head circumference and (biparietal) head breadth as well as standard intellectual measures were available for all subjects. One hundred eighty-eight (18.9 percent) of the children had abnormal head growth. Overall, 68.1 percent of these children were mentally retarded. Since the authors did not report the base rate of mental retardation in their sample, the significance of this proportion of impairment in the microcephalic subgroup is difficult to evaluate.

The proportion of retarded children was lowest in those with microcephaly (small head circumference) and normal somatic growth (52 percent) and those with head breadth deficiency, microcephaly, and somatic growth failure (55.6 percent). The highest proportion of mental retardation was found in those children with microcephaly and somatic growth failure (77.8 percent) and those with head breadth deficiency, microcephaly, and normal somatic growth (85.7 percent). Only the last group differed significantly from the overall mean rate of mental retardation for the subjects with abnormal head growth. The authors of this study concluded that the overall mean rate of mental retardation in microcephaly is less than many previous reports have indicated and that both head circumference and head breadth need to be taken into account in predicting intelligence from head size.

The study by Sassaman and Zartler contained subjects whose microcephaly resulted from a wide variety of etiological factors. The chief conclusion to be drawn from their study is that microcephaly does not have a uniform effect on intelligence. Slightly more than 30 percent of their microcephalic subjects had normal intelligence. Most of these, however, had low average or borderline intelligence. Only 6.4 percent of the microcephalic subjects had average intelligence. Within the subcategories of children, the proportion with average intelligence ranged from 2 percent in those with microcephaly and otherwise normal somatic growth to 22 percent in those with head breadth deficiency and microcephaly with somatic growth failure.

Although it might be tempting to conclude that one can expect some degree of lowered intelligence in microcephaly, especially if physical stature is otherwise normal, some data temper such a conclusion. Several studies reported autosomal dominant microcephaly in which the intellectual level of the subjects is often normal, sometimes despite extremely small head circumference (Burton 1981). Although

Burton's subjects also had small stature, Haslam and Smith (1979) and Ramirez, Rivas, and Cantu (1983) reported cases in which intelligence was sometimes not affected and in which stature was normal. Ramirez, Rivas, and Cantu did find that lowered intelligence was associated with the most extreme degrees of microcephaly.

Rossi et al. (1987) reported an autosomally dominant inherited microcephaly in six Italian families with twenty-one affected members. Physical stature was normal in all but one microcephalic subject. Psychometric measures of intelligence were available for twelve of the subjects. Intelligence was average in all but one subject, with average IQ scores ranging from 90 to 112 (mean, 99.3). Head circumference ranged from 2.1 to 4.7 standard deviations below the mean. Subjects with average intelligence included six with head circumference at least 3 standard deviations below the mean, three of whom had a head circumference more than 4 standard deviations below the mean. Other reports of dominantly inherited microcephaly with normal intelligence have also appeared (Crowe and Dickerman 1986; Leung 1985).

Inherited microcephaly with normal intelligence may not be limited to a dominant mode of inheritance. Teebi, Al-Awadi, and White (1987) reported a large Arab kindred in which eight cases of microcephaly were found. Microcephaly was associated with short stature. Although psychometric data were not reported, intelligence in all of the affected subjects was reported as normal. The authors speculated that their cases were similar to those reported by Seemanova et al. (1985), who also found a type of autosomal recessive microcephaly with short stature and normal intelligence. These subjects, however, also had immunodeficiency and lymphoreticular cancers, unlike those studied by Teebi, Al-Awadi, and White.

Although it is difficult to make a general statement regarding the relationship between microcephaly and intelligence, some tentative conclusions can be drawn. Decreased head size may or may not be associated with lowered intelligence. This finding alone must indicate that small head size by itself does not affect intelligence. The presence of subgroups of microcephalic persons who typically have normal intelligence is sufficient to rule out a causal relationship between head size and intellect. The only disclaimer that must be made for this conclusion is that reports of even average intelligence in small samples of microcephalic subjects do not rule out the possibility that their intelligence is lowered relative to what it might have been without microcephaly. However, in the sample reported by Rossi et al. (1987), the socioeconomic and educational level of the families of the index cases indicated that the average intelligence scores that were found were within expectation for their group. The normal intelligence found by Sells (1977) in schoolchildren with small head size also militates against any straightforward relationship between diminished head size and lowered intelligence.

Although normal intelligence has been reported only in subjects with inherited microcephaly, it cannot be concluded that "true" microcephaly does not affect intelligence while secondary microcephaly does. These terms themselves are confusing, since they have been used variously to indicate differences between inherited versus environmentally caused microcephaly and microcephaly without associated abnormalities versus microcephaly with associated abnormalities. One must agree with Cowie (1987) that *true* or *primary microcephaly* includes a number of genetic disorders. Some of these seem to affect intelligence, but others do not.

Many conditions that affect head size also affect intelligence. In some conditions of dominantly inherited microcephaly with normal stature, only head size may be affected. There may also be recessively inherited conditions that affect head size and stature but not intelligence. The majority of conditions, either genetic or environmental, that result in reduced head size also impair intelligence. This implies a variety of pathological processes that affect the developing brain, in terms of not only its volume but also those structures that support intellectual development.

Warkany, Lemire, and Cohen (1981) described some of the brain abnormalities that may be found in microcephaly. There is generally a reduction in the size of the frontal lobes, which corresponds to the receding forehead reported by a number of investigators (Baraitser 1985; Kloepfer, Platou, and Hansche 1964; Salmon and Lindenbaum 1978). The smallness of the occipital lobes may leave the cerebellum uncovered. Ventricular dilatation may also occur, reducing brain volume from the inside. Simplified convolutional patterns are often observed, and one microcephalic brain may show pachygyria, macrogyria, and microgyria. Heterotopic cells are also often observed. Associated malformations of the corpus callosum, cerebellum, and brainstem may also be found. Warkany, Lemire, and Cohen also stated that it is not possible to separate "true" microcephaly from other microcephaly on the basis of these anatomical abnormalities.

All of the above lead to a conclusion that agrees with that of Cowie (1987): in general, microcephaly reflects a pathological change in brain structure, usually occurring in early fetal life, with the effect on intelligence most likely dependent on the extent and type of underlying abnormality. It can be added that reduction in brain size without such structural abnormality, as may occur in some genetic conditions or even as a result of normal variation, does not affect intelligence.

Recently, Lynn (1992) challenged the above conclusions. Citing evidence from no fewer than fifteen studies of head size and intelligence, dating from 1906 to 1990, and all involving normal adult or child samples, he demonstrated a typical correlation of about 0.14, which was statistically significant in every case. Johnson (1991) also reviewed the head size/intelligence studies and concluded that not only is head size positively correlated with intelligence in the normal population but also brain size is probably even more highly related to intelligence. He also speculated that brain size and intelligence may be related to the same gene.

Johnson's conclusions regarding brain size and intelligence seem to be borne out by recent studies by Willerman et al. (1991, 1992). These authors used magnetic resonance imaging to measure brain size separately from the skull, meningeal coverings, and intrahemispheric fissure in normal college students. Measures of brain size were correlated with IQ and Graduate Record Examination (GRE) scores. After adjusting for body size, the correlation between IQ and brain size was .51, which the authors speculated was an overestimate because they had deliberately selected students with especially high and low IQs for their study. Most interesting, the correlation was smaller for women than for men, a finding that was followed up in their second study.

In their second study, Willerman et al. (1992) looked at not only brain size but also differences between right and left hemisphere size in both men and women. These measures were related to Verbal and Performance IQ and to differences between Verbal IQ and Performance IQ. In men, but not in women, brain size was positively correlated with both Verbal and Performance IQ. Asymmetry, in favor of a larger left than right hemisphere, was associated with higher Verbal than Performance IQ in men and with higher Performance than Verbal IQ in women. Willerman et al. suggested that women's brains are organized differently from men's and that the crucial variable related to intelligence in women may be axonal transfer of information, which may be enhanced because of either more fibers or more myelin around the fibers. The reason for this being more crucial for intelligence in women is that the brain may be less lateralized in terms of function, so brain areas relevant to processing any particular type of information (in this case, nonverbal) may be more distributed between the two hemispheres than in the case of men.

The data of Willerman et al. (1992) are intriguing. Though their conclusions are speculative and based on a small set of data, they suggest that the relationship between brain size and intelligence is not the same for men and women. This certainly does not make it any easier to draw a simple conclusion regarding the question of whether brain size affects intelligence. For the time being, it seems safest to conclude that brain size and intelligence are related, in men at least, and that brain size can be smaller without affecting intelligence in some cases of genetically small head size and perhaps in women compared to men. With regard to the question of whether small brain size causes lowered intelligence, we can say only that the question is more complicated than it might seem. There is still no positive indication that such a causal relationship exists, and there are some studies that imply that it doesn't.

Velocardiofacial Syndrome

In 1978, Shprintzen et al. identified a syndrome among children with cleft palate that also included cardiac anomalies, characteristic facies, and learning disabilities. Although its identification as a syndrome is fairly recent, it is now recognized as perhaps the most common syndrome of clefting (Shprintzen et al. 1985). The original report by Shprintzen et al. (1978) described twelve children, eleven of whom were characterized as having specific learning disabilities in the areas of abstract reasoning, mathematics, and visuomotor skills. The twelfth child had delays in motor development. IQ scores ranged from 78 to 104, with all but two children having IQs in the normal range. Sensorineural or conductive hearing loss was present in five cases. Analysis of the familial transmission patterns in a sample of thirty-nine cases indicated a most likely autosomal-dominant genetic basis for the disorder (Shprintzen et al. 1981).

It is not clear why learning disabilities should be associated with the other features of the syndrome. Shprintzen et al. (1981) established that neither hypoxia (secondary to airway obstruction) nor the congenital heart anomalies present in the syndrome could account for the cognitive impairment. In the series examined by Shprintzen et al. (1981), thirty of thirty-nine subjects had conductive hearing loss and ten of sixteen subjects showing intellectual impairment had microcephaly.

Golding-Kushner, Weller, and Shprintzen (1985) administered intellectual and language tests to twenty-six patients with velocardiofacial syndrome. There was an inverse relationship between IQ and age, with the deterioration in IQ with increasing age being attributed to a weakness in abstract reasoning skills that affected tests appropriate for older children more than those for younger children. Visuomotor skills were impaired in all subjects. On the Illinois Test of Psycholinguistic Abilities, rote skills such as auditory-sequential memory were intact, whereas auditory and visual association, both requiring more abstract reasoning skills, were impaired. In reading, matching letters and recognition skills were unimpaired but comprehension was poor. The authors also reported a characteristic personality profile consisting of bland affect, poor social interactions, and impulsive and disinhibited behavior.

The velocardiofacial syndrome is an interesting congenital and probably genetic anomaly. The presence of midline facial abnormalities, suggestive of interruption of the developmental process during early pregnancy, and learning disabilities that usually do not include mental retardation (Shprintzen and Goldberg 1986) is perplexing. However, even the coincidence of cardiac and facial anomalies is not clearly explainable in this syndrome. Further work on careful delineation of the cognitive pattern in this syndrome and its possible relationship to associated symptoms such as hearing loss and microcephaly needs to be carried out. A dissociation of abstract reasoning from less abstract cognitive processes could provide interesting data for theories of cognitive development.

4

Toxic Influences and Infections

As with other topics in this book, there is some arbitrariness in the delineation of a chapter on toxic influences and infections. In our society, not only does the risk of encountering an environmental toxicant covary with socioeconomic factors but also the effects of such toxicants may interact with other adverse effects of low socioeconomic status to produce an overall negative result (Dietrich et al. 1989). Thus, prematurity, low birth weight, and other risk factors may themselves be the result of toxic influences and also potentiate the effects of such influences. Additionally, genetic factors, even as broad as gender or maternal susceptibility, may influence susceptibility to infections as well as birth weight and prematurity (Gualtieri 1987).

The range of negative influences that might be examined is quite large. The choice of which to cover has depended primarily on the availability of a reasonable body of literature and secondarily on the importance of the influence in terms of the number of children affected. Those influences that will be examined include alcohol; environmental lead, mercury, and polychlorinated biphenyls; ionizing radiation; and human immunodeficiency virus.

Environmental Toxicants

Lead

The effects of human exposure to lead have been studied in terms of growth, behavior, and timing of exposure (pre- or postnatal). With increasing detection and reduction of environmental sources of lead, particularly since the change to unleaded gasoline, research has focused on ever lower levels of exposure to lead.

The evidence in favor of a negative influence of lead exposure on growth is meager. Needleman et al. (1984) failed to find an association between prenatal lead exposure and either birth weight or gestational age. Similarly, Greene and Ernhart (1991) found no association either between cord maternal blood levels and birth weight or between preschool blood lead levels and preschool size indices. One of the few instances of a significant association between prenatal lead exposure and birth weight was reported by Dietrich et al. (1987). In fact, they were unable to detect independent effects of prenatal lead exposure on birth weight and gestational age.

The evidence with regard to negative effects on cognitive development is more consistent. Two reports from the U.S. Environmental Protection Agency (1986, 1989) indicated that Bayley Mental Development Index (MDI) scores (Bayley 1969) may be depressed from two to eight points by prenatal exposure to lead at relatively low levels. Dietrich et al. (1991) reported a similar finding using the Kaufman Assessment Battery for Children (K-ABC) administered at four years of age. Umbilical cord lead levels were related to four-year cognitive development, but only in subjects from the poorest families. Neither maternal blood concentrations of lead nor postnatal blood levels in the children were related to overall cognitive development. However, postnatal lead levels were related to specific indices of visuospatial and visuomotor integration.

Although it has not been difficult to obtain positive correlations between pre- or even postnatal blood levels and IQ, the relationships are reduced considerably or even disappear when such other factors as birth weight, socioeconomic status, and race are taken into account. This has provoked a dilemma with regard to the true relationship between lead exposure and cognitive development. The dilemma stems from the methodological problem of how to control environmental or constitutional variables that may interact with lead exposure to potentiate or reduce its effects on cognitive development. Since none of the variables in question is under experimental control, the only available controls are statistical. Multiple regression analyses can isolate direct effects of lead exposure that are independent of other variables but not indirect effects that are mediated by them. Indirect effects can be tested only by using various statistical modeling procedures, none of which is particularly conclusive.

Dietrich et al. (1987) attempted to find a solution to this dilemma using a sophisticated but complex structural equation modeling procedure. Their sample included 185 predominantly African American expectant mothers recruited from an area of Cincinnati known to pose risks from environmental exposure to lead. Variables recorded included maternal blood lead levels; infant blood lead levels at ten days, three months, and six months after birth; obstetrical and perinatal complications and data; socioeconomic status; and the quality of the home environment.

Dietrich et al. found that three-month lead levels were strongly predictive of six-month Bayley mental and motor scores, but only among the white children in the sample. In the multiple regression prediction of Bayley scores, prenatal exposure to lead was not predictive of cognitive or motor scores, but birth weight and gestational age were. Using structural equation modeling, the investigators determined that prenatal lead exposure was related to both low birth weight and shortened gestational age, which were, in turn, related to six-month cognitive and motor scales. This result was not confined to either racial subset of the sample.

A very suggestive finding reported in the Dietrich et al. study involved what the authors referred to as a "dynamic relationship" between postnatal exposure to lead and behavioral development. Higher lead levels at six months were positively related to Bayley MDI and, particularly, Psychomotor Development Index (PDI) scores at six months. Also, higher Bayley scores were related to increases in lead levels between three and six months. The authors offered the explanation that more developmentally advanced infants are more likely to expose themselves to sources of lead because of their greater mobility and better visuomotor coordination.

Davis et al. (1990) analyzed the types of cognitive impairment that seem to result from exposure to lead. Their analysis was based on the results of both human and animal studies. They pointed out that numerous studies had shown that Bayley mental scores are more highly related to lead exposure than are motor scores. This was seen as an indication that more complex cognitive processes were more affected by lead exposure than were simple motor skills. On the other hand, they speculated that such impairment in cognitive function could be secondary to more basic deficits in maintaining attention and regulating the level of behavior. Such a hypothesis fits the evidence available from animal studies of exposure to lead.

Both animal and human studies show a dose-response relationship between the level of lead exposure and the degree of behavioral impairment. In humans, greater concentrations of lead in the blood are related to greater decreases in IQ scores (U.S. Environmental

Protection Agency 1986). It is disturbing, however, that the levels at which behavioral effects in humans are now being detected were considered "safe" several years ago and, in fact, were average U.S. blood levels at that time (Mahaffey et al. 1982). Davis et al. (1990) questioned whether a lower threshold for behavioral effects of lead exposure really exists.

Despite the somewhat pessimistic speculations of Davis et al., positive findings put some perspective on the problem. First, the average blood levels of lead in the United States have, in fact, decreased considerably over the years. Just as important, it is not clear how long the negative influence of early exposure to lead persists. The Cincinnati study found that negative cognitive effects of early exposure to lead persisted only in those children from the most adverse environments. Bellinger et al. (1987) found no effect of prenatal exposure to lead on cognitive abilities at five years, despite earlier negative effects in the same cohort. Presumably, there is an effect of the level of early exposure to lead on the persistence of adverse effects. Such a relationship was found in rats (Cory-Slechta 1988).

Polychlorinated Biphenyls and Methyl Mercury

Polychlorinated biphenyls (PCBs) and methyl mercury are environmental hazards whose risk potential became known through public health disasters, which probably do not represent the more usual low-level risk that affects the larger public. PCBs are no longer used in industry, but for more than forty years (until the mid-1970s) they were, and with little thought to the toxic effects that might result from their haphazard disposal. It is known that they resist physical or biological breakdown and that they show up in human tissue, but the normal route for human exposure is not clear.

Some sources of PCBs are substantial enough to allow an examination of their toxic effects in humans. In a somewhat similar fashion, the toxic effects of human exposure to methyl mercury in utero have been observed, primarily at high levels of exposure. Disastrous exposure levels due to grain contamination in Iraq (Amin-Zaki et al. 1974) and fish contamination in Japan (Matsumoto, Koya, and Takeuchi 1965) provided much of the data on toxic effects.

Major studies of the toxic effects of pre- and postnatal exposure to PCBs have centered around disastrous exposures in Japan in 1968 and Taiwan in 1979, as well as more chronic exposure to contaminated fish in the Great Lakes and industrial exposure in North Carolina (Tilson, Jacobson, and Rogan 1990). In both Japan and Taiwan, cooking oil, in which PCBs used to decolorize the oil resulted in contamination, exposed thousands to high levels of PCBs and other chemicals. Among those exposed were some pregnant women and many young children. In both the Japanese and Taiwanese groups, the children exposed in utero were small for gestational age, showed dark pigmentation of the skin, nails, and gums, and, in most instances, had lowered IQ. Most interesting, the findings from the Taiwanese group revealed similar effects, including lowered IQ, in children born to exposed mothers up to six years after acute exposure (Rogan et al. 1988). This finding indicates that PCB levels in mothers may not decrease appreciably over time and would lead to the expectation that repeated low-level exposures could have cumulative effects. In fact, given what is known regarding the biological processing of PCBs and the results of studies of body accumulations in both humans and animals (Tilson, Jacobson, and Rogan 1990), this is certainly the case.

The children exposed in Taiwan were followed up to six years of age. Compared to matched controls, they showed deficits averaging four to seven points lower on the Bayley mental and motor scales, the Stanford-Binet at preschool age, and the WISC-R Performance IQ at school age (Rogan et al. 1988). Lower-level chronic exposure in mothers eating contaminated fish in Michigan or exposed from work in North Carolina showed greater effects on motor development at early ages (Gladen et al. 1988; Jacobson et al. 1984). This may have been at least partly due to the focus on motor skills in the early assessment devices that were used. Jacobson et al. (1985) found deficits on a visual memory task in infants in the Michigan group, suggesting that the effects were not limited to motor abilities.

In animals, the most typical effect of prenatal exposure is hyperactivity, although this may be either preceded or followed by stages of hypoactivity in some animals (Tilson, Jacobson, and Rogan 1990). Cognitive effects have also been studied in animals. Bowman, Hieronimus, and Allen (1978) demonstrated that rhesus monkeys exposed in utero and for three postnatal months through nursing were deficient on discrimination reversal tasks. Levin, Schantz, and Bowman (1988) found deficits on delayed spatial alternation in monkeys tested four to six years after exposure. More complex cognitive abilities have not been systematically examined in humans, but the animal data point to the likelihood that deficits could be present in these areas.

The massive exposure of Japanese citizens to toxic levels of methyl mercury from fish in the contaminated Minamata Bay led to the naming of acute methyl mercury poisoning as Minamata disease (Masumoto, Koya, and Takeuchi 1965). The behavioral effects of the high levels of intrauterine exposure in this instance tended to be severe. Harada (1977) reported severe intellectual impairment, delayed motor development, and delayed language. The effects of intrauterine exposure after the ingestion of contaminated grain by women in Iraq were more varied. Delays in motor development were prominent (as in Japan), but there were also delays in intellectual development (Marsh 1987).

Because of the nature of the exposures that have yielded most of the data on the behavioral effects of methyl mercury in humans, dose effects have been difficult to determine. Marsh (1987) and Cox et al. (1989) used analysis of maternal hair strand levels of methyl mercury to determine threshold levels for clinical symptoms (chiefly delayed walking) in offspring. A maternal hair strand level of 20 ppm, which translates into a fetal brain dose of 1 ppm, seemed to be a threshold for motor effects. There is some evidence that the threshold for cognitive effects may be lower (Kjellstrom et al. 1986). In animal studies, cognitive and sensory tests proved more sensitive than motor measures in detecting low levels of intrauterine exposure (Burbacher, Rodier, and Weiss 1990).

A fair amount of work has established the neuropathological effects of exposure to methyl mercury in utero. In both humans and animals, brain size is diminished, with smaller gyri and larger sulci. In humans and especially nonhuman primates, ectopic cells and, in the cortex, extreme disorganization of cells and layers have been found (Burbacher, Rodier, and Weiss 1990). Disorders of the migration of cortical cells, of course, date at least some of the effects to the eighth to fifteenth weeks of gestation.

The actual risks for cognitive impairment after early exposure to methyl mercury are difficult to assess. Certainly, the lack of a sufficient number of cognitive studies at low levels of exposure limits any definitive statement regarding effects. Additionally, as pointed out by Burbacher, Rodier, and Weiss (1990), low-level exposures could produce subclinical effects that become apparent only when other factors, such as aging, affect brain functioning. Finally, it is possible that the toxic effects of exposure to methyl mercury through the ingestion of contaminated fish may be lessened by the presence of increased levels of selenium (Burbacher, Rodier, and Weiss 1990; Hansen, 1984). Methyl mercury and selenium levels tend to covary in fish (Freeman, Shum, and Uthe 1978), which may mean that the source of toxic influences is an important factor in determining their effects (Burbacher, Rodier, and Weiss 1990).

Ionizing Radiation

The greatest information regarding the effects of radiation on the developing brain comes from the atomic bomb blasts at Hiroshima and Nagasaki. The extreme dosages involved in such a disaster produced definite evidence of teratogenic effects, but generalizations are limited to situations in which the typical doses are considerably less.

The evidence that radiation exposure results in lowered IQ is quite clear. Not only was there an overrepresentation of severely mentally retarded children after prenatal exposure in Japan but also, within some of the ranges of gestational age at which the exposure occurred, the relationship between dosage and IQ was approximately linear (Otake, Yoshimaru, and Schull 1987; Schull, Otake, and Yoshimaru 1988). In addition to these IQ effects, long-term follow-up of the children's school performance indicated essentially the same linear relationship with exposure dosage as had been found with IQ (Otake et al. 1988).

The most dramatic and provocative finding from the Japanese follow-up studies concerns the timing of exposure to radiation. At the time of exposure, pregnancies were at all of the stages from conception to birth. Effects on both IQ and school performance, however, were nonexistent in children exposed before the eighth week or after the twenty-sixth week of pregnancy (Schull, Norton, and Jensh 1990). The most sensitive period was from the eighth through the fifteenth weeks, the time of maximum neuronal migratory activity. The mechanisms by which migratory errors may be produced is not known. The various fates that may result from migratory errors were delineated by Nowakowski (1987) and are discussed in chapter 1. In discussing the effects of ionizing radiation, in particular, Schull, Norton, and Jensh (1990) raised several possibilities with regard to the causation of migratory errors. If either the glial cells that guide migratory neurons are destroyed or the cell surface phenomena that allow neurons to move along the glial paths are altered, migratory errors occur. They pointed out that glial cell death should result in a later decrease in the formation of myelin, which has not been found, a fact that decreases the likelihood of this possibility. If either dendritic arborization or some other factor affecting the likelihood of neural connections (i.e., synaptogenesis) were affected, this might alter the survival of neurons related to specific migratory periods, since competition for synaptic sites seems to be a major factor in neuron survival. Finally, direct influence on neuron death could have a similar effect in terms of altering the level of competition among migratory neurons and the eventual elimination of migratory errors. In rats, both fewer neurons and reduced dendritic branching have been observed after exposure to radiation (Konermann 1986; Schneider and Norton 1980).

A clear finding from the Japanese studies was that lowered IQ was associated with reduced head size (Schull, Norton, and Jensh 1990). Sixty percent of the children with severe mental retardation had head sizes two or more standard deviations below the mean for the entire sample. Ten percent of those with small head sizes were severely retarded (Wood, Johnson, and Omori 1965; Wood et al. 1966).

The most likely exposure to the developing fetus is through diagnostic X-ray during pregnancy. Schull, Norton, and Jensh (1990) were not able to estimate a threshold level for teratogenic effects during the critical eighth- to fifteenth-week gestational period in their analysis of Japanese findings. However, the typical exposures considerably exceeded those used in diagnostic X-ray examinations. In the less sensitive sixteenth- through twenty-fifth-week gestational period, the lower threshold of 0.5 Gy still exceeds X-ray levels (Neumeister 1978). Unfortunately, the absence of a lower threshold in those exposed during the most sensitive period mainly indicates that we do not know from these data how risky diagnostic X-ray examinations might be.

Some data are available from follow-up studies of children exposed in utero during maternal X-ray examination. Most of these have failed to yield evidence of an increase in mental retardation or at least have failed to yield convincing evidence. Granroth (1979) found an increase in birth defects in mothers who had undergone pelvic X-ray examinations, but it is not clear that the types of defect found (e.g., anencephaly, hydrocephaly) could be related to the time of X-ray exposure. Neither Neumeister (1978) nor Meyer, Tonascia, and Merz (1976) found an increase in mental retardation in the children of mothers who had undergone diagnostic X-ray examinations.

Cranial Irradiation for Cancer

The use of cranial irradiation to treat childhood acute lymphoblastic leukemia (ALL) has considerably increased the survival rate of children with this disorder. However, reports of intellectual decline after radiation therapy for the disease have added a disturbing element to the otherwise promising picture of outcome (e.g., Eiser 1980; Meadows et al. 1981; Moses 1981; Stehbens and Kisker 1984).

Cousens et al. (1988) conducted a much-needed meta-analysis, using thirty IQ comparisons from twenty different studies addressing the question of IQ changes after cranial radiation therapy in ALL. Twenty-eight of the thirty comparisons showed a negative effect on IQ. The mean effect size was about nine to ten Full-Scale IQ points on the WISC-R.

Several variables were correlated with the magnitude of the effect size. Younger children showed a more negative effect of radiation, especially if they were four years of age or younger. The amount of time between the irradiation and the IQ measurement was also related to IQ differences: the longer the elapsed time, the lower the IQ. This effect was independent of the age at which the child received treatment. A final moderator variable was whether the control group was composed of healthy children or nonirradiated cancer patients. The difference between treated and nontreated children was greater if the control group was healthy. However, the mean difference between irradiated and nonirradiated cancer patients was still about six or seven IQ points.

Younger children showed a greater negative effect of radiation therapy on IQ than did older children. IQ differences increased as the time from the therapy increased, particularly after about three years. These findings are concordant with a hypothesis of a permanent alteration in brain functioning that has a cumulative effect related to impaired learning.

Fetal Alcohol Syndrome

Fetal alcohol syndrome (FAS) was identified by Jones et al. in 1973. They described eight children whose mothers were chronically alcoholic. The children exhibited a similar pattern of pre- and postnatal growth abnormalities, distinctive facial characteristics, limb deformities, and heart defects. The syndrome was formally named by Jones and Smith (1973), who added three more cases and described the brain pathology in one, who had died and come to autopsy. The neuropathological findings of the case included defects in neural migration, agenesis of the corpus callosum, enlarged ventricles, and only partial cortical development. Delayed development was noted in all of the surviving patients.

The conclusion that high consumption of alcohol during pregnancy causes a characteristic pattern of physical and behavioral deficits in the children of such pregnancies has not gone unchallenged (Plant 1985). To examine the cognitive aspects of the syndrome, one must address several pertinent questions: Does such a syndrome exist, regardless of whether or not it is related to the consumption of alcohol? Is the consumption of alcohol during pregnancy related to cognitive deficits in the offspring, regardless of whether or not it produces the fetal alcohol syndrome? Are cognitive deficits in the children of mothers who drink related linearly to the degree of alcohol consumed or do they appear only with excessive drinking? Can the mechanisms responsible for cognitive deficits in the children of mothers who drink during pregnancy be identified? The answers to some of these questions are clearer than others. Some are beyond the scope of this chapter. Although all are touched on occasionally, our main effort is to identify the cognitive characteristics associated with either fetal alcohol syndrome or excessive maternal drinking during pregnancy, with some excursion into the question of the brain abnormalities that may be involved.

Although an association between the consumption of alcohol during pregnancy and adverse effects on the offspring was hypothesized some time ago (e.g., Sullivan 1899), most of the association was related to pregnancy outcomes such as spontaneous abortion or stillbirth. In 1968, Lemoine et al. reported on abnormalities observed in 127 children whose parents were alcoholic. Abnormalities were found in 20 percent of the children. These included peculiar facies, heart defects, limb malformations, cleft palate, delayed development, and below-average IQ. These characteristics resembled what has since come to be known as the fetal alcohol syndrome, but it required the papers by Jones et al. (1973) and Jones and Smith (1973) to focus on the syndrome as a diagnostic entity. Since then, the number of case reports of FAS has mushroomed. In 1984 Abel abstracted thirty-five case studies, describing 277 children, published between the time of the Jones et al. study and 1979. Plant (1985) added nine studies published between 1980 and 1983, describing another 277 children. The fact that more than 550 cases have been reported in the literature over a ten-year period lends support to the notion that an identifiable syndrome exists.

Jones and Smith (1975a) identified fifteen features of the FAS which were present in 18–100 percent of their cases. These included pre- and postnatal growth deficiency, developmental delay, craniofacial features (such as short palpebral fissures, microcephaly, epicanthal folds, maxillary hypoplasia, micrognathia, and cleft palate), limb deformities (such as joint anomalies, altered palmar crease patterns, and fine motor dysfunction), cardiac defects, anomalous external genitalia, and capillary hemangiomata. Several authors observed that children may exhibit varying degrees of the syndrome. This led to the development of scales to classify children as having mild, moderate, or severe degrees of the syndrome (Majewski 1978; Rosett and Weiner 1984). The cognitive level has been found to be inversely related to the severity or number of physical symptoms seen (Majewski 1978), especially facial dysmorphic features (Streissguth, Herman, and Smith 1978).

Majewski (1978) rejected the idea that FAS constitutes a "syndrome" in the ordinary sense. Part of his objection concerned his view that the label "syndrome" should be reserved for genetic disorders. He also objected that maternal consumption of alcohol may have an effect on a number of developing biological systems and that the severity of the effect is merely additive. None of the symptoms of FAS is specific to the effects of alcohol; they occur in other disorders with a variety of causes. Nevertheless, the full-blown syndrome in severe cases is usually regarded as nearly pathognomonic for maternal abuse of alcohol during pregnancy, thus deserving the designation of a syndrome. More in line with this view, Rosett (1980) recommended that a constellation of symptoms be present to confirm a diagnosis of the syndrome. The criteria, taken from Clarren and Smith (1978), required signs in each of three areas: (1) pre- or postnatal growth retardation; (2) the involvement of the central nervous system; and (3) facial dysmorphology. Even proponents of the syndromic nature of FAS have admitted that the so-called characteristic facial features required for a diagnosis of the syndrome are difficult to identify, especially in infants. The classic descriptions of the syndrome were developed by dysmorphologists skilled in making fine observations and distinctions with regard to physical features. For this reason, Rosett and Weiner (1984) favored the Clarren and Smith (1978) criteria but also recommended the use of Majewski's (1978) quantitative scale of individual symptoms.

There is some controversy regarding the actual role of alcohol in producing FAS. Similar groupings of symptoms have been noted in children of mothers who took anticonvulsants (Hill 1976) and mothers with phenylketonuria (Lipson et al. 1981). Zuckerman and Hingson (1986) pointed out that, even in their own studies, which established the prevalence of FAS, maternal consumption of alcohol is so closely tied to the use and abuse of other drugs that it may not be correct to single out alcohol as the etiological agent. Plant and Plant (1988) went so far as to suggest that the syndrome may have been misnamed, since to focus on alcohol may give "undue primacy to a variable, alcohol, which is only a part of a constellation of factors affecting the development of the human fetus." In an opposite vein, Streissguth, Barr, and

Martin (1983) extended the search for the kinds of neurobehavioral symptoms found in FAS to children of moderate drinkers who do not show many of the characteristics of FAS. For them, FAS can serve as a model of the effects of alcohol that may, in turn, show up in less-affected children.

Incidence

The incidence of FAS has been difficult to establish. In general, retrospective studies have led to higher estimates than have prospective studies. Jones et al. (1974) found that six of nineteen (32 percent) surviving children of alcoholic mothers had FAS. Taking into account stillbirths, they estimated the incidence of FAS to be 43 percent in the offspring of alcoholic mothers.

In their prospective longitudinal study, Hanson, Streissguth, and Smith (1978) identified 2 infants with FAS (3 percent) born to 63 mothers who drank heavily. An additional 16 cases had "anomalies suggestive of FAS." The mothers in this study were generally middle class, and their drinking behavior was slightly less severe than that reported by some researchers. Sokol, Miller, and Reed (1980) examined computerized records of obstetric and birth history variables in more than twelve thousand pregnancies. Five cases of FAS were identified in 204 pregnancies in alcoholic mothers (2.5 percent). Rosett et al. (1983) found 5 children with FAS among 52 children born to heavily drinking mothers (10 percent). As in the study by Hanson, Streissguth, and Smith, the last two studies found congenital anomalies, without the complete FAS, at a higher rate than FAS in offspring of mothers who were alcoholic.

Plant (1985) used statistical rather than clinical criteria to determine whether FAS appeared as a syndrome in her study of 926 surviving offspring of 1,008 unselected pregnancies. Data on abnormalities were subjected to a factor analysis to determine whether a cluster of symptoms associated together as a possible "syndrome." No such cluster was found, leading to an incidence of 0 out of 263 pregnancies of mothers classified as drinking heavily.

Several studies have examined large cohorts of unselected pregnancies, yielding estimates regarding the incidence of FAS in the general population. These numbers are somewhat less informative, since virtually all cases of FAS occurred in instances of heavy maternal drinking during pregnancy (Rosett and Weiner 1984). Such figures are directly related to the rate of heavy drinking in pregnant women. Nevertheless, the study by Hanson, Streissguth, and Smith (1978) found a rate of 2 cases of FAS in 1,529 pregnancies (0.13 percent). Sokol, Miller, and Reed (1980) observed 5 cases in a total sample of 12,127 pregnancies (0.04 percent). Hingson et al. (1982) found 1 case in 1,690 pregnancies.

Intellectual Functioning

Streissguth (1986) provided a profile of the cognitive abilities of children with FAS. These included mental retardation in the vast majority of cases, with the average IQ being in the mildly retarded range. Other findings included fine motor problems, slow gross motor development, feeding problems, self-stimulation, hyperactivity and short attention span, and ambiguous hand dominance. Streissguth, Herman, and Smith (1978) studied twenty children who were nine to twenty-one years old, all with FAS. The mean IQ was 65, with a range of 15 to 105. Hyperactivity was common, as were feeding problems. Streissguth, Herman, and Smith (1978) also found a negative relationship between IQ and the number of dysmorphic facial features. Golden et al. (1982) examined twelve one-year-old infants with FAS. Mental Development on the Bayley scales was twenty points below that of a control group.

Robinson, Conry, and Conry (1987) studied an isolated Native American tribe in British Columbia to determine the prevalence of FAS and its effect on cognition. Twenty-two of 123 (18 percent) children showed either complete FAS or a partial syndrome meeting two of the three criteria of Clarren and Smith (1978). Full-Scale, Verbal, and Performance IQ were all below those of an age- and sex-matched control group from the same tribe and were mildly retarded to borderline. The authors speculated that Performance IQ may have been more affected than Verbal IQ because the latter is typically lower than the former in Native Americans, as it was in the control group. The two scores were more nearly equal in the FAS subjects.

The stability of intellectual functioning in FAS has been the topic of some interest. Streissguth, Herman, and Smith (1978) found that IQ changed very little in a group of twenty children with FAS over periods of one to four years. Spohr and Steinhausen (1984) found less stability in IQ after three to four years in forty-two children with FAS. The mean IQ for the group increased. However, the increase was due to a small proportion of the children with low normal and average intelligence who improved, while most of the children with either retarded or above-average IQ remained the same. Interestingly, more physiological indices, such as dysmorphic features, neurological symptoms, and electroencephalogram recordings, showed more consistent improvement. Hyperactivity and distractibility remained significant problems after the three- to four-year lapse of time.

Other Cognitive and Behavioral Findings

An important question regarding the syndromic nature of FAS is whether or not the behavioral characteristics reported in different subjects constitute an identifiable pattern. Some of the earlier reports from the Seattle researchers cited a variety of behavioral abnormalities in newborn infants of heavily drinking mothers. Observation of 124 one-day-old infants whose mothers drank heavily indicated that they were more tremulous, slept less, and spent less time engaging in vigorous limb movements than did the infants of mothers who drank lightly or not at all (Landesman- Dwyer, Keller, and Streissguth 1978). At two days of age, infants born to mothers who both smoked and drank during pregnancy were slower to learn operant head turning and sucking responses than were those of mothers who did not do both (Martin et al. 1977). Using correlational procedures, these researchers were unable to show a significant effect of alcohol use by itself. The same group demonstrated abnormalities related to the level of alcohol consumed during pregnancy in the rate of habituation to repeated stimulation and in the level of arousal in a very large sample ($n = 417$) of one- and two-day-old infants (Streissguth, Barr, and Martin 1983).

None of the above studies was restricted to infants with FAS. Rather, they attempted to ascertain whether there was a dose-response relationship between the consumption of alcohol during pregnancy and infant behavior. It is not clear whether the different behavioral abnormalities were observed in the same infants or across different infants. On the other hand, several confounding variables, such as birth weight, sex, and birth order, as well as the effects of use of other substances such as nicotine, were controlled in the studies.

Some suggestion that there are commonalities in the behavioral patterns shown by infants of heavily drinking mothers has emerged from studies carried out in Boston by Rosett and colleagues (Ouelette et al. 1977; Rosett et al. 1983). Poor sucking ability, jitteriness, and decreased time spent sleeping were more common in the two- and three-day-old infants of mothers who drank heavily as opposed to mothers who drank lightly or not at all. Havlicek, Childiaeva, and Chernick (1977) reported similar findings of jitteriness and sleep disturbance in twenty-six infants born to alcoholic mothers, as well as significant electroencephalogram abnormalities during sleep in infants of alcoholic mothers but not nondrinking mothers. Infants with dysmorphological features of FAS were the most deviant. The Seattle studies, in particular, controlled for a variety of factors, other than maternal drinking, that might affect infant behavioral outcome. Such control does not mean that other factors do not have an effect, however. The Seattle and Boston studies sampled from primarily different socioeconomic levels, with subjects from Seattle generally of higher socioeconomic status than those from Boston. Although the findings from the two sets of studies were quite similar, the incidence of FAS was nearly three times as high in Boston as in Seattle. It has also been more difficult to separate the effects of alcohol from those of other drugs in the Boston group, which might reflect the differences in socioeconomic status in the samples. Zuckerman and Hingson (1986) reported that 2.2 percent of their Boston sample of pregnancies had FAS. However, FAS was significantly associated with marijuana use, poor weight gain during pregnancy, and X-ray exposure, but not with alcohol consumption when other variables were controlled.

Several studies examined the long-term behavioral effects of FAS or heavy consumption of alcohol during pregnancy on older children. Streissguth et al. (1980) found that, at eighteen months, higher levels of alcohol consumed during pregnancy were associated with lower scores in the Bayley Scales of Infant Development, especially the Psychomotor scale. Streissguth, Barr, and Martin (1984) found that sustained attention and reaction times in four year olds were both related to the amount of alcohol consumed during pregnancy by their mothers. More recently, Streissguth et al. (1986) found similar decrements in attention and reaction times in seven to eight year olds whose mothers drank during pregnancy. There was a dose-response relationship between the number of drinks per occasion and the behavioral deficits.

Steinhausen, Gobel, and Nestler (1984) conducted follow-up studies of children with FAS. Intelligence and psycholinguistic abilities, as measured by the Illinois Test of Psycholinguistic Abilities (ITPA), both increased over a thirty-six-month period. Several psychiatric symptoms also showed a significant reduction over time, although hyperactivity and anxiety remained problems. Spohr and Streinhausen (1984) reported an increase in IQ and decreasing dysmorphological signs in thirty-six children with FAS who were tested at ages six and eight and one-half years old. Only six children (19 percent) were in normal schools by the age of eight. It was the authors' impression that hyperactivity and distractibility were major factors in preventing the children from attending regular school. Although not a study of FAS per se, Marino et al. (1987) compared thirty children who were seven to eleven years old and nonretarded but learning disabled to thirty normal controls. The learning-disabled children were 7.5 times more likely to have minor physical signs associated with FAS.

The studies reviewed above reveal a fairly consistent picture of cognitive and behavioral abnormalities associated with FAS. These include jitteriness, tremulousness, and sleep disturbances in infancy; lowered IQ, usually in the mildly retarded range; and hyperactivity and attentional problems that persist into school age, even though some symptoms such as IQ, language skills, and even physiological symptoms improve with age. The findings with regard to intelligence may not extend to severely subnormal children, who seem to remain similarly impaired as they grow older (Steinhausen, Gobel, and Nestler 1984). Learning disorders may be a symptoms of FAS at school age. Although children with FAS are the most extreme in terms of impairment, there seems to be a relationship between heavy drinking during pregnancy and cognitive, behavioral, and physiological abnormalities even when FAS is not present.

Neuropathological Findings

Some of the earliest reports on FAS described brain abnormalities in children with the syndrome. Clarren et al. (1978) reported a covering of heteropic neuronal and glial cells over the cortex in four infants with FAS. Two of the infants had enlarged ventricles and small cerebella and one had no corpus callosum or anterior commissure. Hydrocephalus has been reported in several cases of FAS, along with spina bifida in many. The presence of midline facial dysmorphism has been cited by a number of authors as evidence that brain abnormalities dating to development in the first trimester of pregnancy should be the rule in FAS. Defects in neural tube closure and commissural agenesis support this conjecture, but abnormalities are not limited to those that would stem from such an early period. Heterotopic cells might be due, for instance, to aberrant development of migration pathways early in fetal life or to interference with cell loss later.

Studies have shown alterations in the development of dendritic spines on pyramidal neurons in rats exposed to alcohol from the first day of gestation through or beyond birth (Hammer and Scheibel 1981; Lopez-Tejero 1986; Reyes 1983; Schapiro, Rosman, and Kemper 1984; Stoltenburg-Didinger and Spohr 1983). Fabregues et al.

(1985) reported a similar finding in the guinea pig, in which the brain development during gestation is more similar to that in humans than is the rats'. The general finding has been a reduced number of dendritic spines and spines with long, thin pedicles. Ferrer and Galofré (1987) found similar alterations in the appearance of dendritic spines in the brain of a four-month-old human infant with FAS. When the number of dendritic spines was compared to that in the brains of three control infants who had died as a newborn or three or four month old, the number of dendritic spines at any distance of more than 100 μ from the cell body was reduced well below that found in even the newborn.

The reduction in the number and the alteration in the shape of dendritic spines may well turn out to be two of the more robust and important findings with regard to FAS. The animal studies that produced such an effect have generally been those that maintained alcohol exposure throughout gestation, which approximates the typical drinking pattern in alcoholic mothers. Dose-response relationships between exposure to alcohol and the development of dendritic spines have not been established, but it seems conceivable that an effect such as this, which is less dramatic than a lack of structure development or widely aberrant migration errors, could result from alcohol exposure that produced less than the full-blown FAS. There is no evidence that this is the case at present.

Alterations in the development of dendritic spines would be most likely to produce an atypical neuronal circuitry, the effects of which might be subtle or dramatic, depending on its extent. The attentional and learning problems reported in children with FAS or of heavily drinking mothers (Streissguth, Barr, and Martin 1983) might be more likely due to such alterations in neuronal connectivity than gross structural anomalies. Similar findings have been reported in mentally retarded children with other conditions (Huttenlocher 1974; Marin-Padilla 1972; Purpura 1975).

Social Drinking

The effects of social drinking were examined in a prospective, longitudinal study by the Seattle group. Less than 1 percent of the mothers in the study reported alcohol-related problems. Nevertheless, mild impairments were found in infancy, at preschool age, and at school age (Driscoll, Streissguth, and Riley 1990). At eight months of age the differences between alcohol-exposed infants and controls on the Bayley scales were small but statistically significant. By four years of age the differences remained, although the alcohol-exposed children's IQs were within the normal range (Streissguth, Barr, et al. 1989). At age seven similar results were obtained. Alcohol-exposed children also showed deficits in spatial integration and memory, verbal integration and memory, attention and flexible problem solving on a neuropsychological battery and were rated as more distractible by their teachers (Streissguth, Bookstein, et al. 1989).

Social drinking does not produce the severe effects of chronic alcoholism, but it does produce measurable impairment in cognitive functioning. These findings support the other evidence of a dose-response relationship between the level of alcohol exposure and the degree of cognitive deficit. They imply that the effects of exposure to alcohol during gestation may be much more prevalent than studies of FAS have suggested.

Pediatric Acquired Immunodeficiency Syndrome

The first cases of pediatric acquired immunodeficiency syndrome (AIDS) were described in 1983 (Rubinstein et al. 1983). By 1988, infants and children accounted for 1–2 percent of cases of AIDS reported to the Centers for Disease Control (Pizzo et al. 1988). The distribution of children with AIDS follows geographic, socioeconomic, and cultural lines. The majority are from New York, New Jersey, Florida, and California. Children who live in large urban areas are particularly at risk. Fifty-eight percent of the children are African American, 22 percent hispanic, and 20 percent white (Rogers et al. 1987). The vast majority of infected children were infected before or during birth. Eighty percent had a parent infected with human immunodeficiency virus (HIV), usually with AIDS or AIDS-related complex (ARC). Another 18 percent were infected by contaminated blood products (U.S. Department of Health and Human Services 1992).

In most cases, HIV infection is contracted from the mother. Maternal infected blood may be a source of infection during pregnancy or birth. HIV infection has been detected in thirteen- to twenty-week-old fetuses (Jovaisas et al. 1985; Lapointe et al. 1985; Sprecher et al. 1986). It may be acquired during birth by exposure to maternal genital tract infections (Vogt et al. 1987). A less common route of transmission may be through breastfeeding (Ziegler et al. 1985).

The diagnosis of AIDS in children is made in the first year of life in 50 percent of cases and by age three in 82 percent of cases (Rubinstein 1986). The onset of AIDS after HIV infection is generally sooner in children than in adults and sooner in those infected congenitally than in those infected by blood transfusion (Rogers et al. 1987). A variety of diagnoses are relevant to AIDS in children. HIV-infected children who are asymptomatic are referred to as *seropositive*. Because passively acquired maternal HIV antibodies may circulate within the uninfected infant's blood for up to one year, a child under fifteen months of age must have other clinical or laboratory signs of HIV infection to be considered seropositive (Falloon et al. 1989). Symptomatic children who do not meet all of the criteria for AIDS are diagnosed as having ARC. AIDS dementia complex (ADC), a syndrome of subcortical dementia affecting cognitive, motor, and, often behavioral functioning, occurs with increasing frequency at progressively more serious stages of HIV infection in adults. The diagnosis is made less often in children, although cognitive and motor behaviors are nearly always affected. In children, it is less clear that there is a progressive loss of function as opposed to initial and continuing impairment. There is some evidence of progressive deterioration, however, which also shows up on computed tomographic scans (Epstein et al. 1985, 1986).

The clinical-cognitive manifestations of pediatric AIDS and its course have been the subject of several studies. Ultmann et al. (1985) conducted one of the more comprehensive studies of the cognitive manifestations of pediatric AIDS. The sixteen children in the study were diagnosed with either AIDS or ARC and at the beginning of the study ranged in age from six months to six years. Cognitive measures varied, depending on the age of the child, and included the Bayley Scales of Infant Development, the Denver Developmental Screening Test, and the Stanford-Binet Intelligence Scale.

The majority of the children showed delays in cognitive and motor skills. Only one child, who was in the ARC category, had a normal IQ. Thirteen children with AIDS regressed after the onset of opportunistic infections. The most profound delays were in the development of motor skills.

Fourteen months after the initial assessment, a follow-up evaluation was conducted (Ultmann et al. 1987). Five of the children had died. Sixty percent of the survivors maintained developmental progress at their below-normal levels. Twenty percent showed some acceleration in cognitive development, and 20 percent decelerated. Nine children showed signs of neurological deterioration, although some of these did not show developmental regression.

Belman et al. (1988) found more consistent evidence of progressive decline in cognitive abilities in sixty-eight infants and children, six weeks to thirteen years old, who were followed for one to forty-eight months. Sixty-two of the children, diagnosed with either AIDS or ARC, followed what was characterized as a subacute but steadily progressive course, which included progressive encephalopathy, long tract signs, cerebral atrophy, white matter attenuation, and, in some patients, calcification of the basal ganglia. The remaining cases showed either a static course or a rapidly progressive one. All of the children showed cognitive impairment, with IQ ranging from 50 to 78 on the Bayley, Stanford-Binet, or Kaufman Assessment Battery for Children. Thirty-four of the children died during the course of the study, with death occurring one to twenty-three months after the onset of neurological disease.

There is some evidence that treatment with azidothymidine (AZT) may improve cognitive functioning, even in seropositive children who are otherwise asymptomatic. Pizzo et al. (1988) provided continuous intravenous infusion of AZT to twenty-one HIV-infected children aged fourteen months to twelve years. Thirteen subjects presented with evidence of encephalopathy at the beginning of treatment. Thirteen subjects were available to be reevaluated. As a group, they showed a mean increase of more than fifteen points in IQ, with all but one subject showing some improvement. Improvements in gait and coordination, receptive and expressive language, and social interaction were also present. Interestingly, improvement occurred also in those children who had not shown evidence of encephalopathy, suggesting that subtle changes in cognitive functioning may be detectable as early signs of a more frank encephalopathy.

At present, the prognosis for HIV-infected children is grim, even more so than that for adults. Children who are infected before or at birth may never develop normal intellectual functioning and remain more helpless and dependent than just their young age would normally make them. The majority already are born into disadvantaged social and economic circumstances and have at least one HIV-infected parent who may be dealing with a debilitating illness. At the same time, new medical treatments may offer some hope for at least longer survival, perhaps with less impairment during a significant portion of their lives. We need further research into the behavioral and social aspects of the disease, as well as into methods for improving the quality of life of these children and their families.

5

The Cognitive Effects
of Premature Birth

The normal length of a pregnancy is considered to be thirty-seven to forty-two weeks (World Health Organization 1948–49, 1961). Normal birth weight is considered to be more than 2,500 grams (World Health Organization 1961). These two categories of normal birth are not always in agreement, however, and an infant may be born from a pregnancy of normal length but weigh less than 2,500 grams (Babson, Behrman, and Lessel 1970). This has led to some difficulty in evaluating the literature on prematurity, since it may be defined by either gestational age or birth weight. Although the majority of researchers currently seem to focus on birth weight, others look at gestational age (e.g., Als, Duffy, and McAnulty 1988). The two variables are highly correlated before thirty-seven weeks gestation but much less so beyond that (Babson 1970; Babson, Behrman, and Lessel 1970). For most studies of very low birth weight (<1,500 grams), the typical gestational age is less than thirty weeks.

In the last forty years the mortality rate for prematurely born infants of low birth weight has dropped considerably. This seems to be true in at least all of the developed countries, including England and Wales (McDonald 1981; Pharoah and Alberman 1981), the United States (Lee et al. 1980), Canada (Dunn 1986), and Sweden (Hagberg, Hagberg, and Olow 1982). It has been less clear, however, whether handicapping conditions, either major or minor, have shown a similar reduction. There have been conflicting reports, with some indicating a very low prevalence of handicap in low-birth-weight survivors (e.g., Stewart and Reynolds 1974) and others indicating relatively higher rates and little decline between the early 1960s and the late 1970s (Horwood et al. 1982). Estimates of major handicap (cerebral palsy or mental retardation) have ranged from 5 to 18 percent and of minor handicap (learning, behavioral, or minor neurological signs) from 5 to 10 percent in children of very low birth weight (Jones, Cummins, and Davies 1979; Knobloch et al. 1982; Stewart, Reynolds, and Lipscomb 1981).

In a child of very low birth weight, it is difficult to assess the effect of prematurity or low birth weight per se because medical complications increase as the birth weight and gestational age decrease. Periventricular-intraventricular hemorrhage, for instance, has been found in about 40 percent of all very-low-birth-weight infants when computed tomography or ultrasound scanning is done (Ahmann et al. 1978; Papile et al. 1978; Tekolste, Bennett, and Mack 1985). Such hemorrhages are often associated with respiratory distress syndrome, which develops in an even larger percentage of very-low-birth-weight infants (Fitzhardinge et al. 1976; Johnson et al. 1974). In addition to hemorrhagic brain lesions, ischemic lesions, particularly periventricular leucomalacia, increase in prevalence with decreasing birth weight (Pape and Wigglesworth 1979).

The Effects of Prematurity on Neonatal Behavior

Despite the difficulty separating the effects of premature birth from the effects of the medical complications that often accompany it, some studies allow us to draw some conclusions regarding the effect of prematurity per se. Als, Duffy, and McAnulty (1988) divided healthy prematurely born and healthy full-term infants into three groups based on gestational age. In the sample of children born prematurely, there was no difference in developmental status at two weeks beyond the *expected* due date between the earliest and latest preterm infants when assessed with a modified Brazelton scale. However, the prematurely born infants scored lower than the full-term infants on all of the categories of the assessment scale. Their finding was similar to that reported earlier by Sell et al. (1980) but contradicted the finding of Paludetto et al. (1982) that healthy preterm infants did as well as healthy full-term infants when measured at "term" age.

Because of the association between very low birth weight and various medical complications, several researchers have attempted to divide prematurely born infants into those who are at "high risk" and those who are at "low risk." Risk status is usually defined as the presence of medical complications associated with neurological sequelae. Emory and Mapp (1988) studied spontaneous sleep startles, which they hypothesized to be a healthy discharge phenomenon dependent on a functioning "central pacemaker" that may also generate the electroencephalogram in neonates. They found that both healthy preterm infants and those with respiratory distress syndrome had fewer sleep startles than did healthy full-term infants. The premature infants with respiratory distress syndrome, however, had even fewer sleep startles than did the healthy preterm infants.

Scanlon, Scanlon, and Tronick (1984) found an interaction between the type of medical complication and the age of assessment in infants of very low birth weight. At age seven days, medical variables related to perinatal asphyxia (e.g., cord pH, duration of oxygen exposure, and lowest partial pressure of oxygen) were the best predictors of developmental status on a modified Brazelton scale. However, at twenty-one days the best predictors were variables related to the degree of prematurity and nutrition (e.g., weight change, peak bilirubin, duration of oxygen exposure). Their findings indicate that the degree of prematurity may affect developmental outcome at early ages but that the birth condition may overshadow other variables in the first week of life.

Both low birth weight and medical complications have been shown to have an effect on developmental status at the *expected* birth date, even when gestational age did not. Piper et al. (1985) studied four groups of infants at forty to forty-one weeks conceptional age. Three groups were preterm infants in the gestational age ranges of twenty-three to twenty-seven weeks, twenty-eight to thirty-one weeks, and thirty-two to thirty-six weeks. The fourth group were full-term infants with and without medical complications.

There were no differences between the preterm groups of different gestational ages or between preterm infants and medically complicated full-term infants on optimality scores on the Prechtl neurological examination. However, when the preterm infants were grouped according to birth weight, those born at less than 1,000 grams had lower scores than those born at more than 1,000 grams. In addition, several medical complications (e.g., bronchopulmonary dysplasia, seizures, and prolonged ventilation), which were more likely to occur in the infants of the lowest gestational age, were associated with lower scores. "Healthy" full-term infants had higher scores than the preterm infants, even when the medically complicated preterm infants were eliminated. However, medically complicated full-term infants were most similar to the preterm infants. The authors concluded that medical complications have a qualitatively similar effect on developmental status in both preterm and full-term infants but are more likely to occur in younger preterm infants.

Emory, Tynan, and Davé (1989) further explored the question of whether medical complications impaired the behavior of preterm and full-term infants when assessed at term age. Using the Brazelton Neonatal Behavioral Assessments, they compared healthy full-term infants, prematurely born infants with respiratory distress syndrome, and infants with neonatal seizures, some of whom were preterm but most of whom were not. On most of the scales, the infants with seizure disorder performed worse than either the full-term infants or the preterm infants with respiratory distress syndrome. The latter two groups did not differ except on the behavioral clusters related to the regulation of state and the persistence of primitive reflexes. These findings, like those cited previously, point to the importance of major medical complications rather than prematurity per se in determining the status of the infant at the time of normal birth.

The Later Development of Prematurely Born Children

Even in the first year of life, preterm infants may have behavioral deficits that decrease their potential for later development. Studies of infant attention responses have shown that infants who actively examine toys have higher scores on other measures of behavioral development and develop at faster rates than do infants who do not (Kopp and Vaughn 1982; Ruff et al. 1984). In both preterm and full-term infants, measures of attention are associated with higher intellectual functioning at later ages (Cohen and Parmelee 1983; Fagan and McGrath 1981; Lewis and Brooks-Gunn 1981). Although some measures of attention have been shown to discriminate between preterm and full-term infants (Kopp and Vaughn 1982; Rose 1983; Sigman and Parmelee 1974) and between neurologically impaired preterm and healthy preterm infants (Spungen, Kurtzberg, and Vaughn 1985), this finding is not always clear. Sigman and Parmelee (1974) and Cohen and Parmelee (1983) found that the average length of time an infant looked at a toy discriminated between preterm and full-term infants at three months of age. However, Landry et al. (1985) and Ruff (1986) found no differences between preterm and full-term infants on this measure at six months of age.

Landry and Chapieski (1988) carried out a detailed study of infants' visual attention at six months of age. They compared full-term infants to preterm infants who were either at high risk (grade III or IV intraventricular hemorrhage and/or bronchopulmonary dysplasia) or at low risk (mild to moderate respiratory distress syndrome with or without grade I or II intraventricular hemorrhage). Infants were tested on the Bayley scales and on measures of visual and physical examination of objects and shifts of attention from one object to another. The full-term and low-risk preterm infants had higher Bayley Mental Developmental Index scores. Their mean length of examination of objects, number of objects examined, and shifts of attention from one object to another were also greater than those of the high-risk preterm infants.

In their longitudinal study of low-birth-weight children up to seven years of age, McBurney and Eaves (1986) found significant differences, compared to full-birth-weight controls, in developmental scores on every scale of the Griffiths exam at three months, six months, one year, and eighteen months. There was a clear linear relationship between birth weight and developmental quotient that was much more marked in infancy than after eighteen months. Within the low-birth-weight sample, those who were of greater gestational age (small for gestational age) had higher developmental quotients than did equivalent-weight infants of shorter gestational age. This was, again, much more marked at the time of the earliest assessments, suggesting that the more mature nervous system has some initial advantage, even at low birth weight. McBurney and Eaves did not "correct" their scores for gestational age. Their finding of an early disadvantage of the infants with shorter gestational age is common and has led many investigators to favor such a correction.

Although shorter gestational age is a relatively good predictor of early cognitive outcome, even when birth weight is controlled, birth weight itself, independent of gestational age, may have a more long term influence on cognitive development in prematurely born children. When prematurely born children are matched for gestational age, those who are born at significantly less than the usual birth weight for their gestational age do less well than those who are born at a weight appropriate for their gestational age.

The majority of studies of prematurely born children who are small for the gestational age have focused on the first year after birth. The results of these studies are fairly uniform: preterm children small for their gestational age are slower in development than are heavier preterm infants (Commey and Fitzhardinge 1979; Fitzhardinge and Pape 1977; Tudehope et al. 1983). Aylward, Verhulst, and Bell (1988) found that birth weight and gestational age were the best, and nearly the only, significant predictors of cognitive, motor, and neurological outcome at forty weeks, nine months, eighteen months, and thirty-six months among a number of maternal and prenatal variables in a sample of 608 preterm infants. When compared to other neonatal status variables (e.g., Apgar score, infections, hyperbilirubinemia), being small for the gestational age became increasingly predictive of cognitive function up to thirty-six months, while most of the other variables decreased in significance as predictors.

Being born small for the gestational age has been the subject of longitudinal research that has followed children up to school age. Neligan et al. (1976) compared three groups of seven-year-old children: normal-birth-weight controls, children of short gestation but appropriate weight for the gestational age, and children born small for the gestational age. The children who were small for their gestational age were further divided into two groups: "rather light for dates" and "very light for dates." Children were assessed with a variety of intelligence, language, visuomotor, motor, and academic achievement tests. On nearly all measures, except the academic (reading) tests, the short-gestation group performed less well than the controls and the "very light for dates" group performed even less well than the group with short gestation but appropriate weight for gestational age. The results of this study illustrate the persistence of the adverse effects of being small for the gestational age, even up to school age. Social class factors, however, were of even greater importance than birth weight in predicting later cognitive development.

More recently, Dunn and others (1986) reported the results of a longitudinal study of low-birth-weight children who were followed up to six and one-half years of age. Birth weight by itself was a significant predictor of intelligence only up to eighteen months of age. At early ages the typical finding of children of greater gestational age performing better than less mature children of the same birth weight was evident at the lowest birth weights up to eighteen months. By eighteen months this finding began to reverse itself and the children who were small for their gestational age, at most birth weights, began to have lower cognitive scores than the children who were of appropriate weight for their gestational age.

Being small for the gestational age is usually considered synonymous with intrauterine growth retardation. Studies that refer to being small for gestational age are essentially studies of intrauterine growth retardation. However, one must be quite careful in interpreting the results of such studies. The difficulty lies in the method of reporting results. Some studies held birth weight constant and defined being small for gestational age as being born at a greater gestational age than peers of similar birth weight (e.g., Dunn 1986). Other studies held gestational age constant and defined being small for gestational age or having intrauterine growth retardation as being of lesser birth weight than peers of similar gestational age (e.g., Neligan et al. 1976).

If both lower birth weight and shorter gestational age are negatively related to early cognitive development, when birth weight is held constant the infant who is small for the gestational age will show an advantage over the infant who is of appropriate weight for the gestational age because the former is less premature. On the other hand, if gestational age is held constant, the infant who is small for the gestational age will show a disadvantage compared to the infant who is of appropriate weight for the gestational age because the former is smaller.

Studies that refer to intrauterine growth retardation tend to vary the birth weight and hold gestational age constant. For example, Matilainen, Heinonen, and Siren-Tiusanen (1988) held gestational age constant and compared children of different birth weights on cognitive indices at five years of age. Based on differing birth weights, they divided preterm children into those born at weight appropriate for the gestational age and those born with normal body length but birth weight more than two standard deviations below the mean (intrauterine growth retardation). They also included healthy, full-term controls.

At age five years the infants with intrauterine growth retardation scored significantly lower than the full-term controls on nonverbal intelligence (Leiter International Performance Scale), vocabulary, and human figure drawing. On none of the measures did the preterm children of appropriate weight for the gestational age differ from the full-term controls.

Delays in brain growth do not just occur prenatally in preterm children. Even in preterm children of appropriate weight for the gestational age, there is evidence that postnatal growth is delayed in a large percentage of children. Astbury et al. (1986) followed 235 preterm children of appropriate weight for the gestational age up to two years of age. At two years the distributions of weight, length, and head circumference all differed from normal, with an excess in the lower percentiles. This was true to a much greater extent for weight and length than for head circumference. Poor growth, as defined by poor weight gain, was a good predictor of delays in gross- and fine-motor development at two years.

Hack and Breslau (1986) also studied the relationship between postnatal growth and intelligence in preterm children of appropriate weight for the gestational age. They found that head circumference measured at eight months was the best predictor of Stanford-Binet IQ at three years of age. Using a path model, they determined that head circumference at eight months had a direct effect on IQ, whereas neonatal risk factors had an indirect effect, expressed through head circumference. Neurological impairment had both indirect effects, expressed through head circumference, and direct effects on IQ.

It is clear that postnatal growth is associated with subsequent intellectual and motor development in preterm infants of appropriate weight for the gestational age. The association is even more striking in preterm children who are small for the gestational age. Babson (1970) found that preterm infants who are small for the gestational age showed less "catch-up" growth than infants of appropriate weight for the gestational age during the first year. Fitzhardinge and Steven (1972) reported that 35 percent of preterm children who were small for the gestational age were at or below the third percentile for height at six years of age. Fancourt et al. (1976) used ultrasound to determine that, when growth failure began to occur in utero before twenty-six weeks of gestation, preterm children who were small for the gestational age had lower developmental quotients at four years of age.

Dunn, Hughes, and Schulzer (1986) studied preterm children who were of appropriate weight for the gestational age, full-term children who were small for the gestational age, and full-term, full-birth-weight children. Their data indicated that weight, length, and head circumference in both preterm children of appropriate weight for gestational age and full-term children small for the gestational age began at lower levels at birth than in the full-birth-weight, full-term children (although the preterm children were no different from the full-term, normal-birth-weight children when equated for conceptional age). All of the children showed maximum growth velocity during the first year. However, at six and one-half years the preterm children of appropriate weight for gestational age and the full-birth-weight full-term children were relatively close to each other, whereas the full-term children who were small for the gestational age lagged behind on all three measures.

Intellectual and neurological measures at six and one-half years were significantly related to head sizes at birth and at six and one-half years. Head size at six and one-half years was more highly related to intellectual and neurological outcome than was head size at birth. For instance, when considering only those children who were below the tenth percentile at birth, those who had normal head size at age six and one-half were, on the average, nearly thirty points higher in intellectual ability than were those whose head size remained below the tenth percentile. In contrast, body length at birth did not add to the prediction of intellect beyond the ability to predict it on the basis of head size alone. The relationship between head size and IQ remained, even after controlling for differences in social class. Both boys and girls showed a similar relationship between head size and intellect, with the exception that, for boys, extremely large head size was also associated with low intellect. For girls, the positive relationship between head size and intellect was simply linear.

From all of the above results, several conclusions can be drawn regarding gestational age, birth weight, and later psychological development. The degree of medical/neurological complications experienced by the newborn seems to be the primary determinant of the initial developmental status. As some of the problems resolve themselves, the degree of prematurity exerts a stronger influence, although it may not be as powerful a predictor as some neurological complications, such as seizures. Infants who are small for the gestational age experience an additional negative influence. This fact can be obscured during the first twelve to eighteen months if infants who are small for the gestational age are compared to similar-birth-weight infants of appropriate weight for the gestational age. Thus, the degree of maturity of the infant's physiological systems is an important factor, independent of birth weight. Conversely, infants who are small for the gestational age, when compared to heavier infants of similar gestational age, do worse in early development, indicating an independent contribution of birth weight. As development continues into early childhood, the advantage for those children born of longer pregnancies fades and there is a more long-term negative influence on cognitive development associated with being small for the gestational age, even when children who are small for the gestational age are compared to similar-birth-weight children.

As development continues throughout infancy and early childhood, there is generally an early period of "catch-up" growth in both preterm children who are of appropriate weight for the gestational age and preterm children who are small for the gestational age. By school age, the former are close to the norm on most growth indices, whereas the latter tend to remain small. The most crucial growth indicator, in terms of cognitive development, is head size. Head size is less affected by intrauterine growth retardation than are body weight or length. However, there is some diminution of head size in infants who are small for the gestational age, and head size at birth has some predictive significance for later cognitive development. Of greater importance than head size at birth is head growth. Failure to increase head size to reach normal values is highly associated with lower intellect in childhood.

Whereas the studies cited above focused on separating the effects of gestational age, birth weight, and intrauterine growth retardation on rather global measures of cognitive development, other studies examined cognitive abilities in greater detail while focusing less on separating the influence of one predictive variable from another. Klein et al. (1985) matched forty-six very-low-birth-weight (<1,500 grams) five year olds, all of whom were free of neurological problems and had normal intellect, to full-birth-weight classmates. All of the children were given a battery of intellectual, cognitive, and visuomotor tests. Significant differences between the very-low-birth-weight children and their matched controls were found only on measures of visuospatial and visuomotor abilities. Intellectual, auditory, and language measures did not yield differences between the two groups. The authors speculated that the visual and motor systems may be more vulnerable to the effects of prematurity than the auditory-language systems.

Largo et al. (1986) examined language development in considerable detail in a group of prematurely born children compared to healthy, full-term children. The language being studied in this group of Swiss families was Swiss-German. In terms of medical complications, the preterm group was generally at high risk.

The mother of each child maintained a record of the exact date at which each of twenty-five stages of language development was reached. Laboratory observations of each child's language behavior were also made at ten intervals up to sixty months. At age five, each child was assessed with three subtests from a Swiss-German version of the ITPA and was given a test of speech articulation.

When neurologically impaired preterm children were excluded, the preterm children generally lagged behind the full-term children in reaching all stages of language development. However, the differences between the groups were significant in only two instances. At age five years, preterm girls performed significantly worse than full-term girls on two of the ITPA subtests. There were no differences between preterm and full-term boys. Similarly, preterm girls showed more articulation defects than did full-term girls, but differences between full-term and preterm boys were not significant. Both birth weight and gestational age were positively correlated with language development and language ability at five years in the preterm group. When the neurologically impaired preterm children were compared to the full-term controls, the differences were more pronounced and occurred especially on the articulation measure.

The study by Largo et al. (1986) is perhaps the most elaborate yet reported in terms of language assessment. A number of positive correlations between the stage measures and the static five-year measures offer some support of the validity of the former measurement procedures. However, the differences between non–neurologically impaired preterm and full-term children were not striking, although they were consistently in the right direction. This lends some support to the idea that language development may be less vulnerable to the effects of prematurity than is visuomotor development. In addition, when neurological disorder does affect language, it has a stronger effect on articulation than on other, more cognitive aspects of language.

In the longitudinal study carried out by Dunn, Hughes, and Schulzer (1986) in Vancouver, significant differences in intelligence were found at all ages up to six and one-half years when low-birth-weight and full-birth-weight children were compared. The relationship between IQ and birth weight was linear at all ages. Interestingly, at age six and one-half years the only WISC-R subtests that did not show a significant difference between low-birth-weight and full-birth-weight children were Coding and Mazes, which are the most motoric subtests. For that matter, the Draw-a-Person test also produced no significant differences at either four years or six and one-half years. Repetition of sentences, however, which is clearly a language and memory task, produced significantly lower scores for the low-birth-weight children at age six and one-half years.

The performance of the low-birth-weight children on the Bender Visuo-Motor Gestalt was significantly worse than that of the full-birth-weight children, even when IQ, socioeconomic status, and sex were controlled. Within the low-birth-weight group, both the Draw-a-Person and the Bender Gestalt were significantly worse in those children with abnormal neurological findings.

At age four years an extensive examination of communication skills was carried out with all of the children in the study. Low-birth-weight children performed significantly worse than full-birth-weight children on seven of twenty language measures. Six of the seven were expressive rather than receptive. In addition, the low-birth-weight children did significantly worse on a measure of speech articulation at age six and one-half years.

Prematurity and low birth weight affect all areas of cognitive development all the way up to school age. The pattern of the effects is less clear, although visuomotor ability, as in copying designs, is the most consistently impaired skill. Language also is impaired, although the effects seem to be harder to demonstrate. Expressive language skills are more often impaired than are receptive language skills, and speech articulation is especially vulnerable. Although cognitive impairment is possible to demonstrate even when neurologically impaired preterm children are excluded from studies, it is clearly the case that the prognosis is worse for IQ, language, and visuomotor skills if neurological impairment is present.

Medical Complications and Cognitive Development in Prematurely Born Children

Prematurely born infants are known to be at increased risk for a variety of medical complications. In general, the risk of serious complications increases with the degree of prematurity. As noted earlier, this relationship makes it quite difficult to assess the influence of low birth weight or short gestational age as a risk factor by itself, separate from the medical complications associated with it.

Medical complications may be divided into three broad categories: (1) conditions that may lead to brain injury (e.g., infection, asphyxia), (2) evidence of brain injury (e.g., intraventricular hemorrhage), and (3) symptoms of brain injury (e.g., seizures). The assumption is that the common pathway by which medical complications affect cognitive development is through injury to the brain. Such an assumption is an oversimplification, since there are other ways in which cognitive development may be affected by medical problems. Chronic sickness during infancy, for instance, might restrict the child's access to early stimulation. Even when neurological disorder is present, as in cerebral palsy, it is difficult to separate the effect of impairment in sensorimotor experience from the effect of the brain injury underlying the motor systems.

Despite the above caveats, it is interesting to examine what is known of the relationships between medical complications and cognitive development in preterm children. The theoretical assumption that prompts such a search for these relationships is that of a "continuum of reproductive casualty" (Knobloch and Pasamanick 1960). Those conditions that increase the risk for death or major handicap, when present to a lesser degree, increase the risk for minor handicaps, including cognitive and learning disabilities. Stewart and Hope (1988) reported figures on mortality and morbidity, with the latter defined as major or minor neurodevelopmental disorders, as a result of various degrees of periventricular hemorrhage. The same relationships that were found between hemorrhage characteristics (size, location, and associated complications) and mortality were found between hemorrhage characteristics and morbidity. Although these results are quite strikingly in accord with the continuum of reproductive casualty hypothesis, even these seemingly clear-cut relationships can be questioned. Hemorrhagic lesions and ischemic lesions are often present together in the brain of a preterm infant. Although the relationships between each of these types of lesion and mortality may be roughly similar, recent studies have shifted the presumed cause for neurodevelopmental impairment to ischemic lesions, particularly cystic periventricular leucomalacia (Hansen et al. 1989; Stewart and Hope 1988).

Studies Involving Multiple Predictor Variables

As reviewed earlier, Scanlon, Scanlon, and Tronick (1984) found that the birth condition of the infant was the best predictor of developmental status in extremely premature infants at one week but that variables related to the degree of prematurity and nutrition were better predictors of developmental status at three weeks of age. The authors recorded twenty-five variables, including birth demographics and physiological variables, about forty-five infants who weighed between 750 and 1,500 grams at birth. They used stepwise multiple regression procedures to examine the predictive ability of each variable with regard to total scores on a modified Brazelton exam. At seven days after birth, the best predictors of developmental status were umbilical vein pH, duration of oxygen exposure, and lowest partial pressure of oxygen. At twenty-one days after birth, the best predictors were the duration of oxygen exposure, weight changes since birth, peak bilirubin level, and initial body temperature. Variables such as birth weight and gestational age exhibited higher correlations with developmental status at twenty-one days than at seven days. These results were interpreted as indicating that variables related to asphyxia and the neonate's initial medical condition were more important at one week and variables related to the degree of prematurity became more important at three weeks.

Low et al. (1985) followed 364 preterm and full-term infants for one year. All infants were at risk because of fetal-newborn complications. Perinatal, obstetric, demographic, and environmental variables were recorded for each infant and used to predict outcome. Outcome was defined as the presence or absence of major or minor cognitive or motor deficits at one year. The Bayley scales and the Uzgiris and Hunt scale were used to define deficits. Neonatal complications were classified as those related to gestational age, birth weight, congenital anomalies, fetal hypoxia, respiratory complications, infections, and newborn encephalopathy. All of these variables were significantly related to the one-year outcome. Variables related to parental socioeconomic status, quality of the home environment, and maternal and obstetric complications were not related to outcome. Using stepwise multiple regression, they found that only the presence of newborn encephalopathy made a significant independent contribution to the prediction of deficits. When newborn encephalopathy was excluded from the analysis, respiratory complications, infections, and hypoxia added to the prediction of deficits. Apparently, birth weight and gestational age expressed their effects only through other variables related to the infant's medical condition at birth.

A major problem in determining the best predictors of developmental status from among a number of medical variables is that many of them are correlated with one another. Multiple regression procedures may underestimate the predictiveness of some variables because of high intercorrelations between the variables. Pederson et al. (1988) tried to overcome this problem by using factor analysis to reduce a number of medical, environmental, and demographic variables to a smaller number of orthogonal factors. Fifteen variables were reduced to four factors. One factor represented the infant's degree of prematurity and medical status (gestational age, birth weight, number of days in the hospital, severity of respiratory distress, and a summary morbidity score based on the presence and severity of twenty common diseases and pathological states of preterm infants). A second factor comprised seven- and twelve-month measures of maternal sensitivity and the quality of stimulation in the home environment. The third factor contained variables related to the parental occupation and education. A fourth factor represented one- and five-minute Apgar scores.

After reducing the fifteen variables to four factors, the investigators used each factor plus a score based on the number of developmental delays on the Denver Developmental Screening test administered at seven months to predict the Bayley Mental Developmental Index and PDI at one year. All four factors and the number of delays on the Denver test were predictive of the developmental status at twelve months.

The results of Pederson et al. emphasize the fact that developmental outcome in preterm infants may be as highly related to variables in social environment as to medical complications. Other authors have found similar results (Dunn 1986; Neligan et al. 1976). This finding prompted Sameroff and Chandler (1975) to speak of a "continuum of caretaking casualty" to capture the idea that there is an interaction between the infant's physiological condition and the quality of the environment in which he or she is raised. Both must be taken into account in predicting the development of a prematurely born child.

In the study by Neligan et al. (1976), social factors and demographic variables were less important in the more severely impaired children. Other authors found similar results (e.g., Dunn 1986). There is reason to think that this may apply also to the baby of extremely low birth weight. Pederson et al. (1988) examined infants with birth weight less than 2,501 grams with a mean birth weight of 1,672 grams. Neligan et al. (1976) used a sample of children whose mean birth weight in the lightest group was 2,397 grams. Dunn (1986) divided study children into various categories of low birth weight. The upper limit for birth weight was 2,500 grams, but the majority of children fell into the category of birth weight between 1,500 and 2,000 grams. All of these studies, which found a strong influence of social factors, involved primarily "heavier" low-birth-weight babies.

Several studies have examined the predictors of development in infants of very low (<1,500 grams) or extremely low (<1,000 grams) birth weight. Mortality is greatly increased in infants of extremely low birth weight. Hirata et al. (1983) studied very tiny infants who had weighed between 501 and 750 grams at birth. Only twenty-two out of sixty (37 percent) survived. Of the survivors, twelve (67 percent) were without any impairment, two (11 percent) were neurologically impaired and mentally retarded, and four (22 percent) were of borderline or below-average intelligence at six years.

In a study of similar-birth-weight children who were born at less than 800 grams, Bennett, Robinson, and Sells (1983) reported a neonatal mortality of 80 percent. Of the sixteen surviving infants, thirteen (81 percent) had no major neurological handicap and only one had below-normal intelligence at six months to three years of follow-up. In this study, Apgar scores at one and five minutes were the best predictors of later outcome. In the study by Pederson et al. (1988), Apgar scores were minimally predictive of developmental outcome and comprised a factor that was separate from other medical variables. This led Pederson et al. to question the usefulness of Apgar scores in predictive studies of long-term outcome. It may well be that, as birth weight decreases and the likelihood of neurological damage increases, the Apgar, as an indicator of the newborn's immediate state, may be a more powerful predictor of later development.

Skoutelli et al. (1985) examined the power of perinatal medical problems (twenty obstetric and thirty-one neonatal) in predicting three-year neurodevelopmental outcome in infants who had weighed less than 1,001 grams at birth. From a sample of sixty infants, twenty-nine (43 percent) survived the neonatal period.

Factors related to survival were more clearly identified than factors related to neurodevelopmental outcome in survivors. Obstetric factors were related to neither survival nor outcome. The variable most related to survival was acidosis. In addition, gestational age, five-minute Apgar score, time on ventilatory support, hypoxia and hypercapnia, and severe grades of periventricular hemorrhage were all related to survival. Fifty percent of the surviving infants were neurologically normal and had average developmental quotients on the Griffiths exam. Another 38 percent had normal developmental quotients with minor neurological signs. Only 17 percent were handicapped in a major way. When the completely normal 50 percent were compared to the 50 percent with any evidence of handicap, the Apgar score at five minutes was the best predictor of outcome. Although this finding supports the validity of the Apgar as a predictor of developmental outcome in infants of extremely low birth weight, it does not particularly support the idea that cognitive outcome in surviving children is related to the same factors as is survival itself.

The conclusion of virtually all of the authors of studies of extremely-low-birth-weight infants has been that, when an infant survives, the prognosis is remarkably good for a normal cognitive outcome. Although this is true to some extent, it is primarily in contrast to the high mortality rate in this group that rates of major handicap of 10–20 percent look good. There clearly is some discontinuity between 50–80 percent mortality rates and 10–20 percent handicap rates in surviving children. However, before discarding the continuum of reproductive casualty hypothesis, one must remember that most of the outcome studies used rather gross measures of cognitive outcome and relatively short follow-up periods. More extensive studies, like those of Neligan et al. (1976) and Dunn (1986), as well as others to be reported later, found a higher incidence of learning and other minor problems than of more gross developmental retardation.

A somewhat more detailed description of outcome was provided in a study by Siegel et al. (1982). Their study included eighty infants of very low birth weight (<1,501 grams) and sixty-eight full-term infants matched on various demographic variables. Survival rates were reported separately for birth weight categories above and below 1,000 grams. They differed markedly, with survival rates above 80 percent for those infants born at more than 1,001 grams and below 40 percent for those born at 1,000 grams or less. Of the eighty preterm survivors, ten had some form of severe handicap, including blindness (four), cerebral palsy (seven), and severe developmental delay (two). These infants were excluded from further analyses.

To predict development at two years, the investigators used variables related to neonatal medical complications, maternal characteristics, and socioeconomic status to predict cognitive development (Bayley Mental Developmental Index), motor development (Bayley PDI), and language development (Reynell Developmental Language Scales). Using stepwise multiple regression, they predicted the Bayley scores at two years by a combination of socioeconomic status, maternal smoking, and birth asphyxia (one-minute Apgar score of less than 5). Essentially the same variables predicted language development. Despite a more differentiated outcome measure in this study compared to many others, language, cognitive, and motor development were predicted by essentially the same variables, representing socioeconomic status, maternal health, and the condition of the infant at birth.

Largo et al. (1989) also looked at cognitive, neurological, and language development as separate outcome variables in a follow-up study that was carried out for seven years. Subjects were 346 preterm infants. Ninety-seven of the children were followed until seven years, with developmental assessments performed periodically up to that time. Two hundred and forty-nine children were tested once at five years. Predictor variables included optimality ratings on prenatal, perinatal, and postnatal medical variables, gestational age and birth weight, and a score of minor congenital anomalies recorded at the five-year examination.

The pregnancy, birth, and postnatal optimality scores were significantly correlated with Verbal and Performance IQ on the WISC-R and with psycholinguistic scores on the ITPA, but only for boys and not consistently across the two samples. Minor congenital anomalies were related to the results of the neurological examination but not to intellectual or language test results. Interestingly, birth weight and, even more so, gestational age were more highly related to the intellectual and psycholinguistic measures than were the three perinatal optimality scores.

This study provided one of the longest follow-up periods, the most complete set of predictor variables, and some of the most sophisticated outcome measures. The results, although sometimes statistically significant, were not particularly striking or consistent.

Those studies using multiple predictors of developmental outcome have provided fairly consistent results. Obstetric factors do not seem to have a powerful influence on later development in preterm children. When studies involve a wide range of birth weights and gestational ages, and particularly if the typical birth weight is not too low, socioeconomic status and the quality of the home environment are as predictive as most perinatal medical complications. With decreasing birth weight in samples in which infant mortality is high, those variables related to the infant's immediate medical status at birth (e.g., asphyxia, infections) assume increasing importance in predicting cognitive outcome. Those studies that separated intellectual from language development did not show different variables to be related to outcome in the two domains.

Studies of Particular Medical Complications

Some studies have focused on developmental outcome in children with periventricular-intraventricular hemorrhage. In an interesting study of the development of visual attention in preterm infants with and without intraventricular hemorrhage, Landry et al. (1985) examined the ability to shift attention to a new stimulus in seven-month-old infants. Attention measures such as these have been shown to be predictive of later intelligence (Fagan and McGrath 1981; Lewis and Brooks-Gunn 1981). Landry et al. compared preterm infants of less than 1,700 grams birth weight with respiratory distress syndrome and no intraventricular hemorrhage and those with both respiratory distress syndrome and intraventricular hemorrhage. Also included were full-term control infants.

When presented with a novel stimulus, the infants with both respiratory distress syndrome and intraventricular hemorrhage were slower to shift their attention to the new stimulus than were either the infants with respiratory distress syndrome but no hemorrhage or the full-term controls. There were no differences between the groups on measures of the duration of attention to a stimulus. These results were as predicted by the authors, who hypothesized that intraventricular hemorrhage, particularly with posthemorrhagic hydrocephalus, should affect "cognitive lower-level motor skills" involved with moving the focus of attention.

A variety of factors related to intraventricular hemorrhage have been studied in terms of their effect on developmental outcome. One factor is the severity of the hemorrhage. Papile et al. (1978) developed a grading system for hemorrhage severity: grade I refers to bleeding confined to one or more germinal matrices, grade II refers to germinal matrix bleeding that has ruptured into the lateral ventricles but with no ventricular swelling, grade III includes swelling of the lateral ventricles, and grade IV includes dilated ventricles with extension of the hemorrhage into the adjacent brain parenchyma. Although both grade III and grade IV hemorrhage include ventricular dilatation, continued expansion of the ventricles constitutes a progressive hydrocephalus, the presence of which has also been the subject of study in terms of its effect on developmental outcome.

There is a fair amount of evidence that the more severe grades III and IV intraventricular hemorrhages are associated with poor developmental outcome (Papile, Munsick-Bruno, and Schaefer 1983; Papile et al. 1978; Tekolste, Bennett, and Mack 1985; Williamson et al. 1982). Both the likelihood of cerebral palsy and that of mental retardation increase similarly in patients with the more severe grades (Papile, Munsick-Bruno, and Schaefer 1983; Williamson et al. 1982). In fact, in the studies reported by Papile et al. and Williamson et al., the majority of abnormal outcomes in grades III and IV intraventricular hemorrhage involved both cerebral palsy and mental retardation.

Conclusions regarding the effects of intraventricular hemorrhage on cognitive development are not so clear cut as some of the earlier research, cited earlier, would indicate. Landry et al. (1984) attempted to separate the effects of intraventricular hemorrhage from those of respiratory distress syndrome and bronchopulmonary dysplasia, both of which are often associated with intraventricular hemorrhage. In addition, they included children with posthemorrhagic hydrocephalus. Comparisons of Bayley scale scores between groups were made at six, twelve, and twenty-four months.

At six months the infants with respiratory distress syndrome with or without intraventricular hemorrhage were generally normal on the Bayley scales and performed significantly better than did infants with bronchopulmonary dysplasia or hydrocephalus. Similar results were obtained at twelve months. By twenty-four months the groups with bronchopulmonary dysplasia and hydrocephalus continued to show poorer outcomes, although the groups with respiratory distress syndrome with or without intraventricular hemorrhage also showed an increase in the percentage of cognitively impaired children. Despite this, the mean Bayley scores for the children with respiratory distress syndrome increased from six to twenty-four months, while those of the groups with bronchopulmonary dysplasia and hydrocephalus tended to remain the same and below the normal range. A crucial factor in predicting poor outcome for the group with bronchopulmonary dysplasia was a lengthy hospitalization. Interestingly, in this study there was no relationship between the severity of the hemorrhage and the cognitive outcome.

Some studies have indicated that intraventricular hemorrhage has a more adverse effect on motor than on cognitive development. Landry et al. (1984) found fairly substantial discrepancies between Bayley Mental Developmental Index and PDI scores; the Mental Developmental Index scores were higher in all of the groups except those with bronchopulmonary dysplasia. Garfinkel et al. (1988) found that grades III and IV hemorrhage was more highly associated with motor and focal neuromuscular impairment than with mental impairment in preterm infants during infancy and, to a lesser extent, in childhood. Language delays were also associated with grade III and IV hemorrhage in childhood. On the other hand, Landry, Schmidt, and Richardson (1989) found no differences in communication skills of two year olds related to the severity or presence of intraventricular hemorrhage.

More recently, there has been evidence that negative outcomes attributed to intraventricular hemorrhage may more likely be due to periventricular leucomalacia, an ischemic lesion in associated white matter areas. Sostek et al. (1987) evaluated premature infants born at birth weights of less than 1,750 grams at one and two years. Infants who exhibited intraventricular hemorrhage were classified using Papile's grades of severity. At age one year, Bayley Mental Developmental Index scores were significantly lower for those who had grade IV hemorrhage than for those who had grades I–III hemorrhage. Motor development (Bayley PDI and neurological exam) was significantly lower in those infants with either grade III or IV hemorrhage than in those with grades I or II or no hemorrhage. At two years the relationships between intraventricular hemorrhage and developmental outcome were diminished. The only significant predictor of two-year developmental status was one-year developmental status. The authors concluded that intraventricular hemorrhage has limited predictive value after one year with regard to cognitive status. They cited evidence that cognitive development may be more related to periventricular leucomalacia as one possible reason for their findings. However, their use of a multiple regression model may have obscured relationships between intraventricular hemorrhage and two-year cognitive development. By using stepwise procedures and entering one-year developmental status as a variable in the prediction equation, they eliminated only the direct effects of intraventricular hemorrhage on two-year developmental status. Any indirect effects that were expressed through earlier developmental outcomes would have been taken into account in the correlation between one- and two-year cognitive variables. A more appropriate model to have used would have been a path model that hypothesized relationships among intraventricular hemorrhage, one-year developmental status, and two-year developmental status. In effect, Sostek et al. showed that intraventricular hemorrhage does not directly affect two-year developmental status over and above its influence on earlier development, not that it does not affect two-year developmental status at all.

Sostek et al.'s suspicion that periventricular leucomalacia may be more important than intraventricular hemorrhage has been voiced by other authors. Stewart and Hope (1988) discussed the historical evolution of computed tomography and ultrasound imaging techniques that led to an emphasis on the more easily visualized intraventricular hemorrhage lesions during the early 1980s. Only quite recently has sufficient attention been paid to the often less markedly dense echodensities on ultrasound that were present in the periventricular region and that signaled the early changes of periventricular leucomalacia. At the same time, autopsy studies of severely impaired preterm infants often showed cystic lesions in the periventricular region that were the eventual outcome of the ischemic effects of periventricular leucomalacia (Wigglesworth 1984).

The data reported by Stewart and Hope (1988) summarize studies carried out by Stewart and colleagues during the mid-1980s. The overall findings, based on follow-up of 342 preterm infants studied by ultrasound scanning, were that small, uncomplicated intraventricular hemorrhages carried very little risk of increasing the likelihood of neurological or cognitive handicap, measured between one and two years. The risk increased dramatically with the presence of ventricular dilatation, hydrocephalus, or cerebral atrophy. In the latter category, those infants with evidence of cystic periventricular leucomalacia had an 80 percent likelihood of major neurodevelopmental handicap and a 100 percent likelihood of either major or minor handicap. Stewart, Thorburn, and Hope (1983) estimated that intraventricular hemorrhage accounted for approximately 19 percent of neurodevelopmental disorders diagnosed by eighteen months, whereas ischemic lesions accounted for up to 66 percent of impaired infants.

In a study that used an alternative to ultrasound or computed tomographic scanning, van Bel et al. (1989) used Doppler ultrasound to examine the relationship between the velocity of blood flow in the anterior cerebral artery and later developmental outcome. Those preterm children who showed major neurodevelopmental handicap at age two years had changes in cerebral blood flow velocity (higher pulsatility index and peak systolic velocity), which were interpreted as due to increased compliance of the vascular bed in the periventricular white matter. Although ultrasound evidence of periventricular leucomalacia was present in only a portion of the handicapped children, the authors speculated that periventricular leucomalacia was the chief cause of the increased compliance of the vascular bed of the white matter. Intraventricular hemorrhage, which was visualized with greater surety than periventricular leucomalacia, was not highly related to outcome.

In probably the most detailed examination of the effects of cystic periventricular leucomalacia, Hansen et al. (1989) studied thirty-five infants with cystic parenchymal lesions, identified by ultrasound, for developmental status at two years. Sixteen infants had bilateral cystic lesions, and all sixteen were severely handicapped in terms of Bayley Mental Development Index and PDI scores below the normal range. Of the nineteen children with unilateral lesions, eight had no handicap, seven had severe handicap, and four had motor deficits but normal cognitive outcome. Using stepwise multiple regression analysis, the investigators found that the type of cyst, head circumference at six to eight months, and neurological findings at six to eight months accounted for the majority of the variance in the Bayley mental and motor scores at two years. The correlation was somewhat higher for motor than for mental scores. Although hydrocephalus was associated with poor outcome, intraventricular hemorrhage was not.

Hansen et al. (1989) reviewed other studies that provided similar data on mental and motor outcome associated with cystic lesions. By adding cases from several studies, they determined that 88 percent of infants with bilateral lesions develop motor deficits and 65 percent have severe cognitive deficits. In contrast, 51 percent of infants with unilateral lesions have motor deficits and 23 percent have cognitive deficits. Graham, Levene, and Trounce (1987) reported that parietal-occipital lesions had a worse prognosis than frontal lesions. However, Hansen et al. found no relationship between the location of the lesion and outcome in their series. Fawer, Diebold, and Calame (1987) also reported a relationship between the site of the cystic periventricular leucomalacia and outcome. In eighty-two preterm infants they found no relationship between isolated intraventricular hemorrhage or posthemorrhagic hydrocephalus and developmental outcome on

the Griffiths scale at eighteen months. Frontal periventricular leucomalacia was also associated with normal outcome, but frontal-parietal
and frontal-parietal-occipital periventricular leucomalacia was associated with poor outcome (development quotient < 80).

The chief problem with virtually all of the studies in this area is that
follow-up has generally been only from one to three years. Although
it seems likely that the link between periventricular leucomalacia and
severe handicap (including cerebral palsy) would remain with longer
follow-up, it is not clear that the negative findings with regard to
intraventricular hemorrhage and severe handicap at young ages
imply a similar lack of a relationship between intraventricular hemorrhage and milder handicaps in childhood.

Although uncomplicated intraventricular hemorrhage does not
seem to increase the risk of neurological handicap at early ages, posthemorrhagic hydrocephalus has consistently been implicated as a
good predictor of handicap (Hansen et al. 1989; Landry et al. 1984;
Papile et al. 1978; Stewart, Thorburn, and Hope 1983). Fernell et al.
(1987) conducted a study in a total population series that included all
infants born prematurely who developed infantile hydrocephalus.
The predominant cause was posthemorrhagic hydrocephalus, which
was verified in 31 percent of the cases and suspected in another
25 percent. The most crucial variable associated with neurodevelopmental handicap was a clear-cut onset of hydrocephalus. Seventy-
eight percent of survivors with clear-cut onset were neurologically
handicapped. A more insidious onset was associated with better outcome. Fernell et al. also found an association between gestational age
and hydrocephalus in predicting outcome. All infants born at less
than twenty-eight weeks gestational age who developed hydrocephalus were severely multiply handicapped. Stellman and Bannister
(1985) found a somewhat similar result in a similar sample of prematurely born children who developed hydrocephalus secondary to
intraventricular hemorrhage. Late onset of intraventricular hemorrhage was associated with a poorer prognosis at ages nine to eighteen
months on the Griffiths exam.

Some investigators have followed children with intraventricular
hemorrhage to later ages. The available results do not clearly confirm a hypothesis of an increase in minor cognitive and learning problems among those children who escaped major disability. In fact, in a
study that followed 171 preterm children until age four and evaluated
them on a variety of cognitive and neurological tests, similar levels
of both major and minor impairment were found in children with
uncomplicated intraventricular hemorrhage and no intraventricular

hemorrhage (Costello et al. 1988). Both major and minor impairment increased substantially with evidence of ventricular dilatation, hydrocephalus, or cerebral atrophy. Most interesting, however, was that the impairments associated with abnormal ultrasound scans were largely neurological; there was no evidence that cognitive impairment could be predicted in infants who were free of neurological impairment.

An even more surprising finding was reported by Papile, Munsick-Bruno, and Lowe (1988). In a long-term follow-up of children with grades III and IV intraventricular hemorrhage, there was a decrease in the percentage of handicapped children and an increase in the percentage of children with a normal outcome between ages two and eight years old. The number of subjects who remained in the study for that length of follow-up was quite small, but the results were dramatic. Twelve children had grade III hemorrhage involving ventricular dilatation. At age two years only 16 percent were normal. Forty-two percent had major and 42 percent had minor handicaps. At eight years old 42 percent were normal. Twenty-five percent had major and 33 percent had minor handicaps.

With grade IV hemorrhage, including ventricular dilatation and extension into the parenchyma, the results were even more dramatic. At age two years 17 percent were normal, 8 percent had minor handicaps, and 75 percent had major handicaps. At age eight years 25 percent were normal, 67 percent had a minor handicap, and only 8 percent had a major handicap. The greatest improvement was in cognitive scores, rather than being fewer deficits shown by the neurological examination.

These results are both striking and puzzling. The very negative outcomes reported at earlier ages with grade III or IV intraventricular hemorrhage seem to diminish with age. It is not clear whether more subtle deficits are left over. Neither is it clear whether the lower grades of hemorrhage, which do not show an increase in handicap over no hemorrhage, even in early childhood (Papile, Munsick-Bruno, and Schaefer 1983), result in greater problems at school age when learning disabilities might be detected.

Some recent studies have shed some light on these issues, although the picture is not markedly clearer. Van de Bor et al. (1993) evaluated 304 surviving children out of an original cohort of 484 infants with very low birth weight. All of the children had been screened for intraventricular hemorrhage at birth. One hundred forty had had hemorrhage, and seventy-three of these had died by age five, when the follow-up study was conducted. Outcome evaluation on the surviving children had been previously conducted at age two. When the children were five years old, they received a comprehensive evaluation of mental development, neurological status, vision, hearing, motor skills, and speech and language.

At age five, 85 percent of the children had a disability, defined as abnormal performance on any of the developmental measures. Handicap was defined as an interference with adaptive abilities because of the disability; twenty-seven (8.9 percent) had a major handicap, and twenty-three (7.6 percent) had a minor handicap. Seventeen (5.6 percent) who were not neurodevelopmentally handicapped at age two were handicapped at age five. Thirty-five (11.5 percent) were handicapped at age two but not at age five.

Children with grades I and II hemorrhage had more disabilities (42 percent) and handicap (26 percent) than did those without hemorrhage, who had 24 percent disability and 13 percent handicap. Those with grades III and IV hemorrhage had 35 percent disability and 29 percent handicap. A remarkable finding, reminiscent of that of Papile, Munsick-Bruno, and Lowe (1988), was that, with grades III and IV hemorrhage, seven out of seventeen children had major handicap at age two but only four children had major handicap at age five. Three children went from major handicap to no handicap between ages two and five. When the data were adjusted for other confounding medical complications (e.g., birth weight, gestational age, peak bilirubin level, seizures, bronchopulmonary dysplasia, socioeconomic status), intraventricular hemorrhage significantly increased the risk of disability at age five years but the increased risk of handicap was nonsignificant. In addition, there were no differences between grades of hemorrhage in terms of increased risk.

The most detailed study of the cognitive effects of intraventricular hemorrhage in older children was conducted by Selzer, Lindgren, and Blackman (1992). They evaluated twenty five-year-old children who had had hemorrhage at birth but were free of significant health or developmental difficulties through age thirty months. These children were matched to twenty children from the same birth cohort who were equivalent on gender, birth weight, ventilatory assistance, and maternal education but who had not experienced hemorrhage. Another group of seventy children without perinatal problems or prematurity and matched with the high-risk samples on demographic variables served as a normal control. In the hemorrhage group were nine children with grades I or II hemorrhage, eight with grades III or IV hemorrhage, and three with other types of intracranial hemorrhage.

All of the children in the study were given a comprehensive neuropsychological test battery at age five years. This battery consisted of thirteen measures in areas of verbal ability, perceptual-motor ability, and preacademic ability. In addition, the Color Span Test, a measure of short-term memory for color names presented in different stimulus and response modalities (visual-visuomotor, visual-verbal, verbal-visuomotor, and verbal-verbal), was given.

On the neuropsychological measures, the normal control group outperformed the two clinical groups on the verbal and preacademic measures. Only the group with hemorrhage was significantly worse than the normal control group on the perceptual-motor measures. On the Color Span Test, the hemorrhage group was significantly worse than the normal control group and the perinatal problems group on the visual-verbal subtest and was worse than the normal control group on the verbal-visual subtest, but none of the groups differed on the subtests that used the same input and output modalities. The pattern of responses on this test indicated that the subjects with hemorrhage had a particular problem with cross-modal memory tasks, which the authors hypothesized might interfere with later development of academic skills. The authors also hypothesized that a specific deficit in intermodal processing of information in the hemorrhage group might be due to interference with white matter pathways.

Subjects with either mild or severe intraventricular hemorrhage were compared across the neuropsychological measures. Only on the perceptual-motor measures did the severe-hemorrhage group perform worse than the mild-hemorrhage group. However, the small number of subjects may have limited findings on the other measures.

This was the most detailed examination of cognitive functioning in children with intraventricular hemorrhage. Those children with significant developmental difficulties had been screened out of the study, which would limit the findings to fairly subtle ones. However, it is clear that intraventricular hemorrhage can contribute to mild deficits, particularly in perceptual-motor and intermodal integration tasks, even when no major handicap is present.

Learning Disabilities in Prematurely Born Children

The relationship between premature birth and the medical risk factors associated with it and academic learning disabilities is not clearly established. In her review of studies conducted up to the mid-1980s, Cohen (1986) cited a variety of methodological issues that have prevented the emergence of clear-cut findings. Some methodological issues, such as the lack of control groups or the confounding of social class with prematurity, make results difficult to interpret. However, the chief issues are simply that very few studies have followed prematurely born children to school age and that studies that have done so have usually used impressionistic measures of learning problems rather than standardized tests.

Although she followed children only to age five, Siegel (1983) provided particularly pertinent information regarding the likelihood of the development of learning disabilities in prematurely born children. The children in her study included forty-four preterm children and a full-term control group. In addition to recording demographic variables, maternal risk factors, and perinatal risk factors, Siegel gave infant tests at ages four, eight, twelve, eighteen, and twenty-four months; the Reynell Scales of Language Development at ages two, three, and four years; and the Stanford-Binet Intelligence Scale at age three years.

At age five years all of the children were given the Satz Kindergarten Screening Battery for reading problems (Satz and Fletcher 1982). This battery is a valid predictor of later reading disability when administered to kindergarten children. It consists of the Peabody Picture Vocabulary Test, a measure of receptive vocabulary; the Beery Developmental Test of Visuo-motor Integration, a design copying task (Beery 1967); a Finger Localization test; Alphabet Recitation; and a Recognition-Discrimination test, which requires visual-perceptual matching of designs.

Significant differences were found between the preterm and full-term children on the Beery Visuo-motor Integration, the Recognition-Discrimination test, and Alphabet Recitation, but not on the Peabody Picture Vocabulary Test or the Finger Localization test. Demographic variables (socioeconomic status and parental education), maternal risk, and perinatal risk all significantly predicted impairment on the Satz battery. Language functioning on the Peabody Picture Vocabulary Test was more highly related to socioeconomic factors, whereas perceptual-motor functioning was more highly related to perinatal risk factors. Infant tests and the early language and intelligence tests were also related to both language and perceptual-motor functioning on the Satz battery.

Although Siegel's (1983) findings do not directly identify learning problems in prematurely born children, they do show a continuity between early risk factors, early cognitive development, and five-year-old functioning in areas related to the development of later reading problems. That perinatal risks are more highly related to perceptual-motor delays is similar to findings reported elsewhere. The Satz

Battery, however, is generally used for prediction by taking a weighted composite of all of the scores (Satz and Fletcher 1982) rather than by using the results of each component separately. The relationship between prematurity and only some components of the battery may not be predictive of reading problems.

Landman et al. (1986) looked at the relationship between minor neurological signs and measures of visual-perceptual, fine motor, gross motor, cognitive, language, quantitative, and preacademic functioning in normal four and five year olds. Although their subjects were not prematurely born, their results are relevant to the question of how delays in visual-perceptual or fine motor skills are related to other cognitive abilities in children that age. They found that minor neurological signs were related to impairment in visual-perceptual, fine motor, and gross motor skills but not to other cognitive, language, quantitative, or preacademic skills. These findings raise some questions about the relevance of Siegel's (1983) results to academic learning problems.

Further evidence that visual-perceptual and visuomotor abilities may be impaired in prematurely born children without affecting other cognitive skills was provided by Klein (1988). She studied sixty-two preterm children of very low birth weight at age five years. These represented all of the available surviving neonatal intensive care unit graduates from a one-year period in one hospital who were in regular education classrooms. Normal classmates matched on race, sex, and age were enlisted as controls. All children were given a battery of intelligence, visuomotor, and psychoeducational tests as well as a behavior-rating scale, completed by the teacher. Significant differences were found on measures of visuomotor ability, spatial relationships, and quantitative concepts but not on measures of intelligence, language, or auditory skills. That quantitative concepts were impaired suggests that a likely area of academic difficulty would be in mathematics.

Studies of preschool or kindergarten children are suggestive with regard to learning disabilities but hardly conclusive. The ideal study requires that prematurely born children be followed until they are far enough along in school that the inability to learn academic material will be obvious. Vohr and Garcia Coll (1985) followed forty-two infants of very low birth weight for seven years. Children were assessed yearly for neurological status, at one year for developmental status on the Bayley Scales of Infant Development, at three to five years on the Stanford-Binet Intelligence Scale, and at seven years on the Stanford-Binet, the Beery Developmental Test of Visuo-motor Integration, the Reading subtest from the Wide Range Achievement Test, and the

Picture Completion and Block Designs subtests from the WISC-R. At the one-year neurological assessment, the children were classified as normal, suspect, or abnormal.

The children classified as normal at one year generally retained their classification at seven years, as did those classified as abnormal. The suspect group tended to shift either up or down in classification. The abnormal group improved in intellectual ability as they got older, although their ability remained lower than that of those classified as normal. Of major interest was the finding that the children classified as normal at one year had average IQ scores and average reading scores at seven years, despite impaired visuomotor skills on the Beery Test of Visuo-motor Integration. In fact, visuomotor integration was poorer than reading in all three groups at age seven. In the suspect and abnormal groups, however, reading was impaired relative to IQ, in one-half or more of the children. Thus, when no evidence of neurological damage was present, subtle deficits were confined to visuomotor skills but not reading. On the other hand, when evidence of neurological damage had been present, both visuomotor and reading problems were likely to remain, even when intelligence improved to within the normal range.

Hunt, Cooper, and Tooley (1988) found a relationship between perceptual-motor impairment and learning disabilities in prematurely born children of very low birth weight. One hundred eight children of very low birth weight, followed until age eight, were tested with intellectual, visuomotor, and academic achievement tests. Those children who had normal intelligence and no difference between Verbal IQ and Performance IQ scores on the WISC-R had a low incidence of learning disabilities (defined as a discrepancy between IQ and achievement on the Wide Range Achievement Test). The incidence of learning disabilities was also low for children with either low IQ or low Verbal IQ compared to Performance IQ. However, in those children with either low Performance IQ compared to Verbal IQ or low visuomotor scores on the Bender Gestalt test compared to their IQ, learning disabilities were found in 30–35 percent. Unfortunately, the authors did not differentiate learning problems in one academic area from those in another, so it was not possible to determine whether impaired visual-perceptual or visuomotor skills were associated with problems in reading, spelling, or arithmetic. Interestingly, when the children were classified as to outcome (no problems, mild problems, or moderate to severe problems), a combination of neonatal illness ratings and socioeconomic status was highly successful in predicting outcome. Cohen et al. (1982) found similar results in an eight-year follow-up of preterm children. Factors associated with the parents' socioeconomic status were highly predictive of intellectual, visuomotor, and reading problems. Neonatal medical complications were less predictive, but newborn neurobehavioral measures were predictive of eight-year-old test results and interacted with social factors to determine outcome.

Probably the most complete and clear-cut study of learning problems in children with very low birth weight was conducted by Klein, Hack, and Breslau (1989). Sixty-five children of very low birth weight were followed to age nine years and matched with sixty-five full-term controls who were their classmates. An extensive battery of cognitive, visuomotor, and academic achievement tests was administered to all of the children. Results were analyzed both for the whole sample and for just those forty-three subjects who had normal intelligence. Within the total sample, significant differences between the children with very low birth weight and the controls were found on nearly all of the measures except those that reflected purely auditory and language skills. Children with very low birth weight performed more poorly than did controls in reading and arithmetic.

When only those children with normal IQ were examined, the differences between the children with very low birth weight and controls were much less. Differences in IQ remained, as did those on visuomotor and fine-motor tasks. However, cognitive differences were confined to visual and quantitative tasks and, in the academic area, were confined to arithmetic. Because there were IQ differences between the children with very low birth weight and controls, even in the subgroup with normal IQ, regression techniques were used to partial out the effects of IQ on math achievement. The results of this analysis showed that children with very low birth weight were deficient in mathematical ability, relative to controls, even when the effects of IQ were removed.

The study by Klein, Hack, and Breslau (1989) is of major importance because the children with very low birth weight were compared to matched full-birth-weight control children, because the outcome measures included a wide battery of well-standardized tests, and because IQ differences were controlled. Their finding of deficits in visual-perceptual, visuomotor, and motor skills is similar to those of nearly all previous studies. The finding that academic learning problems were confined to arithmetic in the normal IQ group is most interesting. Previous studies focused primarily on reading problems, and the results were inconsistent. When reading problems were found, they most often were in subjects with lower IQ or obvious neurological problems. On the other hand, visuomotor or visual-perceptual deficits were found routinely in children with otherwise normal outcome. Arithmetic problems were associated with visual-perceptual impairment in some studies of learning-disabled children (Rourke and Finlayson 1978; Rourke and Strang 1978; Share, Moffitt, and Silva 1988; White, Moffitt, and Silva 1992).

Rourke (1989) in particular stressed this association and speculated that it might be related to the destruction of white matter, particularly in the right hemisphere. Although not invoked as a primary explanation by Rourke, the evidence presented earlier regarding the type of damage to which the premature brain is most susceptible (i.e., intra-ventricular hemorrhage and/or periventricular leucomalacia) implicates white matter areas more often than gray matter (Wigglesworth and Pape 1978). As Rourke pointed out, there is evidence that the ratio of white matter to gray matter is greater in the right hemisphere than in the left (Goldberg and Costa 1981), so a destructive neurological process that affected white matter more than gray matter might resemble right- more than left-hemisphere dysfunction. This is an attractive theoretical explanation for the preponderance of visual-perceptual and arithmetic problems over language problems after early brain injury.

6

A Follow-up Study of Prematurely Born Children: *Intellectual, Visuomotor, and Academic Abilities*

We recently completed a seven-year follow-up study of children born prematurely (Katzir 1992). Our overall aim was to determine whether such indications of early brain injury as degree of prematurity, respiratory distress, and asphyxia would predict intellectual, visuomotor, and academic abilities at school age. We were also interested in determining whether, if such influences were present, they would show their effect primarily by influencing early cognitive development or they would continue to directly affect abilities at school age.

Subjects

Subjects included all of the children admitted to the neonatal intensive care unit (NICU) at San Diego Children's Hospital between 1980 and 1989 with a birth weight of less than 2,500 grams. All survivors who were discharged from the NICU were followed for evaluation at six months, one year, two years, three and one-half years, and five years. The subject pool for the assessment of mathematical abilities included only those children who had undergone a complete set of developmental evaluations through age five years. Of these children,

We are indebted to Kristen Gist, Director of the Newborn Follow-up Clinic at Children's Hospital and Health Center in San Diego, California, for access to the children in this study and to their early medical and developmental data, as well as for her invaluable assistance in planning the study.

all of those who had an episode of intraventricular hemorrhage were selected as candidates for the study. Seventy-three children met these criteria. Of these, thirty-one were located and tested as part of the study, twenty-four had either moved from the area or could not be located. Eight children were excluded from the study because of mild to severe mental retardation and/or severe physical disability. One child was excluded because of deafness and another because he didn't speak English. Eight children's parents declined to participate for various reasons. An additional seventeen children who did not have intraventricular hemorrhage but who otherwise met the same criteria regarding birth weight and the availability of follow-up data were randomly selected from the pool of children who fell into this category.

Procedures

All subjects were tested at the Developmental Evaluation Clinic at Children's Hospital of San Diego. The WISC-R, WRAT-R, and Test of Early Mathematics Ability (TEMA) (Ginsburg and Baroody 1983) were part of a larger battery of cognitive tests administered by either of two doctoral candidates in clinical psychology. The entire battery of tests took approximately four hours to administer and was divided into two sessions. The WISC-R was administered during the first session; the WRAT-R and TEMA were administered one week later. Each child's parents were seen in a follow-up session in which the results of the tests were explained to them.

Medical Variables

The staff of the Developmental Evaluation Unit recorded medical variables in the patients' charts at the time of the infant's discharge from the NICU. Where they had initially been recorded as continuous variables, medical variables were converted to dichotomous variables before being entered into the factor analysis.

The following medical and demographic variables were recorded for each subject while he or she was in the NICU.

Socioeconomic Status.   The Hollingshead and Redlich (1958) single-factor scale, which yielded a seven-point scale based on the occupation of the chief breadwinner of the family, was recorded for each child. For the purposes of the factor analysis, the scores were divided at the median into low and high socioeconomic status.

Apgar Score at One Minute.   Apgar scores include ratings of 0 to 2 on five characteristics of the newborn: heart rate, respiratory effort, muscle tone, response to stimuli, and color. Scores were recorded in the medical chart using the 10-point Apgar rating scale (Apgar 1953). For the purposes of the factor analysis, the scores were converted into low (4 or less) and high (5 or more).

Apgar Score at Five Minutes.   Scores were recorded and converted using the same procedure as for the one-minute Apgar score.

Gestational Age.   Gestational age was determined using the Dubowitz examination (Dubowitz, Dubowitz, and Goldberg 1971) and was recorded in the medical chart. The Dubowitz examination estimates the gestational age of the infant based on twenty-one clinical signs and is correct within two weeks 95 percent of the time. For the purposes of the factor analysis, the gestational ages were divided into less than thirty-one weeks and thirty-one weeks or more.

Birth Weight.   Birth weight was recorded, in grams, in the medical chart at the time of birth. For the purposes of the factor analysis, the birth weights were divided into less than 1,504 grams and 1,504 grams or more.

Multiple Births.   The birth of more than one infant from the same pregnancy was recorded as either yes or no, regardless of whether of twins, triplets, and so forth or of whether the other children survived.

Being Small for Gestational Age.   Being small for gestational age was determined by the tables provided by Battaglia and Lubchenko (1967). Data were recorded as yes or no.

Asphyxia.   Asphyxia was determined by an Apgar score of less than 5 at one minute or less than 7 at five minutes or by clinical judgment on the basis of need for resuscitation in the delivery room. Asphyxia was recorded as yes or no.

Infection.   Infection was recorded if there was sepsis of any kind based on a positive culture at any time during the stay in the NICU. Infection was recorded as yes or no.

Respiratory Distress Syndrome.   Respiratory distress syndrome was recorded as severe (mechanical ventilation or continuous positive airway pressure), mild-moderate (oxygen by hood only), or none. For the purposes of the factor analysis, the data were converted to presence or absence.

Intraventricular Hemorrhage.   Intraventricular hemorrhage (IVH) was determined by ultrasound of the head performed daily for the first week. IVH was recorded according to the grading system of Papile et al. (1978) as: I, germinal matrix hemorrhage; II, extension into the ventricles but without ventricular dilatation; III, ventricular dilatation; or IV, bleeding into the brain parenchyma. The determination was made by the neonatologist or radiologist. For the purpose of the factor analysis, the presence of each of the grades of IVH was recorded as yes or no.

Hydrocephalus.   Hydrocephalus, an increased accumulation of cerebrospinal fluid within the ventricles, was recorded on the basis of ultrasound as either present or absent.

Apnea of Prematurity.   Apnea, a temporary cessation of breathing, was recorded on the basis of a diagnosis of more apnea or bradycardia, a slowing of heart rate, than normal. Apnea was recorded as yes or no.

Patent Ductus Arteriosus.   Patent ductus arteriosus, the abnormal persistence of communication between the main pulmonary artery and the aorta after birth was detected symptomatically and verified by ultrasound. It was recorded in terms of the treatment as spontaneous resolution, surgical ligation, or medication. If more than one treatment was utilized, it was recorded in terms of the more severe treatment.

Chronic Lung Disease.   Chronic lung disease was recorded as present or absent if the infant required oxygen for more than twenty-eight days.

Seizures.   Seizures were recorded if seizure activity, supported by electroencephalogram findings, was present before discharge from the NICU.

Meconium Aspiration.   The signs of the newborn's having aspirated the fetal feces, such as meconium staining of the amniotic fluid or the neonate itself, were recorded as a diagnosis made by the delivering physician at delivery.

Necrotizing Enterocolitis.   Necrotizing enterocolitis, involving ischemia of the intestinal tract and bacterial infection of the intestinal mucosa, was recorded as a diagnosis in the NICU.

Cerebral Palsy.   Cerebral palsy was recorded as a diagnosis made by the neurologist before age two and was recorded as present or absent whether or not symptoms seemed to resolve at a later age.

Hyperbilirubinemia.   Hyperbilirubinemia is an excess of bilirubin, the orange or yellowish pigment in bile, in the blood. A bilirubin count of 10 to 12 or more (for the infant with very low birth weight) was recorded as the presence of hyperbilirubinemia.

Length of Stay.   The length of stay was recorded as the number of days in tertiary care.

Retinopathy of Prematurity.   Retinopathy of prematurity was recorded simply as present or absent based on neonatal diagnosis.

Persistent Fetal Circulation.   Persistent fetal circulation (persistent pulmonary hypertension of the newborn) was recorded on the basis of a medical diagnosis placed in the medical chart during the stay in the NICU.

Because many of the medical variables were correlated with one another and because of their large number, a principal components factor analysis was conducted to reduce the medical variables to a smaller number of independent factors. Factor scores from this data-reduction procedure, rather than the scores on the individual medical variables, were used as independent variables in all further analyses.

Developmental Assessments

All subjects were given the Bayley Scales of Infant Development at six months, one year, and two years of age. Infants were brought to the Developmental Evaluation Clinic by their mothers, and testing was conducted by the developmental psychologists employed by the clinic. Mental and Psychomotor Developmental indices were computed using the age in months, corrected for prematurity.

At age three and one-half and five years, each subject was tested individually with the Stanford-Binet, Form L-M. The examiner was usually the same person who had previously administered the Bayley scales to that child. IQ scores were computed using the normative tables for the child's chronological age.

Subjects were also tested at age five years with the Beery Developmental Test of Visual-Motor Integration by the same staff of the Developmental Evaluation Clinic.

Mathematical Ability

Standard scores on the TEMA and the WRAT-R were used as the measures of mathematical achievement. Because these tests measure different aspects of mathematical skill, separate analyses were conducted using each as a dependent variable.

Mathematical disability was defined in two ways: (1) mathematical disability versus no mathematical disability, and (2) mathematical disability versus generalized learning disability versus no learning disability. Children whose standard score on the WRAT-R Arithmetic test was one standard deviation (15 points) or more below their seven-year-old WISC-R Full-Scale IQ were classified as mathematically disabled, regardless of their scores on other WRAT-R subtests. Children whose standard score on the WRAT-R Arithmetic subtest was one standard deviation or more below their WISC-R Full-Scale IQ but whose reading scores were not, were defined as having a specific mathematical disability. Children whose standard scores on the WRAT-R Arithmetic test were one standard deviation below their WISC-R Full-Scale IQ and whose WRAT-R Reading test scores were also one standard deviation below their Full-Scale IQ were defined as having a generalized learning disability. Children whose WRAT-R Arithmetic test score was within one standard deviation of their WISC-R Full-Scale IQ were defined as not mathematically disabled.

Data Analysis

The initial set of medical variables was too large, given the small sample size, and there was a high likelihood of multicollinearity among the variables. Both of these considerations mandated some form of data reduction to a smaller set of orthogonal predictor variables. The availability of a much larger data set ($n = 951$), consisting of all of the low-birth-weight infants who survived for any length of time in the NICU at San Diego Children's Hospital and Health Center covering a period of ten years (1980–89), allowed us to conduct an exploratory factor analysis to determine a smaller set of latent variables (factors) that could be used as independent variables. These factors yielded a set of factor scores for each subject, representing the extent to which each latent variable, or factor, represented by a set of variables was present for that subject.

Using data from all surviving subjects who had been available for assessment at each successive age level up to five years, we performed a series of multiple regression analyses to determine the predictive value of each previously assessed variable on each variable assessed later in time. Thus, demographic variables were first used to predict the medical factors. Then the demographic and medical factors were used to predict the six-month developmental assessments. Next, the demographic variables, medical factors, and six-month developmental assessments were used to predict the twelve-month assessments, and so on. The resulting regression coefficients from each analysis were then used to construct a path diagram of the relationships between earlier variables and later variables up to the five-year visuomotor and intellectual assessments.

To predict mathematical achievement and mathematical disability, we performed a series of stepwise multiple regression analyses using data from the forty-eight subjects who were followed until school age. Predictor variables were blocked into groups based on the age of the assessment and entered separately by blocks. The variable with the highest correlation within each block was entered first, the one with the next largest partial correlation was entered next, and so on. Any variable that was retained at one age level was then entered as the first variable, along with the variables from the block from the next younger age level. With regard to the prediction of subtype of mathematical disability, the procedure used was stepwise discriminant function analysis but was otherwise the same in terms of order of entry of the variables. The regression coefficients from the analyses were then placed in the path diagram along with those from the larger samples at younger ages.

Results

Description of the Sample

Original Birth Sample ($n = 951$)
A total of 951 infants met the criteria of weighing less than 2,500 grams at birth and having available information regarding their med-

ical complications at birth. Attrition through mortality, severe handicap, geographic relocation, and other factors, as well as a decreasing number of subjects who had reached each successive age level, resulted in smaller numbers at each time of assessment after birth. Descriptive data regarding demographics and medical variables (except sensory loss and cerebral palsy, which were diagnosed any time within the first two years) were recorded while the infants were in the NICU and include all 951 infants.

As indicated in table 6.1, the original sample of 951 infants was primarily caucasian and middle class and nearly 55 percent male. The mean gestational age was thirty-one weeks, and the mean birth weight of 1,504 grams indicates that about one-half of the sample fell into the category of very low birth weight (the median birth weight was 1,474 grams). The most prevalent medical complications were respiratory distress syndrome, apnea, asphyxia, patent ductus arteriosus, chronic lung disease, and hyperbilirubinemia. Less than 8 percent of the sample were small for gestational age.

Respiratory distress syndrome occurred in over 60 percent of the infants, apnea in nearly 50 percent, and asphyxia in over one third. All of these complications are associated with IVH, and IVH of one grade or another occurred in 26.5 percent of the sample. Over one-half of the infants with IVH had grade I, while the other cases were nearly evenly distributed among grades II, III, and IV. Hydrocephalus occurred in 6.3 percent of the infants.

The primary symptoms of brain injury, seizures and cerebral palsy, occurred in 7.5 percent and 11 percent of the infants, respectively. Between 3 and 6 percent of the infants had hearing or vision loss. Of the sample 18.7 percent were products of a multiple birth.

This sample may be compared to that reported by Dunn (1986), for which extensive data are available. Although the children in Dunn's study tended to be heavier than those in this study, the range of birth weights was similar. Of the data reported, very similar percentages were reported for multiple births (20 percent), cerebral palsy (8.1 percent), seizures (4.2 percent), visual defects (4.8 percent), and hearing loss (3.6 percent). The main difference between Dunn's data and those from the present sample was the much smaller percentage of infants small for their gestational age in this sample (7.8 percent) compared to that of Dunn (24 percent). Since Dunn reported no infants small for gestational age below thirty weeks gestational age, which is near the median of the present sample, this may account for the difference.

Table 6.1   Descriptive Statistics: Birth Sample ($n = 951$)

Variable	Range	Value	Percentage	Mean	SD
Gender	0–1	1 = male	54.7		
		0 = female	45.3		
Socioeconomic status	0–7	1 = high 7 = low		4.482	1.952
Race	0–1	1 = white	64.6		
		0 = nonwhite			
Age of mother (yr)	14–42			27.165	5.519
Gestational age (wk)	22–42			31.269	3.830
Birth weight (g)	482–2,495			1,504.46	530.226
Apgar 1 min	0–10			4.838	2.714
5 min	0–10			6.706	2.575
Length of hospital stay	1–611			33.620	58.356
Multiple birth	0–1	1 = yes	18.7		
		0 = no	81.3		
Small for gestational age	0–1	1 = yes	7.8		
		0 = no	92.2		
Asphyxia	0–1	1 = yes	37.3		
		0 = no	62.7		
Infection	0–1	1 = yes	16.2		
		0 = no	83.8		
Respiratory distress syndrome	0–1	1 = yes	61.5		
		0 = no	38.5		
Hydrocephalus	0–1	1 = yes	6.3		
		0 = no	93.7		
Apnea	0–1	1 = yes	48.8		
		0 = no	51.2		
Patent ductus arteriosus	0–1	1 = yes	32.0		
		0 = no	68.0		
Chronic lung disease	0–1	1 = yes	22.0		
		0 = no	78.0		
Seizures	0–1	1 = yes	7.5		
		0 = no	92.5		
Meconium aspiration	0–1	1 = yes	1.7		
		0 = no	98.3		
Necrotizing enterocolitis	0–1	1 = yes	5.0		
		0 = no	95.5		

Table 6.1   (continued)

Variable	Range	Value	Percentage	Mean	SD
IVH					
I	0–1	1 = yes	13.8		
		0 = no	86.2		
II	0–1	1 = yes	4.1		
		0 = no	95.9		
III	0–1	1 = yes	5.2		
		0 = no	94.8		
IV	0–1	1 = yes	3.4		
		0 = no	96.6		
Persistent fetal	0–1	1 = yes	5.2		
circulation		0 = no	94.8		
Retinopathy of	0–1	1 = yes	4.5		
prematurity		0 = no	95.5		
Hyperbilirubinemia	0–1	1 = yes	20.3		
		0 = no	79.7		
Cerebral palsy	0–1	1 = yes	11.3		
		0 = no	88.7		
Visual handicap	0–1	1 = yes	5.4		
		0 = no	94.6		
Hearing loss	0–1	1 = yes	3.4		
		0 = no	96.6		

Note: IVH, intraventricular hemorrhage.

In general, the original sample of 951 infants seemed to be representative of prematurely born infants in terms of medical complications, particularly if their low mean birth weight is taken into account.

School-age Sample

Table 6.2 gives the percentage, means, and standard deviations for the forty-eight children followed until school age. The group was primarily caucasian, male, and middle class; 37.5 percent were twins. The mean birth weight and gestational age were within the range of infants with very low birth weight. Over one-half of the sample had respiratory distress syndrome. Over 40 percent had apnea or asphyxia. Approximately one-third had patent ductus arteriosus, chronic lung disease, or IVH-I. IVH-II, IVH-III, and IVH-IV were present in 14.6 percent, 12.5 percent, and 4.2 percent of the sample, respectively. Hydrocephalus was present in 12.5 percent of the sample. In terms of symptoms of brain injury, over 20 percent of the sample had cerebral palsy and 2.1 percent had seizures.

Table 6.2   Descriptive Statistics: School-age Sample ($n = 48$)

Variable	Range	Value	Percentage	Mean	SD
Gender	0–1	1 = male	62.5		
		0 = female	37.5		
Socioeconomic status	0–7	1 = high		3.534	0.233
		7 = low			
Race	0–1	1 = white	87.5		
		0 = nonwhite	12.5		
Age of mother (yr)	22–37			27.730	4.059
Gestational age (wk)	24–35			29.652	2.713
Birth weight (g)	660–2,220			1,268.965	409.811
Apgar					
1 min	1–10			4.983	2.436
5 min	1–10			7.300	2.071
Length of hospital stay (d)	4–144			38.432	30.200
Multiple birth	0–1	1 = yes	37.5		
		0 = no	62.5		
Small for gestational age	0–1	1 = yes	6.3		
		0 = no	93.8		
Asphyxia	0–1	1 = yes	41.7		
		0 = no	58.3		
Infection	0–1	1 = yes	8.3		
		0 = no	91.7		
Respiratory distress syndrome	0–1	1 = yes	56.3		
		0 = no	43.8		
Hydrocephalus	0–1	1 = yes	12.5		
		0 = no	87.5		
Apnea	0–1	1 = yes	58.3		
		0 = no	41.7		
Patent ductus arteriosus	0–1	1 = yes	29.2		
		0 = no	70.8		
Chronic lung disease	0–1	1 = yes	31.3		
		0 = no	68.8		
Seizures	0–1	1 = yes	2.1		
		0 = no	97.9		
Meconium aspiration	0–1	1 = yes	0.0		
		0 = no	100.0		
Necrotizing enterocolitis	0–1	1 = yes	6.3		
		0 = no	93.8		

Table 6.2   (continued)

Variable	Range	Value	Percentage	Mean	SD
IVH					
I	0–1	1 = yes	33.3		
		0 = no	67.7		
II	0–1	1 = yes	14.6		
		0 = no	85.4		
III	0–1	1 = yes	12.5		
		0 = no	87.5		
IV	0–1	1 = yes	4.2		
		0 = no	95.8		
Persistent fetal	0–1	1 = yes	2.1		
circulation		0 = no	97.9		
Retinopathy of	0–1	1 = yes	8.3		
prematurity		0 = no	91.7		
Hyperbilirubinemia	0–1	1 = yes	8.3		
		0 = no	91.7		
Cerebral palsy	0–1	1 = yes	20.8		
		0 = no	79.2		
Age at assessment				7.3 yr	1.05

Note: IVH, intraventricular hemorrhage.

Differences between the Birth Sample and the School-age Sample

A comparison of tables 6.1 and 6.2 shows that the sample selection procedures for the school-age sample resulted in subjects with a higher proportion of medical complications than in the original sample. The mean socioeconomic status of the school-age sample was higher than that in the original sample and the proportion of noncaucasian infants was lower. There was a slightly higher percentage of boys in the school-age sample.

In the school-age sample both the mean birth weight and the length of pregnancy were lower than in the original sample. There were twice the percentage of twins. The length of hospital stay averaged five days more in the school-age group. Infections, hydrocephalus, persistent fetal circulation, and hyperbilirubinemia occurred twice as often in the school-age sample. Apnea and chronic lung disease occurred more often. Asphyxia, respiratory distress syndrome, and being small for gestational age were similar for the two groups.

Because the selection procedures emphasized IVH, the school-age group had three times the proportion of IVH-I, II, and III. The prevalence of IVH-IV was similar between the groups. The symptoms of brain injury (seizures and cerebral palsy) occurred at three and two times the rates, respectively, in the school-age sample.

The school-age sample was clearly a more impaired subgroup of the original birth sample in terms of both early medical complications and later symptoms of neurological damage, despite the fact that these children had higher socioeconomic status. There is little doubt that this represents the selection criteria, which emphasized the presence of IVH and regular participation in follow-up assessments, as well as willingness to come in for the lengthy school-age assessment. It may also reflect a greater likelihood for the parents of children with problems to be motivated to have their child assessed at school age. The two deliberate selection biases that were operating were the effort to obtain subjects with IVH and an effort to obtain twins. The latter bias was simply the result of the greater ease of obtaining two subjects at one time. However, since both biases were present, this could increase the correlation between these two variables in the school-age sample.

An assumption of the study is that the relationships between early medical complications and later cognitive development and academic skills are the same, regardless of the sample size and regardless of the overrepresentation or underrepresentation of any particular problems, since all of the relationships were determined within the samples and, at each successive year of assessment, including school age, the sample was composed of only members of the original birth sample. This is a longitudinal study with a decreasing number in the cohort at each successive year, rather than a cross-sectional study of different samples at different years.

Selection biases prohibit conclusions regarding the *likelihood* of having any particular problem at school age as a result of being a member of the original birth sample. For instance, if medical complications increase the likelihood of developing mathematical learning problems, then such learning problems should be overrepresented in the school-age sample. Because of this, comparisons to a control group to determine the effects of prematurity on school-age learning difficulties would be meaningless.

Reduction of the Number of Medical Complications by the Use of Factor Analysis

Data were recorded on twenty-five medical variables, which included cerebral palsy as the only variable recorded after the child left the NICU and excluded hearing loss and visual handicap (but not retinopathy of prematurity) because they were recorded at later ages. Three considerations dictated that these twenty-five variables be reduced before being used in the multiple regression analyses: (1) There was a likelihood of high correlations among several subsets of the variables (e.g., birth weight and gestational age; Apgar at one minute and Apgar at five minutes), which would have introduced excessive multicollinearity among the predictor variables. (2) As the sample size decreased with each successive year of the study, the ratio of predictor variables to the number of subjects increased. Since medical variables, demographic variables, and all prior developmental assessments were used as predictor variables in each multiple regression analysis, the increasingly high variable/subject ratio would be expected to increase the likelihood of making type I errors. (3) Factor scores, representing each subject's score on a latent variable, which was estimated by the presence of positive scores on several correlated medical variables, would be expected to be more reliable indicators of the presence of the latent variable than would be single scores on the original variables.

Scores from all 951 infants, each of whom met the criteria of complete data on all medical complication variables and had a birth weight of less than 2,500 grams, were included in the factor analysis. Before conducting the factor analysis, all variables were converted to dichotomous variables. These conversions included conversions of respiratory distress syndrome and patent ductus arteriosus to presence or absence, as recorded in table 6.3. The length of hospital stay was converted to above or below the median, and Apgar scores were converted to above or below 5. Gender, socioeconomic status, race, and age of the mother were considered demographic variables and not included in the analysis.

A principal components analysis of the medical variables yielded ten factors with eigen values greater than 1.0 and accounted for 65 percent of the variability within the data set. Factors were then rotated using a varimax procedure to achieve maximum separation between the factors, with the resulting factor structure as shown in table 6.4. Factors are listed in order of the size of their eigen values and named according to the authors' impression of the underlying variable expressed by the factor. The factor analysis was exploratory, and no conditions regarding the factor structure or number of factors were imposed before the procedure.

Factor 1.   Factor 1 seems to represent the degree of prematurity. The highest loadings are from the birth weight and gestational age. Apnea is known to show an increase in incidence and severity with decreasing gestational age (Fanaroff and Martin 1983). Higher scores on this

Table 6.3 Factor Structure of Medical Complications (*n* = 951)

Medical Variable	Factor									
	1	2	3	4	5	6	7	8	9	10
1. Prematurity										
Birth weight	.816									
Gestational age	.809									
Apnea	−.688									
2. Brain Injury										
IVH-IV		.841								
Cerebral palsy		.673								
Hydrocephalus		.643								
Seizures		.524								
3. Asphyxia										
Apgar 1 min (low)			.900							
Asphyxia			.896							
Apgar 5 min (low)			.524							
4. Persisting Neonatal Illness										
Patent ductus arteriosus				.657						
Chronic lung disease				.638						
Length of hospital stay				.520						
Persistent fetal circulation				.453						
5. Absence of Severe IVH										
IVH-I					.954					
No IVH					−.799					
6. IVH-III										
IVH-III						.916				

	1	2	3	4	5	6	7	8	9	10
7. Small for Gestational Age										
Small for gestational age							.734			
Respiratory distress syndrome							-.616			
Meconium aspiration							.502			
8. Toxicity/Infection										
Hyperbilirubinemia								.697		
Infections								.688		
Necrotizing enterocolitis								.450		
9. IVH-II										
IVH-II									.907	
10. Multiple Birth										
Multiple birth										.875
Percentage of variance	14.7	8.3	7.3	6.1	5.7	5.5	4.6	4.6	4.3	4.2

Note: IVH, intraventricular hemorrhage.

Table 6.4   Factor Scores for the Birth and School-age Samples

Factor	Birth Sample		School-aged Sample	
	Mean	SD	Mean	SD
1. Degree of prematurity	.335	.249	.514	.412
2. Brain injury	.071	.175	.099	.191
3. Asphyxia	.227	.339	.341	.372
4. Persisting neonatal illness	.299	.264	.276	.165
5. Absence of severe IVH	.437	.166	.344	.234
6. IVH-III	.052	.221	.125	.334
7. Small for gestational age	.237	.172	.208	.190
8. Toxicity	.138	.218	.076	.157
9. IVH-II	.041	.198	.146	.357
10. Multiple birth	.187	.390	.375	.489

Note: IVH, intraventricular hemorrhage.

factor would represent less prematurity. It is of considerable interest that the degree of prematurity is represented by a factor by itself, since virtually all of the medical complications are known to increase in incidence with greater prematurity. Apparently, the generally low birth weight of the entire sample allowed other medical complications to show variability independent of birth weight and gestational age.

Factor 2.   Factor 2 seems to represent the presence of brain injury. IVH-IV and hydrocephalus are both mechanisms by which brain injury can occur, and cerebral palsy and seizures are symptoms of such injury. It is somewhat curious that only IVH-IV loads on this factor, when many studies have treated IVH-III or IVH-IV as similar forms of hemorrhage in terms of their effect (e.g., Garfinkel et al. 1988).

Factor 3.   Since asphyxia was diagnosed using the Apgar scores, it is not surprising that it is found on the same factor as the one- and five-minute Apgar scores. One- and five-minute Apgar scores also represented a separate factor in the study by Pederson et al. (1988). In their study it was a better predictor of early development than of later development. However, Bennett, Robinson, and Sells (1983) found one- and five-minute Apgar scores to be the best predictors of three-year developmental status in infants with extremely low birth weight.

Factor 4.   Factor 4 is somewhat difficult to characterize. Patent ductus arteriosus and persistent fetal circulation both represent immaturity of the neonatal circulatory system. Chronic lung disease and length of hospital stay represent the failure of the newborn to gain its healthy status quickly after birth. The factor seems to represent persisting neonatal poor health and is related to immaturity of the circulatory system. For purposes of simplicity, it was named persisting neonatal illness.

Factor 5.   Factor 5 represents either no IVH or IVH-I. No IVH loads negatively because of the method of scoring, since it represented a score of 0 rather than 1 on any of the IVH variables. In terms of correlations with other variables, the presence of this factor indicates that IVH-I is similar to having no IVH at all.

Factor 6.   IVH-III defined a separate factor by itself. However, hydrocephalus loaded .570 on this factor, although it was assigned to factor 2, where it had a higher factor loading (.643). Since both IVH-III and IVH-IV involve ventricular dilatation, it would be expected that hydrocephalus would be associated with each.

Factor 7.   Factor 7 includes being small for gestational age and having respiratory distress syndrome as well as meconium aspiration. The negative loading of respiratory distress syndrome is somewhat difficult to explain, yet it is substantial. Respiratory distress syndrome occurred in the majority of the sample (62 percent), whereas being small for gestational age occurred very seldom (7.8 percent). There are a number of reasons for assuming that being small for gestational age might be associated with longer gestational ages, and, in fact, the correlation of factor 7 with gestational age is .214. That factor 7 might measure an aspect of maturity of the newborn could explain the negative loading of respiratory distress syndrome, which is known to increase with decreasing gestational age (Mannino and Merritt 1986).

Factor 8.   Factor 8 includes the mixed effects of bilirubin toxicity and infections.

Factor 9.   Factor 9 was defined by the presence of IVH-II.

Factor 10.   Multiple birth defined a separate factor. The vast majority of multiple births were twins, which, it should be remembered, were overrepresented in the school-age sample.

Correlations between Factors

Table 6.5 presents the correlations between the factors for the original birth sample. Substantial correlations existed between several factors. Factor 5, representing no IVH or IVH-I, was negatively correlated with each of the more severe IVH factors and positively correlated with factor 4 (persisting neonatal illness). Factor 4 was also positively correlated with factor 2 (brain injury). Several other correlations were significant but quite small.

The correlations between the factors in the school-age sample are presented in table 6.6. Each of the substantial correlations found in the birth sample, except that between factors 4 and 5, was at least significant in the school-age sample. In addition, factor 10 (multiple birth) was significantly correlated with factors 1 (degree of prematurity), 4 (persisting neonatal illness), and 9 (IVH-II). Only the correlation with factor 4 was positive. Factors 3 (asphyxia) and 9 (IVH-II) were also significantly correlated in a positive direction.

The primary purpose of assessing the correlations between factors was to determine if multicollinearity between predictor variables would be a problem in the multiple regression analyses. Although there is no clear-cut way to determine this in advance, it seemed that, should it be a problem, it would occur with factor 5 (absence of severe IVH) because of its high correlations with the factors representing the presence of IVH-II, III, or IV.

Prediction of Cognitive and Intellectual Development Up to Five Years of Age

Consistency of Developmental and Intellectual Assessments

Table 6.7 presents the intercorrelations between the developmental assessments on the Bayley scales and the intellectual assessments on the Stanford-Binet from six months to five years of age. Only one correlation coefficient is below .5. In fact, the correlation between the six-month Bayley MDI and the five-year Stanford-Binet is .505, which is considerably higher than the .21 reported for normal children by Bee (1989). The lowest correlation (.466) is between the six-month Bayley PDI and the five-year Stanford-Binet. This reflects a uniform tendency for Bayley mental scores at all ages to be more highly correlated with Stanford-Binet IQ than are Bayley motor scale scores.

The correlations from one successive test to the next are remarkably high. Interestingly, the correlations from one mental scale to another and from one motor scale to another at successive age levels

Table 6.5 Correlations between Factors: Birth Sample ($n = 951$)

Factor	1	2	3	4	5	6	7	8	9	10
					Factor					
1	1.00									
2	-.074	1.00								
3	-.088[a]	.168[c]	1.00							
4	-.176[c]	.313[c]	.152[c]	1.00						
5	.142[b]	-.581[c]	-.171[c]	.286[c]	1.00					
6	-.099[a]	.217[c]	.079	.170[c]	-.619[c]	1.00				
7	-.039	.093[a]	-.015	.192[c]	-.071	.041	1.00			
8	.008	.110[a]	.078	.177[c]	-.073	.000	-.003	1.00		
9	-.074	.081	.077	.106[b]	-.525[c]	-.058	.051	.046	1.00	
10	-.023	.073	-.086	-.057	.035	-.018	-.020	-.063	.001	1.00

[a] $p < .05$.
[b] $p < .01$.
[c] $p < .001$.

Table 6.6 Correlations between Factors: School-age Sample ($n = 48$)

Factor	1	2	3	4	5	6	7	8	9	10
					Factor					
1	1.00									
2	-.022	1.00								
3	.079	-.010	1.00							
4	-.121	-.342[a]	.065	1.00						
5	.011	-.388[b]	-.191	.126	1.00					
6	-.119	.140	-.090	-.16	-.496[c]	1.00				
7	-.096	-.003	.056	.121	.125	-.149	1.00			
8	.031	-.077	-.191	-.189	.045	.248	-.205	1.00		
9	.083	.047	.259[a]	-.027	-.658[c]	-.102	.125	-.183	1.00	
10	-.297[a]	-.136	-.051	.318[a]	.093	.163	.193	.122	-.288[a]	1.00

[a] $p < .05$.
[b] $p < .01$.
[c] $p < .001$.

Table 6.7 Correlations between Developmental and Intellectual Assessments

	6-mo MDI (637)	6-mo PDI (636)	12-mo MDI (460)	12-mo PDI (455)	24-mo MDI (317)	24-mo PDI (307)	3.5-yr IQ (198)	5-yr IQ (122)
6-mo MDI	1.00							
6-mo PDI	.841	1.00						
12-mo MDI	.807	.737	1.00					
12-mo PDI	.714	.755	.767	1.00				
24-mo MDI	.631	.599	.767	.629	1.00			
24-mo PDI	.661	.683	.747	.811	.636	1.00		
3.5-yr IQ	.597	.552	.740	.590	.862	.601	1.00	
5-yr IQ	.505	.466	.614	.532	.784	.523	.798	1.00

Note: All correlations are significant at $< .0005$. Numbers in parentheses, number in group. MDI, Mental Development Index; PDI, Psychomotor Development Index.

Table 6.8   Mean Scores on Developmental and Intellectual Assessments

Assessment	n	Mean	SD
6-mo Bayley MDI	637	93.620	17.944
6-mo Bayley PDI	636	98.398	19.665
12-mo Bayley MDI	460	96.020	20.820
12-mo Bayley PDI	455	88.332	21.267
24-mo Bayley MDI	317	96.557	25.444
24-mo Bayley PDI	307	87.689	20.422
3.5-yr Binet IQ	198	93.444	23.779
5-yr Binet IQ	122	97.624	19.398

Note: MDI, Mental Development Index; PDI, Psychomotor Development Index.

are generally higher than those from mental scale to motor scale at the same age. This would indicate that the two scales are measuring different aspects of development despite their high intercorrelations.

Results of Developmental Assessments at Each Age

Table 6.8 provides the means and standard deviations for the developmental and intellectual assessments at each age level. Mental scale scores were quite stable and remained within the average range at all times, varying no more than about four points from six months to five years. Motor scale scores dropped about 10 points from six to twelve months and remained at the lower level through twenty-four months. This finding is in line with previous research showing a greater negative effect of prematurity and medical complications on motor development than on other aspects of cognitive development. As mentioned in the discussion of the intercorrelations between assessments, Stanford-Binet IQ scores were more highly related to and more consistent with mental scale scores.

Correlations of Demographic and Factor Scores with Developmental and Intellectual Assessments

Table 6.9 shows the correlations of the factor scores and demographic variables with the developmental and intellectual assessments at each age. The demographic variables, except gender, showed a pattern of increasingly high correlation as age increased. From 24 months onward, the correlations between IQ and race, socioeconomic status, and age of mother remained higher than before twenty-four months.

The factors representing medical complications showed a fairly substantial consistency in their correlations with developmental and

Table 6.9 Correlations of Factor Scores and Demographic Variables with Developmental Assessments at Each Age

Variable	6-mo MDI (637)	6-mo PDI (636)	12-mo MDI (460)	12-mo PDI (455)	24-mo MDI (317)	24-mo PDI (307)	3.5 yr IQ (198)	5-yr IQ (122)
Gender	−.004	−.036	−.052	−.066	−.047	−.055	.041	−.050
Socioeconomic status	−.119[c]	−.103[a]	−.175[c]	−.138[b]	−.320[c]	−.238[c]	−.331[c]	−.317[c]
Race	.110[b]	.115[c]	.113[a]	.100[a]	.273[c]	.132[a]	.312[c]	.265[c]
Age of mother	.040	.016	.063	.026	.182[b]	.103	.294[c]	.205[a]
Factors								
1	.062	.037	.029	.072	.165[b]	.088	.035	.040
2	−.490[c]	−.498[c]	−.550[c]	−.530[c]	−.435[c]	−.596[c]	−.412	−.420[c]
3	−.127[b]	−.064	−.153[b]	−.120[a]	−.204[c]	−.183[b]	−.265[c]	−.216[a]
4	−.299[c]	−.356[c]	−.372[c]	−.371[c]	−.345[c]	−.306[c]	−.287[c]	−.273[c]
5	.294[c]	.303[c]	.338[c]	.312[c]	.235[c]	.306[c]	.207[c]	.093
6	−.141[c]	−.148[c]	−.169[a]	−.137[b]	−.102[a]	−.126[a]	−.177[b]	−.150
7	−.174[c]	−.198[c]	−.143[b]	−.132[a]	−.139[b]	−.167[c]	.011	−.001
8	−.099[a]	−.099[a]	−.095[a]	−.103[a]	−.149[b]	−.124[a]	−.081	.054
9	−.099[a]	−.110[a]	−.080	−.085	−.092	−.061	−.055	−.039
10	.060	.038	.016	−.006	.023	.021	−.014	−.008

Note: Numbers in parentheses, number in group. MDI, Mental Development Index; PDI, Psychomotor Development Index.

[a] $p < .05$.
[b] $p < .01$.
[c] $p < .005$.

intellectual assessments from one age to another. Factors 5, 7, 8, and 9 were clearly more highly correlated with early assessments than with later assessments. Factors 2, 3, 4, and 6 retained the size of their correlations at least through age five years, although only factors 2, 3, and 4 were significant at five years because of the smaller sample size.

Factor 2 (brain injury) is unique in having correlations in the .4 to .6 range throughout the age range of the assessments. Factors 3 (asphyxia) and 4 (persisting neonatal illness) showed a similar but somewhat less consistent pattern with lower correlations. It seems reasonable to assume that these factors represent negative influences on intellectual development that persist throughout early childhood.

It is of some interest that factor 1 (degree of prematurity) and factor 10 (multiple birth) showed very little correlation with intellectual development at any age. The single exception is a significant correlation between degree of prematurity and the Bayley mental scale at twenty-four months. Bayley scores were corrected for prematurity from six months through twenty-four months, and this may explain the lack of significant correlations at younger ages. The correction may be insignificant at twenty-four months. Clearly, however, the medical variables are more highly related to intellectual development than is the degree of prematurity, per se.

Prediction of Developmental and Intellectual Levels using Multiple Regression

The results of the series of multiple regression analyses are shown in table 6.10. At each age, all previous assessment results were entered along with the demographic variables and medical factors to predict the developmental assessment scores.

The demographic variables were generally poor predictors of the factor scores. The strongest prediction was a negative association between being caucasian and factor 2 (brain injury). Low socioeconomic status was negatively associated with persisting neonatal illness and IVH-II. With the exception of a positive association between being male and twelve-month Bayley motor scale performance, the demographic variables made their strongest direct contribution in predicting twenty-four-month Bayley scores. Race, socio-economic status, and gender were all significant predictors of twenty-four-month Bayley mental scale scores. Socioeconomic status also predicted twenty-four-month Bayley motor scores. Thereafter, there were no significant contributions of demographic variables to the prediction of Stanford-Binet scores.

Table 6.10   Multiple Regression Predictions of Medical Factors, Developmental Assessments, and IQ Up to Five Years

Factor	Bayley MDI		Bayley PDI		Stanford-Binet IQ	
	6 months		*6 months*		*3.5 years*	
1						
$R = .106$	.548		.578		.985	
$R^2 = .106$	.300		.334		.801	
p = n.s.	<.0001		<.0001		<.0001	
	Factor 2	$-.54^d$	Factor 2	$-.53^d$	24-mo IQ	$.61^d$
	Factor 5	$-.29^b$	Factor 5	$-.31^d$	12-mo IQ	$.19^a$
2						
$R = .145$	Factor 9	$-.20^c$	Factor 9	$-.22^d$	Factor 3	$-.10^b$
$R^2 = .021$	Factor 6	$-.19^b$	Factor 6	$-.21^c$	Factor 10	$-.08^a$
$p < .005$	Factor 4	$-.12^c$	Factor 4	$-.19^d$		
Race = $-.144^b$	Factor 7	$-.10^b$	Factor 7	$-.11^c$		
	12 months		*12 months*		*5 years*	
3						
$R = .125$	.836		.797		.895	
$R^2 = .016$	.699		.635		.802	
$p < .056$	<.0001		<.0001		<.0001	
	6-mo MDI	$.58^d$	6-mo PDI	$.46^d$	3.5-yr IQ	$.76^d$
	Factor 2	$-.19^d$	6-mo MDI	$.23^d$	Factor 2	$-.18^a$
4						
$R = .164$	Factor 4	$-.09^b$	Factor 2	$-.20^d$	Factor 8	$.11^a$
$R^2 = .027$	Factor 4	$-.10^b$				
$p < .001$			Gender	$.08^b$		
SES = $.131^a$			Factor 10	$-.06^a$		
	24 months		*24 months*			
5						
$R = .092$	.816		.856			
$R^2 = .008$	.666		.733			
p = n.s.	<.0001		<.0001			
	12-mo MDI	$.65^d$	12-mo PDI	$.52^d$		
	Race	$.17^d$	Factor 2	$-.24^d$		
6						
$R = .047$	12-mo PDI	$.13^a$	12-mo MDI	$.23^d$		
$R^2 = .002$	SES	$-.09^a$	SES (low)	$-.08^a$		
p = n.s.	Factor 1	$-.09^a$				
	Gender	$-.08^a$				
7						
$R = .030$						
$R^2 = .008$						
p = n.s.						

Table 6.10   (continued)

Factor	Bayley MDI	Bayley PDI	Stanford-Binet IQ
8			
$R = .103$			
$R^2 = .011$			
$p =$ n.s.			
9			
$R = .122$			
$R^2 = .015$			
$p < .05$			
Age of			
mother $= .11^a$			
SES $= -.10^a$			
10			
$R = .118$			
$R^2 = .014$			
$p < .05$			

Note: MDI, Mental Development Index; PDI, Psychomotor Development Index; n.s. not significant; SES, socioeconomic status.
[a] $p < .05$.
[b] $p < .01$.
[c] $p < .005$.
[d] $p < .001$.

The factor scores were good predictors of the six-month Bayley mental and motor scores and showed similar patterns of associations with each. In both cases, factor 2 (brain injury) had a substantially stronger association than the other factors, followed by the other three IVH factors and then by persisting neonatal illness and being small for gestational age.

Brain injury and persisting neonatal illness added further to the prediction of twelve-month Bayley scores. At twenty-four months the degree of prematurity emerged, for the first time, as a significant predictor of Bayley mental scores. Its lack of contribution at earlier ages may have been due to the Bayley scores being corrected for prematurity. Brain injury remained a fairly strong predictor of twenty-four-month Bayley motor scores but not mental scores. It was also a significant predictor of five-year Stanford-Binet IQ.

Factor 3 (asphyxia) added significantly to the prediction of three and one-half year Stanford-Binet IQ and had not been a significant predictor of any earlier variables. Multiple birth also contributed to the prediction of three and one-half year IQ as well as to the twelve-month Bayley motor scores.

The best predictor of each developmental assessment was the previous developmental assessment. Twelve-month Bayley scores were strongly predicted by six-month Bayley scores. Only the mental score from six months predicted the mental scale at twelve months, whereas both the mental and motor scales from six months predicted the twelve-month motor scale. At twenty-four months the mental and motor scales from twelve months added to the prediction of the mental scale, although the twelve-month mental scale was the much stronger predictor. The results were similar for the twenty-four-month motor scale, where both twelve-month Bayley scales added to the prediction, but the motor score was the stronger predictor.

The three and one-half year Stanford-Binet was predicted by both the twenty-four-month Bayley mental scale and the twelve-month Bayley mental scale. Evidently, these two earlier assessments do not carry the same information, despite their substantial correlation. The twenty-four-month Bayley motor scale was not a significant predictor of three and one-half year Stanford-Binet IQ. At age five only the three and one-half year Stanford-Binet, among the earlier developmental assessments, was a significant predictor of IQ on the five-year Stanford-Binet. The regression equation for five-year IQ accounted for 80 percent of the variability in IQ scores.

Path Diagram of Cognitive and Intellectual Development
Figure 6.1 shows the results of the multiple regression analyses in the form of a path diagram. For purposes of simplification, the medical-variables are divided into degree of prematurity (factor 1), brain injury (factor 2), and other medical complications (factors 3 to 10). The squared multiple correlation (R^2) is shown for each dependent variable, indicating the amount of variance accounted for by the prediction equation. Only those variables that contributed directly or indirectly to the prediction of five-year Stanford-Binet IQ were included in the diagram. Thus, twenty-four-month Bayley motor performance is not included because it made no contribution.

Only two variables had a significant effect on five-year Stanford-Binet IQ: three and one-half year Stanford-Binet and the brain injury factor. The three and one-half year Stanford-Binet was, in turn, predicted by the twenty-four- and twelve-month Bayley mental scale scores and medical factors 3 (asphyxia) and 8 (toxicity). Twenty-four month Bayley mental scale scores were predicted by twelve-month Bayley mental and motor scores, by degree of prematurity, and by gender, race, and socioeconomic status. The two twelve-month Bayley

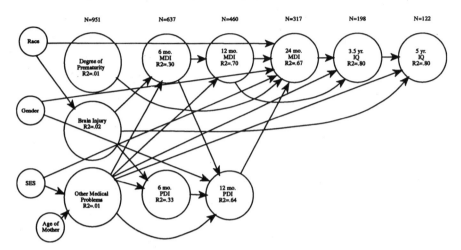

Figure 6.1   Path diagram for the development of five-year IQ. *MDI,* Mental Development Index; *PDI,* Psychomotor Development Index; *SES,* socioeconomic status.

scores were predicted by the six-month Bayley scores and by medical factors 4 (persisting neonatal illness) and 10 (multiple birth). Brain injury was a significant predictor of twelve-month Bayley mental scores. Finally, the six-month Bayley scores were predicted almost identically by brain injury as the strongest factor and a combination of medical factors 4 (persisting neonatal illness), 5 (absence of severe IVH), six (IVH-III), 7 (small for gestational age), and 9 (IVH-II). Race and socioeconomic status made small contributions to the prediction of factors 2 and 9, and the age of the mother contributed slightly to the prediction of factor 9 (IVH-II).

Taken as a whole, the path diagram shows that most of the medical factors exert their major influence on the earliest developmental assessments and account for about a third of the variability in six month Bayley scores. The Bayley mental and motor scales at six and twelve months seem both to assess abilities relevant to the development of the skills measured by the twenty-four-month Bayley mental scale. The early Bayley assessments do seem to measure different abilities, since some medical variables exert a significant influence at six months and others do at twelve months. However, other than the degree of prematurity, whose effect may have been obscured by correcting the Bayley scores for degree of prematurity, the medical factors exert their influence on twenty-four-month Bayley mental scale scores indirectly by influencing earlier mental and motor development. At twenty-four months, the Bayley mental scale is more influenced by social variables than were earlier Bayley scores, perhaps because of its having more verbal content or perhaps because of the waning influence of medical problems.

Although most of the effect of medical and demographic variables on three and one-half year Stanford-Binet IQ is indirect through the twenty-four-month Bayley mental scale, the twelve-month Bayley mental scale adds additional predictive power, perhaps as a more direct measure of the influence of some medical factors on cognitive development. There is also a small contribution from asphyxia and toxicity, which had not contributed to earlier developmental scores.

By age five, nearly all of the effects of earlier medical problems, demographic influences, and cognitive development are reflected in the contribution from the three and one-half year Stanford-Binet IQ. Only the brain injury factor continues to make a direct, independent contribution to the IQ score.

Prediction of Visual-Motor Ability at Five Years of Age

Scaled scores on the Beery Developmental Test of Visuo-motor Integration at five years were available for only the forty-eight children in the school-age sample. The mean scaled score was 7.66 (SD, 3.137), which is nearly one standard deviation below the normative mean of 10. Table 6.11 shows the correlations of the Beery with the demographic variables, medical factors, and developmental assessments before five years. The significant correlations with socioeconomic status and medical factors 2 (brain injury), 5 (absence of severe IVH), and 6 (IVH-III) were statistically significant. All of the developmental assessments except the six-month Bayley motor scale were significantly correlated with the Beery.

Because of the small number of subjects, not all of the variables could be entered in a multiple regression equation to predict Beery scores. Even when only those variables that showed significant simple correlations with the Beery were entered, the high correlations between the predictor variables yielded a highly significant regression equation with a multiple R of .71 but no individually significant predictors.

The same variables, with one exception, were then entered into a stepwise multiple regression analysis. Factor 5 was removed from the analysis because of its high correlations with factors 2 and 6 and because it represented absence of severe IVH, which was redundant

Table 6.11   Correlations of Demographic Variables, Medical Factors, and Developmental Assessments with the Beery Test at Age Five Years

Variable	Correlation	p
Gender	.039	n.s.
Socioeconomic status	−.245	<.05
Race	.104	n.s.
Age of mother	.211	n.s.
Factor		
1	.001	n.s.
2	−.476	<.001
3	−.021	n.s.
4	−.035	n.s.
5	.483	<.001
6	−.286	<.05
7	−.022	n.s.
8	.185	n.s.
9	−.220	n.s.
10	.052	n.s.
6-mo MDI	.373	<.01
6-mo PDI	.219	n.s.
12-mo MDI	.473	<.001
12-mo PDI	.386	<.01
24-mo MDI	.508	<.001
24-mo PDI	.513	<.001
3.5-yr IQ	.484	<.001

with factors representing IVH-III and IVH-IV. The order of entry of variables was determined by the size of the partial correlations with the dependent variable. On step 1, the twenty-four-month Bayley motor scale was entered and no further variables contributed a significant increase in the correlation. The correlation for the twenty-four-month motor scale and the Beery was 0.589, with 35 percent of the variability in Beery scores accounted for.

Obviously, several variables were strong predictors of scores on the Beery. Although the multiple regression using all of the significantly correlated variables was more highly correlated with Beery scores than was just the twenty-four-month Bayley motor scale, no particular variable added significantly more predictive power. Factor 2 (brain injury) very nearly achieved entry into the equation and was nearly as good a predictor as the twenty-four-month Bayley motor score.

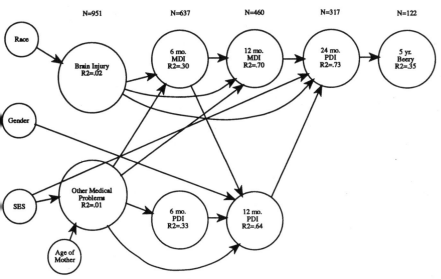

Figure 6.2 Path diagram for the development of visuomotor abilities at five years of age.

Addition of the Results of the Stepwise Multiple Regression Analysis to the Path Diagram
As shown in figure 6.2, most of the variability in the Bayley motor scale at twenty-four months was accounted for by the effects of brain injury, twelve-month motor and mental development, and, to a lesser extent, socioeconomic status. Brain injury in turn affected earlier mental and motor development, as did other medical complications, including the presence of less severe grades of IVH. The influence of brain injury directly on twenty-four-month Bayley motor scores and indirectly through earlier development was substantial.

Five-year visual-motor ability, as measured by the Beery, was directly affected only by the development of psychomotor abilities, as measured by the twenty-four-month Bayley motor scale. Brain injury had its effect indirectly by affecting earlier psychomotor development. The high correlations between the five-year Beery scores and the factors representing brain injury and IVH, however, indicate that both the Beery and earlier motor development are strongly influenced by these factors.

Prediction of Mathematical Achievement

Mathematical achievement was measured using both the Test of Early Mathematics Ability (TEMA) and the Wide Range Achievement Test, Revised (WRAT-R). For the school-age sample the mean standard score on the TEMA was 91.023 (SD, 16.720). The mean score on the WRAT-R was 85.864 (SD, 24.371). The correlations of the demographic variables, medical factors, and developmental assessments are given in table 6.12. Being caucasian and having a higher socioeconomic status are both significantly related to each achievement score. Age of mother shows a significant correlation with the WRAT-R score.

Of the medical factors, factor 2 (brain injury) showed the highest negative correlation with both achievement scores. Factor 3 (asphyxia)

Table 6.12   Correlations with Mathematical Achievement Scores (n = 48)

Variable	TEMA	p	WRAT-R	p
Gender	−.068	n.s.	−.078	n.s.
Socioeconomic status (low)	−.290	<.05	−.346	<.05
Race (white)	.348	<.05	.438	<.01
Age of mother	.256	n.s.	.433	<.01
Factor				
1	−.080	n.s.	−.004	n.s.
2	−.417	<.01	−.452	<.001
3	−.273	<.05	−.233	n.s.
4	−.046	n.s.	.022	n.s.
5	.059	n.s.	.125	n.s.
6	.121	n.s.	.045	n.s.
7	.059	n.s.	−.018	n.s.
8	.039	n.s.	.016	n.s.
9	.002	n.s.	−.122	n.s.
10	−.083	n.s.	−.144	n.s.
6-mo MDI	.294	<.05	.204	n.s.
6-mo PDI	.110	n.s.	.040	n.s.
12-mo MDI	.465	<.001	.545	<.001
12-mo PDI	.451	<.001	.370	<.01
24-mo MDI	.552	<.001	.704	<.001
24-mo PDI	.357	<.05	.522	<.001
3.5-yr IQ	.439	<.01	.561	<.001
5-yr IQ	.549	<.001	.678	<.001
5-yr Beery	.527	<.001	.552	<.001

Note: MDI, Mental Development Index; PDI, Psychomotor Development Index; TEMA, Test of Early Mathematics Ability; WRAT-R, Wide Range Achievement Test, Revised.

is significantly correlated with TEMA scores and nearly so with the WRAT-R scores.

The developmental and intellectual assessments showed higher correlations with both achievement scores with increasing age. At six months of age, only the Bayley mental scale score is significantly correlated with the TEMA. Neither Bayley score showed a significant correlation with the WRAT-R at this age. The twenty-four-month Bayley mental score was as highly correlated with the achievement scores as was the five-year Stanford-Binet IQ.

Stepwise Multiple Regression Analyses of the Mathematical Achievement Scores

Stepwise multiple regression analyses were conducted using each mathematical achievement score as a dependent variable. Predictor variables were entered as blocks, with the two assessments of five year olds (Stanford-Binet IQ and Beery scaled score) entered first. Within a block, the order of entry was determined by the size of the partial correlations with the dependent variable. A criterion of significance at the .05 level was used to permit entry of a variable into the regression analysis. Any variable that was retained at one age level was entered as the first variable along with the variables in the next block, which included all variables measured at the next younger age level. This process was continued until all variables were given an opportunity to enter the regression equation.

TEMA

The five-year Stanford-Binet had the highest single correlation with the TEMA, and no other variables at any age nor any of the medical factors or demographic variables significantly improved the prediction of TEMA scores beyond the use of the five-year IQ alone. Table 6.13 lists the results of the stepwise multiple regression analysis for the TEMA as well as that for the WRAT-R.

WRAT-R

At age five years the Stanford-Binet IQ was correlated .68 with the WRAT-R score and adding the Beery score did not improve the prediction significantly. The five-year Stanford-Binet IQ was retained at age three and one-half years, and at age twenty-four months the Bayley mental score added significantly to the prediction. Both variables were retained in all subsequent analyses, and no other variables were added. The results are listed in table 6.13.

Table 6.13   Stepwise Multiple Regressions for TEMA and WRAT-R

Test		Beta	T	p
TEMA				
Step1: 5-yr Stanford-Binet IQ		.576	4.109	<.0002
Multiple R	576			
$R2$	.332			
p	<.0002			
WRAT-R				
Step 1: 5 yr Stanford-Binet IQ		.449	2.855	<.01
Step 2: 24-mo Bayley MDI		.359	2.281	<.05
Multiple R	.735			
$R2$	.541			
p	<.0001			

Note: TEMA, Test of Early Mathematics Ability; WRAT-R, Wide Range Achievement Test, Revised.

Addition of the Results of the Stepwise Analyses to the Path Diagram
The addition of the results of the stepwise multiple regression analyses of the TEMA to the previously developed path diagram, as illustrated in figure 6.3, was quite simple. The only direct effect on TEMA scores was from the five-year Stanford-Binet IQ. The effects of the demographic variables that were significantly correlated with TEMA scores (socioeconomic status and race) and of significantly correlated medical factors (brain injury and asphyxia) were expressed indirectly through their effects on intelligence.

The addition of the results of the stepwise multiple regression analyses of WRAT-R scores was somewhat more complicated. Both the five-year Stanford-Binet IQ and the twenty-four-month Bayley mental scale scores had direct effects on WRAT-R scores. This indicates that these two measures of mental development were assessing different aspects of cognition. The path diagram for intelligence indicates that brain injury, some medical factors, and aspects of twelve-month Bayley mental scores all have some effect on the development of intelligence after twenty-four months of age. The twenty-four-month Bayley mental scale scores may be more sensitive to social influences (race, socioeconomic status) and less sensitive to brain injury than either earlier or later assessments.

The failure of Bayley motor scale scores or Beery scores to show any direct effect on arithmetic achievement does not confirm the hypothesis that lowered arithmetic scores in prematurely born children are a result of brain injury–induced impairment of visual-motor

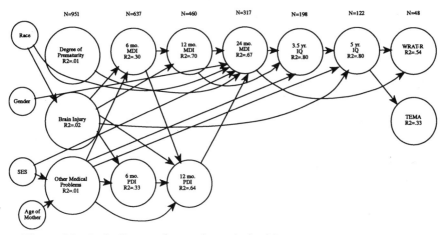

Figure 6.3   Path diagram for mathematical achievement

abilities. In fact, Bayley motor scales do not even exert an indirect influence on intellectual development after twelve months. Although Bayley motor scale scores, Beery scores, and arithmetic achievement scores are all lower than either Bayley mental scale scores or Stanford-Binet IQ, the path diagram does not support a hypothesis that arithmetic achievement is an effect of the lowering of motor or visual-motor abilities. Rather, if brain injury does have an effect on arithmetic achievement at school age, it may be by lowering general intellectual development.

Prediction of Arithmetic Disability

Arithmetic Disability versus No Arithmetic Disability

Subjects whose standard score on the WRAT-R was one standard deviation (15 points) below their Full-Scale IQ on the WISC-R were defined as arithmetic disabled and were compared to subjects whose arithmetic and IQ scores were within one standard deviation of each other.

Table 6.14 shows the means, standard deviations, and significance levels for the two groups on all of the variables, including the TEMA, WRAT-R, and WISC-R. The arithmetic-disabled students had much poorer scores on both the TEMA and the WRAT-R. The WRAT-R scores showed more impairment than the TEMA scores, but the differences between the arithmetic-disabled students and those without an arithmetic disability were highly significant on both measures. The arithmetic-disabled subjects also had lower reading scores on the WRAT-R, but reading scores were not as low as arithmetic scores.

Table 6.14   Mean Scores for Subjects with and without an Arithmetic Disability on All Variables

Variable	No Disability Mean	SD	Disability Mean	SD	p
TEMA	99.958	13.678	79.737	13.127	<.00001
WRAT-R					
Arithmetic	101.440	15.419	65.368	17.929	<.00001
Reading	92.154	23.768	75.526	22.207	<.05
Full-Scale IQ	101.577	13.067	92.211	21.361	n.s.
Verbal IQ	101.808	11.754	95.500	18.894	n.s.
Performance IQ	101.270	14.915	92.222	22.862	n.s.
Gender (male)	57%		73%		n.s.
Socioeconomic status (low)	3.19	1.50	3.94	1.77	n.s.
Race (white)	92%		78%		<.001
Age of mother (yr)	28.46	4.75	26.50	2.68	n.s.
Factor					
1	.526	.454	.474	.339	n.s.
2	.048	.142	.132	.210	n.s.
3	.261	.375	.438	.359	n.s.
4	.269	.157	.303	.178	n.s.
5	.365	.226	.342	.239	n.s.
6	.192	.402	.053	.229	n.s.
7	.192	.193	.211	.199	n.s.
8	.089	.178	.070	.140	n.s.
9	.077	.272	.158	.375	n.s.
10	.346	.485	.474	.513	n.s.
6-mo MDI	95.520	7.545	91.444	4.532	n.s.
6-mo PDI	101.231	11.233	99.611	22.298	n.s.
12-mo MDI	98.654	13.026	83.105	21.298	<.01
12-mo PDI	92.038	16.433	81.000	22.808	<.05
24-mo MDI	96.520	17.362	79.631	17.783	<.01
24-mo PDI	95.196	16.548	80.578	18.748	<.01
3.5-yr IQ	95.800	16.548	89.437	13.569	n.s.
5-yr IQ	97.391	9.529	89.563	13.416	<.05
5-yr Beery	8.577	3.049	6.722	3.102	<.05

Note: MDI, Mental Development Index; PDI, Psychomotor Development Index; TEMA, Test of Early Mathematics Ability; WRAT-R, Wide Range Achievement Test, Revised.

Although the arithmetic-disabled students obtained lower scores on all three WISC-R measures, none of Full-Scale IQ difference reached statistical significance. The mean scores for both groups were within the average range of intelligence on all of the WISC-R measures.

Of the demographic variables, only race showed a significant difference between the two groups. There were a greater percentage of noncaucasians in the arithmetic-disabled group. None of the medical factors differed significantly between the two groups. Most of the differences on the medical factors were in the direction of more medical problems within the disabled group. The variability on the medical factors was quite large, compared to the small mean values, making it difficult to achieve statistical significance on any of these variables.

On the developmental assessments there was no significant difference between the groups at six months, but at twelve months there was a large and significant difference on both the mental and motor scales which continued until after twenty-four months. The differences narrowed on the Stanford-Binet and reached significance only at five years. The arithmetic-disabled subjects were also more impaired on the Beery at five years.

Results of Stepwise Multiple Regression Analyses

A series of stepwise multiple regression analyses were performed using the presence or absence of an arithmetic disability as the dependent variable. The procedure was identical to that used to predict TEMA and WRAT-R scores in that prediction variables were blocked by age of assessment and entered according to the size of the partial correlations with the dependent variable within each block. The order of entry of the blocks was from the most recent to the earliest ages, followed by the medical factors and the demographic variables.

The five-year Stanford-Binet IQ significantly predicted the presence of an arithmetic disability ($R = .355$). Addition of the Beery did not improve the prediction. At the next age level, the addition of the three and one-half year Stanford-Binet also did not add to the prediction. At twenty-four months the mental scale from the Bayley replaced the five-year Stanford-Binet. At twelve months the twelve-month Bayley mental scale replaced the twenty-four-month mental scale. The twelve-month Bayley mental scale remained as the only significant predictor in the rest of the analyses. The results are shown in table 6.15.

Table 6.15 Stepwise Multiple Regression Analysis of Arithmetic Disability ($n = 48$)

		Beta	T	p
Multiple R	.449			
$R2$	.201			
p	<.003			
Predictors:				
12-mo MDI		−.449	−3.259	<.003

Addition of the Results of the Stepwise Multiple Regression Analyses to the Path Diagram

In the path diagram shown in figure 6.4, the only direct effect on the presence of arithmetic disability is the twelve-month Bayley mental scale. What is immediately obvious is that motor and visual-motor assessments do not enter the path for prediction of arithmetic disability. None of the medical factors showed a direct effect on the presence of an arithmetic disability. However, virtually all of the medical complications except degree of prematurity, asphyxia, and toxicity contribute directly to either six-month Bayley mental scores or twelve-month Bayley mental scores, or both. The six-month mental score is the strongest predictor of the twelve-month score.

That mental and intellectual assessments beyond twelve months did not add to the predictive power of the twelve-month Bayley mental scale by itself can be interpreted to mean that early medical problems, as expressed in their effect on early mental development, have a limiting effect on arithmetic skill development despite having less effect on the later development of intelligence.

In terms of the original path model, the current results are considerably different from the model that was hypothesized. It was hypothesized that arithmetic disability would show direct effects of IQ and visual-motor ability as measured by the five-year Stanford-Binet and Beery. Medical factors were hypothesized to operate indirectly, through their influence on these two variables. Clearly, the hypothesized path model does not fit the results. Despite the fact that the arithmetic-disabled subjects were significantly worse on the two variables measured at five years old, this seems to be because they too were affected by the early developmental influences, which were, in fact, more crucial to the development of an arithmetic disability. The fact that the twelve-month Bayley mental scale scores accounted for only 20 percent of the variability between the groups indicates that other

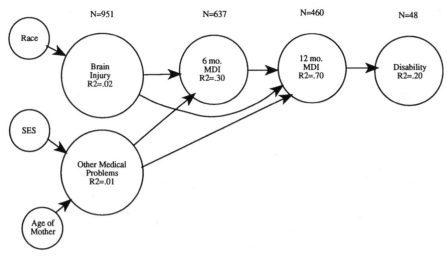

Figure 6.4   Path diagram for the presence of arithmetic disability

factors may play a larger role in determining arithmetic disability or that, perhaps, the definition of disability is too broad and the further division of the disabled group into subtypes would lead to more accurate prediction.

Prediction of Subtype of Arithmetic Disability
The arithmetic-disabled students were divided into two groups: one group was one standard deviation below their Full-Scale IQ in arithmetic only, and the second group was one standard deviation below their Full-Scale IQ in both arithmetic and reading. There were five and fourteen students in the two groups, respectively. Table 6.16 shows the mean scores for the two groups, as well as for the group of twenty-six students who had no arithmetic disability, on all of the variables, including the TEMA, WRAT-R, and the WISC-R. The arithmetic-plus-reading-disabled group scored significantly lower than the no-arithmetic-disability group on the WRAT-R and the TEMA. Although the group with an arithmetic disability only also scored lower than the nondisabled group on both measures, the result was significant only on the WRAT-R. Despite the fact that the group with both arithmetic and reading disability had lower scores on both measures than had the group with arithmetic disability only, the two groups did not differ significantly on either. As expected, there was a large difference between the two arithmetic disability subtypes on the reading subtest from the WRAT-R. Subjects with an arithmetic disability only scored

Table 6.16 Mean Scores for the Arithmetic Disability on All Variables

Variable	No Disability Mean	No Disability SD	Arithmetic Only Mean	Arithmetic Only SD	Arithmetic and Reading Mean	Arithmetic and Reading SD	p	Group Differential
TEMA	99.958	13.678	84.600	11.502	78.000	13.621	.000	(1:3)
WRAT-R								
Arithmetic	101.440	15.419	71.000	24.156	63.358	15.780	.0001	(1:2,3)
Reading	92.154	23.768	93.800	25.411	69.000	17.603	.01	(1:3)
Full-Scale IQ	101.577	13.067	89.800	25.421	93.071	20.735	n.s.	
Verbal IQ	101.807	11.754	97.600	19.165	94.692	19.512	n.s.	
Performance IQ	101.269	14.915	84.200	30.483	95.308	19.839	n.s.	
Gender	57%	80%	71.4%	n.s.	.429	.356	n.s.	
Socioeconomic status	3.19	1.50	3.75	.50	4.00	2.00	n.s.	
Race	92%	80%	78.6%	n.s.	.444	.385	n.s.	
Age of mother	28.46	4.75	26.75	1.50	26.42	3.09	n.s.	
Factor								
1	.526	.454	.600	.279	.429	.356	n.s.	
2	.048	.142	.200	.209	.107	.213	n.s.	
3	.261	.375	.417	.319	.444	.385	n.s.	
5	.365	.226	.400	.224	.321	.249	n.s.	
6	.192	.402	.200	.447	.000	.000	n.s.	
7	.192	.193	.267	.149	.191	.215	n.s.	
8	.089	.178	.000	.000	.095	.156	n.s.	
9	.077	.272	.000	.000	.214	.425	n.s.	
10	.346	.485	.600	.548	.429	.514	n.s.	
6-mo MDI	95.520	7.545	78.400	18.729	96.462	17.567	.05	(2:1,3)

6-mo PDI	101.231	11.233	86.200	14.078	104.769	23.119	n.s.	
12-mo MDI	98.654	13.026	67.800	17.936	88.571	19.972	.001	(1:2)
12-mo PDI	92.038	16.433	67.800	26.169	85.714	20.462	.05	(1:2)
24-mo MDI	96.520	17.362	74.200	23.145	81.571	16.051	.01	(1:2,3)
24-mo PDI	95.196	21.334	66.800	23.921	85.500	14.543	.05	(1:2)
3.5-yr IQ	95.800	16.548	84.250	11.871	91.167	14.128	n.s.	
5-yr IQ	97.391	9.529	84.500	22.898	91.250	9.488	n.s.	
Beery	8.577	3.044	5.400	4.037	7.231	2.682	n.s.	

Note: MDI, Motor Development Index; PDI, Psychomotor Development Index; TEMA, Test of Early Mathematics Ability; WRAT-R, Wide Range Achievement Test-Revised.

within the average range in reading and, in fact, scored slightly higher than the group with no disability. The group with both an arithmetic and a reading disability scored well below normal in reading and nearly as poorly in reading as in arithmetic.

None of the differences on the WISC-R reached significance. The results were quite interesting, however, in the light of Rourke's (1989) theory and his results with similarly subtyped students who were not born prematurely. He reported that Performance IQ is particularly low in students with arithmetic disability only. The same thing was found in this study, but the very small numbers and high variability in scores precluded obtaining statistical significance.

None of the differences on the factor scores reached significance. Without attaching too much importance to insignificant results, it can be observed that the group with both arithmetic and reading disabilities is the most premature and has more asphyxia and, perhaps, mild (grade II) IVH, whereas the group with only arithmetic disability is the least premature and has the most evidence of brain injury and of being small for gestational age. They are also more likely to be twins.

Although the group with an arithmetic disability only tended to have better arithmetic scores than did the group with both arithmetic and reading disabilities, they were generally the lowest group on the developmental measures. None of the individual comparisons between the two disabled groups was significant, however. It is of some interest that the Bayley scales were more sensitive in detecting group differences than were the Stanford-Binet. Either the two tests are differentially sensitive to the skills that are related to arithmetic disability or the cognitive deficits are more prominent at earlier ages.

Stepwise Discriminant Function Analyses of Subtypes of Arithmetic Disability

A series of stepwise discriminant function analyses were performed using membership in each of the three groups (arithmetic disability only, arithmetic and reading disability, and no arithmetic disability) as the dependent variable. The same procedures were used as with the earlier stepwise multiple regression analyses. Predictor variables were blocked according to the age of assessment and entered in order of descending ages, with the medical factors and the demographic variables entered last. To reduce the number of predictor variables, we used only those medical factors on which there was a suggestion of a difference or for which there was a theoretical reason for using the factor. Thus, factors 1 (degree of prematurity), 2 (brain injury),

Table 6.17 Stepwise Discriminant Function Analysis of Subtype of Arithmetic Disability

Step	Variable	Wilks' Lambda	p	Canonical Correlation
1	12-mo MDI	.77463	.0115	
2	Factor 5	.70407	.0166	
3	Factor 1	.64970	.0232	
4	Factor 3	.58660	.0224	
5	6-mo MDI	.53050	.0220	
	Function 1			.6220
	Function 2			.3671

3 (asphyxia), 5 (absence of severe IVH), 6 (IVH-III), and 8 (toxicity) were used.

At age five years the Beery was included in the analysis and the Stanford-Binet IQ was not. At age three and one-half years, no variables significantly predicted group membership and the Beery was retained for entry with the twenty-four-month Bayley scores. Both the mental and motor scores were retained and the Beery was removed. At twelve months the two twenty-four-month scores and the two twelve-month scores were entered. Only the twelve-month mental scale and the twenty-four-month mental scale were retained. At the next age level, the twelve-month mental scale and the six-month mental scale were retained and the twenty-four-month mental scale was removed.

When the medical factor scores were entered, five variables were finally retained in the discriminant function: six- and twelve-month Bayley mental scores, and factors 1, 3, and 5. No demographic variables added to the significance of the prediction from these variables. The results of the final stepwise analysis are presented in table 6.17. The discriminant function was able to correctly classify 76.32 percent of the subjects into their disability groups. The results of this classification are shown in table 6.18.

Addition of the Results of the Stepwise Discriminant Function to the Path Diagram

It is immediately clear from figure 6.5 that neither motor development nor later intellectual development beyond one year makes a significant contribution to the prediction of subtype of arithmetic disability. Although significant differences were found between the groups on mental and motor scores at twenty-four months, the variability in group membership was accounted for more adequately by

Table 6.18   Discriminant Classification of Subtypes of Arithmetic Disability

Actual Group	n	Predicted Group Membership 1	2	3
1. Arithmetic only	4	4 100%	0 0%	0 0%
2. Arithmetic and reading	12	3 25%	8 66%	1 8.3%
3. No disability	22	0 0%	5 22.7%	17 77.3%
Ungrouped subjects	3	0 0%	1 33.3%	2 67.7%
Missing predictor data	7			

the earlier mental measures and some of the medical factor scores. Thus, the predictive power of these later tests and the motor measures was due to their sensitivity to the same variables assessed more precisely by the earlier measures.

Only medical factor 8 (toxicity) does not make either an indirect or direct contribution to the path for subtype of arithmetic disability. Neither factor 1 (degree of prematurity) nor factor 3 (asphyxia) made a direct contribution to the mix or to twelve-month Bayley mental scores. For this reason, they were able to show their influence directly on determining group membership. Factor 5 (absence of severe IVH), on the other hand, did make a direct contribution to the six-month mental score. Since two of the more powerful predictors among the medical variables were expected to be factors 2 (brain injury) and 6 (IVH-III), factor 5 probably carried most of the variability for those two other medical factors because of its negative association with IVH-III and IV. Both were excluded from the final discriminant function.

The hypothesis that medical complications would affect mathematical disability only indirectly through their effect on developmental assessments was not borne out by the results of the study. Later developmental assessments seem to be less sensitive indicators of the underlying neurological problems that result in mathematical disability than are assessments of the medical problems at birth or of mental development in the first year of life.

The hypothesis that medical problems would show their effect through their influence on the development of motor and visuomotor abilities was also not borne out by the results of the study. Neither motor assessments nor visuomotor assessment with the Beery showed

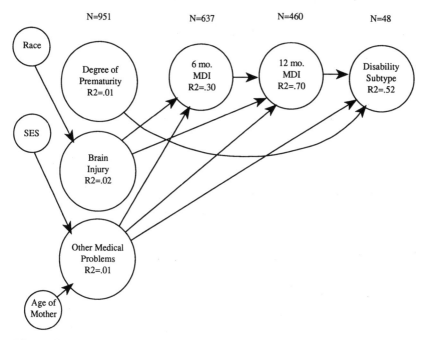

Figure 6.5   Path diagram for subtypes of arithmetic disability

direct effects on subtype of arithmetic disability. These skills do show some association with subtype of mathematical disability, particularly with lower scores occurring in the group with arithmetic disability only. However, they also are not as sensitive indicators as the early medical and mental assessments. Since these variables did not add predictive power to the variables measured earlier, it can be concluded that they do not determine arithmetic disability themselves but rather may be influenced by some of the same early medical problems, as is arithmetic ability.

Conclusions

There were two main hypotheses in the present study: (1) that there would be significant relationships between some medical risk factors and mathematical achievement and disability and between developmental assessments and mathematical achievement and disability and (2) that it would be possible to determine whether the medical risk factors directly affected mathematical achievement and disability or indirectly affected these outcomes through their influence on earlier cognitive and motor development. A third hypothesis involved a proposed path model in which the likelihood of having a mathematical disability would be increased by the indirect effects of brain injury on the development of motor and visuomotor skills. It was hypothesized that this path model would be specifically applicable to children who were disabled in mathematics but not in reading.

With regard to medical risk factors, there were some significant correlations with mathematical achievement at school age. A brain injury factor composed of IVH-IV, hydrocephalus, cerebral palsy, and seizures was significantly correlated with both TEMA and WRAT-R scores at school age. Asphyxia was also related to mathematical achievement on the TEMA. No significant differences between arithmetic-disabled and nondisabled subjects or between subtypes of arithmetic-disabled subjects were found on any of the ten medical factors.

Developmental assessments showed stronger relationships with both mathematical achievement and mathematical disability. Achievement scores were significantly related to developmental assessments at all but the youngest ages. Relationships were stronger with increasing age. Mathematical disability was also related to developmental assessments at nearly all ages, but somewhat more so at younger ages when subtype of disability was being predicted.

The first hypothesis of the study was confirmed, although less so for the medical factors than for the developmental assessments. Brain injury and asphyxia stood out as significantly related to mathematical achievement. Developmental assessments were predictive of both achievement and disability, with different relationships between early and later assessments for each.

The use of path diagrams based on much larger samples at earlier ages allowed confirmation of the second hypothesis. Mathematical achievement was influenced directly by later developmental assessments. In the case of the TEMA, only the five-year Stanford-Binet IQ was a direct predictor of achievement scores. For the WRAT-R, both the five-year Stanford-Binet IQ and the score from the twenty-four-month Bayley mental scale predicted achievement scores directly. However, the path diagrams showed that brain injury had a direct effect on the five-year Stanford-Binet IQ and that it and other medical factors influenced cognitive development at earlier ages. There were strong effects of medical factors on the earliest developmental assessments, which in turn affected later assessments.

Mathematical disability was more directly affected by early cognitive measures and, in the case of subtypes of disability, was affected directly by the degree of prematurity, the presence of asphyxia, and whether or not severe IVH had been present. Later cognitive development was not as important in predicting disability, and it seemed that medical problems affected early mental development most dramatically and that later cognitive measures were not as sensitive to these effects. At the same time, these early effects had a strong influence on determining both the presence and type of mathematical disability. It was possible to predict subtype of disability with 76 percent accuracy based on knowledge of medical problems and cognitive development within the first year.

The third hypothesis was not confirmed at all. Motor development and visuomotor ability at five years had no direct or indirect effect on mathematical disability. Path diagrams completely left these variables out.

The results with regard to the third hypothesis were surprising. The hypothesis was formulated for two reasons. In the first place, a great deal of evidence, which was reviewed in chapter 2, indicated that prematurity and the medical problems associated with it was related to motor and visuomotor disability more often than to other forms of cognitive disability. In the second place, Rourke (1989) assembled a good deal of evidence and proposed a theory to go with it that says that some types of mathematical disability are associated with visuomotor impairment. He described how impairment in visuomotor and visual-perceptual skills can interfere with doing mathematical calculations on a test like the WRAT-R.

This research found many of the same things that have been found by other researchers (e.g., Dunn 1986; Klein, Hack, and Breslau 1989; Landry et al. 1984). The prematurely born subjects as a group tended to fall behind in motor development more than in mental development after the first year. There were strong relationships between medical problems, particularly brain injury and motor development. Motor development, as measured by the twenty-four-month Bayley motor scale, was the only direct predictor of five-year performance on the Beery Test of Visuo-motor Integration. Arithmetic-disabled subjects were poorer on the Beery than were non arithmetic-disabled subjects. Although the groups were too small and variable to achieve statistical significance, subjects with just an arithmetic disability scored worse on the Beery and the WISC-R performance section than did their counterparts with either no disability or a reading disability along with their arithmetic disability.

All of the above findings indicate that the present sample of subjects is similar to other researchers' samples in having a set of results that emphasizes the relationships between brain injury, visuomotor problems, and mathematical disability. The use of a path model, based on multiple regression techniques, however, allowed the finding that knowing how much a subject is impaired in motor abilities or visual-motor abilities does not add anything to the knowledge available from an index of the early medical problems and mental development within the first year in terms of predicting mathematical disability.

An alternative model, based on the data from this study, is that both mathematical ability and visuomotor ability are particularly sensitive to the effects of early brain injury. In fact, visuomotor ability may be more sensitive, since correlations between the Beery and medical factors were stronger and more prevalent than were those between any of the mathematical measures and medical problems. Those children who have a mathematical disability are even more likely to have medical problems, and their mathematical skill development is limited by them. Intelligence, as reflected in developmental or intellectual assessments during childhood, is less directly affected by brain injury and shows the influence of socioeconomic factors more than does either mathematical disability or visual-motor ability. The subgroup of children who are disabled in mathematics will show a disproportionate degree of impairment in visuomotor abilities because the same factors cause both kinds of disabilities. However, no direct link between mathematical disabilities and visuomotor ability may be present.

The results of the study of the prediction of mathematical disabilities bear some relationship to the association between the timing of brain injury and the age of assessment. Early injury had its major effects on the earliest developmental assessments with the Bayley scales. Some medical variables, most notably brain injury, continued to have a direct effect on intelligence, even at five years of age. Direct effects on mathematical disability were limited to the medical factors and the Bayley mental assessments done in the first year. It cannot be said that brain injury and medical problems do not affect the growth of intelligence beyond the first year, since they obviously do. However, in the mathematically disabled subjects, the skills required for arithmetic achievement are, by definition, more impaired than intelligence. Whatever brain impairment lowers cognitive development in the first year seems to exert a limiting effect on arithmetic skill development at school age but does not impair intellectual development to the same degree. This suggests that either early cognitive measures and later mathematical measures require some similar cognitive skills that are required less by later intellectual measures or that the type of cognitive impairment detected by the early developmental assessments is related to the type of cognitive impairment required by arithmetic tests but not to intelligence at school age. A reasonable hypothesis could be that what seems to be substantial cognitive impairment at early ages partially resolves when other variables come into play in determining later intellectual development but that mathematical tasks require more of the basic biological intelligence based on integrity of brain structures, just as had the early developmental assessments.

A more interesting case is presented by the finding that some medical factors (degree of prematurity, asphyxia, and absence of severe IVH) add significantly to the prediction of mathematical disabilities beyond the information provided by the early developmental assessments. It must not be that these medical factors simply affect later cognitive development or else the later cognitive measures, rather than the medical factors, would have been included in the predictive equations. The most obvious conclusion is that these medical factors cause a type of brain impairment that is more related to mathematical tasks than to developmental or intellectual assessments. If this hypothesis is correct, then the further search for the brain mechanisms involved in mathematical problem solving is an important area of research.

In a doctoral dissertation that used essentially the same subjects as were used in the study just reported, Gaines (1991) examined the relationships between perinatal medical problems, infant and childhood developmental assessments, and reading. Her school-age sample differed slightly from ours because of different subjects with data missing on different tests. She also examined the relationships between reading and neonatal medical complications separately from the relationships between reading and developmental assessments. She used multiple regression procedures, but not the path analysis used by Katzir.

Reading achievement was measured in three ways: reading recognition, using the WRAT-R; reading comprehension, using the Peabody Individual Achievement Test-Revised; and phonetic reading skill, using the Word Attack Subtest from the Woodcock Reading Mastery Test-Revised. The best predictor of both reading recognition and phonetic reading ability was the race of the child. Caucasian children read better than did noncaucasians. The degree of prematurity added to the prediction of reading recognition but not phonetic reading ability. Reading comprehension was predicted by medical problems representing persisting neonatal illness and infections.

Gaines analyzed the predictions from early developmental assessments separately from those from medical problems and demographic variables. She found that the later developmental assessments from twenty-four months on were generally the only ones related to reading scores and that the Stanford-Binet scores at five years old (the last assessment done) were the only significant predictors of the reading scores using multiple regression procedures.

Although the medical problems and early developmental assessments were not combined to predict reading scores, Gaines did add the WISC-R Full-Scale IQ scores obtained at the same age as the reading scores (approximately seven years) to the medical and demographic variables to see whether the latter variables added anything to the prediction of reading beyond the effect of intelligence. In fact, the brain injury factor added to the prediction of reading recognition and reading comprehension. Phonetic reading ability was predicted solely on the basis of IQ. Race was no longer a predictor of reading skill when IQ was also one of the independent variables.

Fifty-two percent of the forty-six children in Gaines's school-age sample were reading disabled, with reading recognition scores on the WRAT-R at least one standard deviation lower than Full-Scale IQ on the WISC-R. Although classification of reading disability was based on WRAT-R reading recognition scores, the children thus classified as reading disabled were even more deficient in reading comprehension and phonetic reading compared to the non-reading disabled children.

Using stepwise discriminant function analysis, 67 percent of the children were correctly classified as reading disabled or not reading. disabled on the basis of medical problems and demographic variables. The significant predictors were race, degree of prematurity, socioeconomic status, multiple birth, asphyxia, and gender. Although the developmental assessments were equally successful in predicting subject classification correctly (67 percent), none of the assessments stood out as adding significant predictive utility beyond the others. It should be noted, however, that Gaines averaged the six-month, one-year, and two-year Bayley scores together for this analysis, thereby obscuring whether there were any differences between the Bayley scores at different ages.

Perhaps the most striking finding from Gaines's study was that over one-half of the children had reading scores at least one standard deviation below their IQ scores. This, in itself, suggests that there is a strong relationship between reading disability and prematurity and its complications, because this proportion is considerably higher than that found in the normal population. Medical complications did add to the prediction of reading achievement or reading disability, although demographic variables such as race and socioeconomic status were also good, if not better predictors, unlike the case of mathematical ability or disability. The medical problems did not seem just to lower IQ because they were included along with IQ to predict reading achievement.

7

Language and Visuospatial
Development after Early Brain Injury

The organization of the preceding chapters has been dictated by the assumption that the type of injury to the developing brain is an important factor in determining how cognitive development will be affected. This assumption has serious limitations. The type of injury has been defined in terms of a very vague concept of pathological mechanisms. Genetic disorders, for instance, include gene mutations, chromosome defects, recessive sex-linked disorders, and alterations in chromosome number. Congenital defects do not even really constitute a type in the same sense as genetic, vascular, or infectious disorders, since they could be caused by any of these and have in common only the fact that the development of the nervous system is disrupted in a major way before birth. Toxic disorders comprise an extremely heterogeneous lot that probably overlaps considerably with congenital defects, since our discussion was generally confined to toxic effects in utero. Of course, with infections such as HIV, the major effect probably comes from the continuing influence of the infectious agent after birth.

Perinatal injuries, perhaps surprisingly, may constitute the most homogeneous grouping of disorders because they presume a normally developing brain until the time of the injury and because the injury is a specific insult at a specific time. Even this concept of perinatal injury is probably in error, however, since the retardation of intrauterine growth represents something going wrong early in development and since it is difficult to separate the injury as an event from the environmental context in which recovery from the injury takes place.

Given the above considerations, what purpose can there be in trying to draw any general conclusions from the data provided by a survey of the effects of such a heterogeneous collection of disorders? If the cognitive effects are as heterogeneous as the disorders themselves, then the answer may well be that no general conclusions can be drawn. In fact, we suspect that this is the case, which is why the bulk of this book is devoted to examining each disorder separately. On the other hand, two considerations could make some attempt at synthesizing the findings productive. First, all of the disorders occur early in development. If age itself is a factor in determining the outcome of early brain injury, then there should be some commonality among these various disorders. Second, if there are some common themes in the outcome studies that cross the borders of even some of the disorders, they deserve an attempt at explanation.

Intellectual Development

By far the most common outcome measure used in studies of cognitive development in brain-damaged children is intelligence. There are obvious reasons for this. Intelligence tests would top anyone's list of reliable cognitive measures. They also have at least moderate validity as predictors of adaptive behaviors such as school and job performance. Finally, they are ubiquitously administered as clinical instruments, allowing the investigator to retrieve data when collecting clinical cases in retrospective studies.

Intelligence tests also have limitations. They are obviously restrictive in the range of skills that they assess. As numerous critics have pointed out, intelligence tests place a premium on knowledge gained instructively and, in particular, verbal, declarative knowledge of the type learned in school and in white, middle-class homes. As such, intelligence tests are essentially assessments of the *products* of learning and, especially, of learning those things that are valued by a particular segment of the culture.

Another major problem with intelligence tests, and one that is especially important to the studies surveyed in the earlier chapters, is that they seem to measure different things at different ages. The Bayley Scales of Infant Development, administered at twelve months, and the Wechsler Intelligence Scale for Children, Revised, administered at seven years, share only a small amount of common variance. This immediately provokes a problem in the interpretation of test findings obtained at different ages. Do changes in test scores or in rankings of subjects on test scores represent changes in cognition or changes in what is being measured? No answer to this question is immediately obvious. The theoretical literature on intelligence and cognitive development is not helpful in resolving this issue.

It probably makes the most sense to treat intelligence tests administered in infancy and early childhood as measuring something different from what is measured by those administered at school age. This allows us to examine the relationships between such measures as though they represented different variables. Such a strategy lends some legitimacy to models that treat intellectual skill attained at an early age as a potentially causal variable in predicting intellectual skill attained at a later age.

Given the above point of view, can any generalizations be drawn regarding intellectual development after early brain injury? One clear-cut generalization is that there is at least a rough correlation between the amount of brain damage and later intellectual ability. Various disorders allow some sorts of metric to be established with regard to the extent of brain damage. Microcephaly is a simple illustration of the advantages and disadvantages of using such indices. The measurement of head circumference is a straightforward procedure, and the result can be expressed in standard deviation units above or below a mean value for a particular age or even size of child. In any population that includes pathological subjects, there will be a positive correlation between head size and intelligence (this is also true, but to a lesser extent, in normal populations).

As pointed out in this book and elsewhere (Dorman 1991b), the relationship between head size and intelligence breaks down in some cases of familial microcephaly. This finding actually fits in well with a hypothesis that head size in most pathological cases is related to intelligence because it is an index of the degree of brain damage. If the same relationship between head size and intelligence was found in cases in which no obvious structural brain damage was present, then brain size rather than brain damage would be what is related to intelligence.

Cortical thinning in hydrocephalus is another measure of the extent of brain damage that is related to intelligence. This relationship is not overwhelmingly robust, as it has not always been found. Like head size, the relationship is most straightforward when the cases are most extreme. These are the cases in which the cortical mantle width is thinnest, and in such cases the brain volume has an even stronger relationship with IQ (Shurtleff, Foltz, and Loesser 1973).

The various grades of intraventricular hemorrhage represent degrees of severity that can be translated, at least in a rough fashion, into an index of the extent of the damage. The extension of bleeding into white matter areas is certainly an indication that more of the brain is affected than when the bleeding is confined to germinal matrix tissue. With greater severity, the effects of the hemorrhage are actually secondary because they involve an obstruction of cerebrospinal fluid and hydrocephalus. It seems more unreasonable to argue that this does not represent "more of the brain" being damaged than that it does. The relationship between the severity of IVH and IQ is well documented. A relationship between the extent of brain damage and intellectual impairment is even more convincingly demonstrated when the data on periventricular leucomalacia are added to those on IVH. Periventricular leucomalacia represents an extension of the actual tissue damage into the white matter and as such seems to be even more highly related to intellectual outcome (and physical impairment) than is IVH (Reynolds and Hamilton 1988; Stewart and Hope 1988). Furthermore, bilateral periventricular leucomalacia is associated with greater mental and physical impairment than is unilateral periventricular leucomalacia (Hansen et al. 1989).

In one of the most direct tests of the hypothesis that the amount of brain damage is equal to the amount of cognitive impairment, Levine et al. (1987) used computed tomographic scanning to correlate lesion size and IQ in children with congenital and acquired hemiplegia. The size of the lesion was inversely correlated with Verbal, Performance, and Full-Scale IQ in both congenital and acquired lesions. Nearly all effects of the lesion type or location proved to be secondary to the size of the lesion.

If more of the brain is damaged, then the intellect will be less. The data show this relationship. We should not be surprised. Certainly, Lashley would not have been because he established a similar relationship in rats some sixty years ago (Lashley, 1929). The relationship can best be interpreted as a background limit when examining other relationships. We have no reason to conclude, however, as Lashley did, that there is any incompatibility between this finding and evidence for specific effects of the location of the damage or, for that matter, evidence for plasticity or recovery. On the other hand, by citing the relationship between the extent of the damage and intelligence as a limiting factor, we are saying just that. With enough brain tissue damaged, recovery must be limited and the effects will be generalized.

Language Development

After establishing an overall relationship between the extent of brain damage and intelligence, we must now look at some of the factors that modify this relationship. Two good candidates are that IQ tests are composite measures and thus may obscure more specific effects of damage and that the relationship may depend on the age at which intelligence is assessed.

With regard to specific effects of early brain damage, the question can be asked in two ways: (1) Does early damage to one area of the brain produce different or more or fewer cognitive effects than does damage to another? (2) Is there any selective effect on one or another subset of cognitive abilities regardless of the area of the brain that is damaged? Both of these questions in turn may yield different answers depending on the age at which abilities are assessed.

If we look at school-age outcome, there are two sources of evidence that brain injury can have selective effects. The evidence from genetic disorders is overwhelming with regard to specific cognitive deficits. Williams syndrome and Turner syndrome both comprise clear-cut evidence of impairment in spatial abilities, similar to some focal right-hemisphere lesions in adults. In neither case is it clear what the biological defect really is. Williams syndrome involves an inherited metabolic defect, and Turner syndrome involves a missing X chromosome. Both may affect hormonal influences on the developing nervous system. This, of course, makes it difficult to draw too many conclusions regarding the implications of these disorders. At the least, however, it can be said that visuospatial abilities can be impaired in the developing brain without equal impairment of all cognitive abilities. However, in both disorders, some degree of mental retardation and overall cognitive impairment is involved. It is just that visuospatial abilities are more impaired than other skills.

In some other genetic disorders, such as 47,XYY and Duchenne muscular dystrophy, we find an opposite pattern, with greater impairment of language than of visuospatial abilities. The neurological basis of the cognitive impairment in these disorders is also unclear. However, they too demonstrate persisting selective cognitive impairment, although it is not localizable to any particular anatomical region or age of influence. Of great importance is that these various genetic disorders, taken together, provide evidence of a "double dissociation" between visuospatial and linguistic abilities in the developing brain.

Linguistic abilities and visuospatial abilities evidently can develop with some independence of one another.

Had there been instances of only visuospatial impairment or only language impairment, it would not have been possible to distinguish the situation from one in which some general ability was impaired but more so in one disorder than in another. The reason for this is the familiar resource argument. If two different tasks require different amounts of the same underlying resource (e.g., intelligence, attentional capacity), then the loss of some of that resource may impair one type of task more than the other, leading to an apparent dissociation between the skills required for each. In such cases the dissociation is more apparent than real. One task is simply harder than the other and thus is more impaired by less damage, but they do not require qualitatively different skills.

In the present situation no single resource argument can be made. If one type of task was simply a harder version of the other, we could not find the situation in which impairment was present only or more severely on the supposedly easier task. Thus, these genetic disorders provide convincing evidence that persisting selective impairment in different abilities can date from early childhood.

Do the genetic disorders that involve selective impairment of either visuospatial or language abilities provide evidence against plasticity? After all, there is no evidence that the impairment lessens with age. The answer, however, is no. First, it is not clear that the pathological process is not ongoing (as it is in, for instance, PKU). Second, the impairment in each case is only relatively selective. That is, the overall lower intellect in these disorders implies that the rest of the brain is not functioning at 100 percent efficiency, so its ability to "take over" the more impaired functions may be compromised.

A second area in which selective impairment may be found has been relatively neglected up to this point in our survey. This is the somewhat obvious area of focal cortical lesions. This topic has been neglected because it is not the typical type of early brain damage. However, this is not to say that focal lesions do not occur. As Wigglesworth (1988) pointed out, such lesions are more likely to occur in the full-term brain simply because of the mechanics of cerebral vascular development.

It might seem naive to ask whether early focal lesions result in selective cognitive deficits. After all, it is well known that focal lesions in adults can cause extremely specific deficits, leaving many other cognitive abilities apparently intact. However, the common conception that, as the brain develops, anatomical localization of function becomes progressively "fixed" and that at younger ages it is less fixed (i.e., brain/behavior relationships, at least with regard to localization, are more "plastic") raises the issue of whether focal lesions will produce selective deficits if acquired very early.

The attempt to answer this question has been responsible for a great deal of time and effort on the part of many clinicians and scientists over many years. This is an indication that an answer is not as forthcoming as we might have supposed. There are several reasons for this. First, focal lesions are difficult to verify in living subjects. Even more difficult to verify is that the rest of the brain is intact. In addition, by the time a child is old enough to be examined for, say, language deficits, the lesion is chronic, further events have intervened, and these may involve secondary reactions to the original injury (e.g., seizures).

Subjects with focal lesions have been difficult to recruit and the samples that have been collected have come from different centers and, more important, different years. This last fact has a bearing on not only the outcome measures used and the methods of lesion verification, but also the treatment of the original disorder. A classic example is the observation that most of the evidence for the impairment of language after right-hemisphere lesions comes from the eras preceding the use of antibiotics to reduce systemic infections (Woods and Teuber 1978).

The majority of studies of early focal lesions have centered on the question of whether left-hemisphere lesions impair language development. Although contrast groups often have been composed of children with right-hemisphere lesions, the cognitive task nearly always has been language rather than visuospatial or some other skill. There are probably several reasons for this, although they routinely go unstated. One reason is that groups are often defined in terms of hemiplegia. Such motor impairment creates problems in measuring visuospatial skills, since many measures require drawing ability. Another reason is that, as we shall discuss later, visuospatial ability is often impaired regardless of the site of the lesion, although this could be an artifact, again, of motor impairment. However, hydrocephalus, Williams syndrome, and even cerebral palsy are all syndromes in which visuospatial impairment has been demonstrated on motor-free tasks.

Persisting visuospatial deficits were linked to some anatomical locations in Dennis's studies of both right-hemispherectomy cases and hydrocephalic children with posterior thinning of the cortical mantle

(Dennis 1981; Kohn and Dennis 1974). Children with focal right hemisphere damage show early (before age five) evidence of deficient use of spatial relations in object classification (Stiles-Davis, Sugarman, and Nass 1985) and in drawing ability (Stiles-Davis et al. 1988) and persisting impairment in the perception of spatial orientation and facial recognition (Meerwaldt and van Dongen 1988). Motor skill deficits themselves obviously persist, or we would not have cases of cerebral palsy or hemiplegia. On the other hand, some children apparently recover from motor impairment even when it has been severe enough to warrant a diagnosis of cerebral palsy (Nelson and Ellenberg 1982).

Given these facts, why has the focus been so much on language, rather than motor or visuospatial impairment? Well, motor impairment isn't cognitive impairment, for one thing. Although motor planning *may* be thought of as cognitive, except in higher level tasks such as map route finding, which is impaired in Turner syndrome, it doesn't seem as cognitive as language does. For another thing, since visuospatial abilities are impaired across a variety of disorders, they are presumed to depend on motor exploration (which is often compromised itself in motorically impaired children) and since it can obviously be impaired by subcortical damage, it seems too "fuzzy" to be a candidate for developing theories about plasticity.

Although we must acquiesce with the bulk of the data and consider language as the primary focus of any question regarding early focal injury and persisting cognitive deficits, we also feel compelled to point out a bit of fuzziness in this conceptual framework. Language does have a motor component. As was indicated by our review of perinatal injury studies, much of the evidence for language impairment after such injuries consists of evidence of articulatory impairment, which may be no more "cognitive" than is upper extremity coordination.

Language is confined to neither the left hemisphere nor even the cerebral cortex. The well-known phenomenon of categorical phonetic perception found in both adults and infants may be related more to right- than left-hemisphere processing mechanisms (Molfese 1978; Molfese, Buhrke, and Wang 1985). Some aspects of the visual perception of words that depend on orthographic features also seem to be processed by the right hemisphere (Chiarello 1980). Although controversial, the findings from so-called deep dyslexia cases suggest that some aspects of semantic organization also reside in the right hemisphere (Coltheart 1980).

Generally, it has been concluded that the left hemisphere is required for speech to take place, except in unusual cases of reversed asymmetry. This is not to say that an intact left cortex is sufficient for speech and especially for the production of coherent speech. Crosson (1985) provided a detailed and provocative model of the role of sub-cortical (thalamus, basal ganglia) structures in the production of language. Most intriguing is the role that subcortical pathways, sometimes those likely to be affected by perinatal vascular accidents, have in speech monitoring. Although this is a model of developed language, and not necessarily one that applies to language development, the implication is that language is not localized to any particular anatomical site.

Despite the fact that there is probably no good anatomical reason for assuming that language, at least when conceived as some sort of global skill, would be a victim of selective focal impairment, it is, in fact, what has been most studied. By far the greatest amount of data are available for left-hemisphere lesions, usually collected for different ages of lesion onset and often contrasted to right-hemisphere lesions. These data ought to provide answers to two questions, and perhaps three. The first question relates to whether language impairment depends on the age of lesion onset. The second question relates to whether it matters which hemisphere has the lesion and also if this itself depends on the age of lesion onset. Finally, if follow-up data are collected at a sufficiently distant time from lesion onset, we can ask whether selective language impairment persists and if that too depends on the age of lesion onset.

Woods and Carey (1979) studied twenty-seven patients with left-hemisphere lesions. Eleven had incurred their lesions before their first birthdays and it was "presumed perinatally." Sixteen had incurred their lesions after their first birthdays, with a mean age of lesion onset of 5.7 years. The follow-up evaluation consisted of measures of intelligence and receptive and expressive language on which the lesioned subjects were compared to controls.

Woods and Carey found a striking difference between the early and later lesion groups when the performance of each was compared to that of normal controls. On the various language measures, the later lesioned group performed significantly worse than the normal controls on six of eight tests. Early-lesioned subjects, in contrast, performed more poorly than controls on only a measure of spelling. This seems to be clear evidence that some sort of compensation takes place in the case of early left-hemisphere lesions. Recovery may not be as complete as the results would imply, however, since Woods and Carey also noted that both the early- and late-lesioned groups had lower Verbal IQ scores than did sibling controls.

The finding that less language impairment is present after early left-hemisphere lesions has been replicated several times. In a well-known study, Annett (1973) obtained results that suggested both better preservation of language in subjects with early lesions compared to later lesions and evidence that this might be related to the right hemisphere taking over language dominance from the left. Annett's patients were diagnosed as to the side of injury on the basis of hemiplegia. Eighty-five percent of the patients with left-hemisphere lesions whose onset was after fourteen months and 100 percent with onset after five years showed speech defects. In those subjects with left-hemisphere lesions whose onset was either prenatal or within the first year, only 33 percent showed speech defects. In right-hemisphere lesions, the pattern with regard to age was just the opposite. Speech defects were present in 17 percent of subjects with prenatal lesions, 14 percent of those with perinatal lesions, and none of those with postnatal lesions. Although speech defects were apparent on measures of expressive speech, Verbal IQ differences between groups did not reach significance.

Additional data on hand function showed that the majority of cases with right-hemisphere lesions and speech defects had some impairment of the right hand, indicating that the left hemisphere may also have been affected. Bilateral damage can never be ruled out on the basis of hemiplegia, as illustrated by the case presented by Vargha-Khadem, Watters, and O'Gorman (1985). A six- and one-half-year-old boy with bilateral frontal lesions from birth, verified by computed tomographic scan, showed a left hemiparesis and some trophic changes on the left with perfectly normal right-hand function as well as right handedness.

Annett's data suggest that language may be spared with early left-hemisphere lesions because the right hemisphere is able to take over language abilities at early ages but not later. Annett's findings do not stand in isolation. At least two other studies echoed and even extended her results. Vargha-Khadem, O'Gorman, and Watters (1985) found that, in subjects with left-hemisphere lesions, the incidence of left handedness was greater with earlier age of lesion onset. Their study, like both those of Annett and of Woods and Carey, also found that the earlier the age of lesion onset, the less the impairment of language. Their findings imply a tendency for handedness and language to switch hemisphere in tandem.

The coincidence of hand preference and language dominance residing in the same hemisphere was examined in even greater detail by Satz et al. (1988). They combined data from four samples of patients with left focal brain injury. Speech lateralization was determined by amobarbital injection, dichotic listening, or temporal lobectomy. Subjects were divided into those whose lesion onset was early (less than six years of age) or later (six years or older).

Using the various methods for determining speech laterality, the investigators located speech dominance in the left hemisphere in 41 percent of the subjects with early lesion onset and in 80 percent of the subjects with late lesion onset. Left handedness was present in 62 percent of the subjects with early lesion onset and in 31 percent of the subjects with late lesion onset. Left handedness was present in 22 percent of the early lesion cases who had left hemisphere speech and in 78 percent of the early lesion cases with either right or bilateral speech representation. Bimodal transfer of handedness and speech occurred in 48 percent of the early lesion cases and 9 percent of the late lesion cases. Bilateral speech representation was associated with less transfer of handedness to the left side and was more likely to occur in cases with later, but not extremely late, lesion onset.

A lot of data come out in a rather tidy way in terms of a model of age-limited transfer of both language and handedness from the left to the right hemisphere. The model goes like this: With the earliest lesions, both handedness and speech tend to be transferred to the opposite hemisphere. (In some early lesion cases in which handedness is transferred but speech representation is not, it can be assumed that speech areas are either circumscribed enough not to be affected or that there is some potential for intrahemispheric reorganization.) With somewhat later lesion onset, handedness is less likely to be transferred and speech may be partially transferred, leading to bilateral speech representation. With late lesion onset, neither handedness nor speech is transferred.

The above model, which is really just a description of the results of Satz et al. (1988), hypothesizes an age-related gradient in the likelihood of the transfer of speech from the left to the right hemisphere. The data, when all of the studies are considered, are simply not clear-cut enough to dictate a choice between this model and one of a more circumscribed critical period for speech transfer, such as within the first year, as suggested by the data of Woods and Carey (1979) and Annett (1973).

Aram (1988), reviewing many of the same studies as have been reviewed here, was much less impressed by the data supporting a hypothesis of an age effect on the effects of left-hemisphere lesions on language. Some of her own studies failed to find such an effect (e.g., Aram and Ekelman 1987). However, she herself presented data that provide some support for the age effect hypothesis. Most notably, her data on IQ discrepancies in children with either early (within the first year) or late left- or right-hemisphere lesions indicated that lower Verbal IQ than Performance IQ was found in subjects with late left-hemisphere lesions but not early lesions. Interestingly, she also found that Performance IQ tended to be lower after late right-hemisphere lesions, although late left-hemisphere lesions were associated with a higher Performance IQ than were early left-hemisphere lesions. This latter finding she interpreted as suggesting that early left-hemisphere lesions possibly spare verbal skills at the expense of performance skills, which accords with the hypothesis of interhemispheric transfer of language in the case of early left-hemisphere lesions.

Although appreciating the evidence in favor of a hypothesis that the preservation of speech after early brain injury may be due to inter-hemispheric transfer of speech representation, we must remind ourselves that our original question was whether early brain injury could result in persistent selective deficits in language. The answer to this question is a straightforward yes. Only Woods and Carey (1979) found no persisting language deficits after early left-hemisphere injury. In most instances the percentage of subjects with early injury and persisting language deficits was not trivial. However, the results may be on a continuum, with early lesions causing less language disturbance, which may look like no disturbance if the assessment is either gross or aimed at the wrong aspect of language. For instance, Levine et al. (1987) found that, although Verbal IQ was related to the size of the lesion in both congenital and later acquired lesions, congenital injuries caused less impairment on several Verbal subtests of the WISC-R and on the Peabody Picture Vocabulary Test, Revised. Aram and Ekelman (1987) found no age effects and, what is more surprising, almost no effects at all of either early (before age one) or later unilateral hemispheric lesions on the Revised Token Test. The only effect that they found was that left-hemisphere-lesioned subjects scored worse than did right-hemisphere-lesioned subjects, compared to controls, on those subtests of the Revised Token Test that relied heavily on memory.

It is clear that early focal lesions can produce selective deficits in language (although they may not), that the effects may vary from gross to subtle, and that the age of onset of the lesion seems to be a factor in determining whether or not deficits will be present. Beyond this, it is not possible to make any definitive statement regarding why some lesions produce more or less or no deficit.

Visuospatial Development

Although focal right-hemisphere lesions can produce visuospatial deficits, the relationship to either the site or the age of the injury is less clear than in the case of language. Levine et al. (1987) found no age-of-injury effect when comparing children with congenital versus acquired lesions on visuospatial tasks. It is not clear whether the more confusing findings with regard to early right hemisphere and visuo-spatial deficit are because of the paucity of studies in this area or because the relationships involved are more complex. As mentioned previously, there is clear-cut evidence that right-hemisphere damage in children can produce visuospatial deficits. One of the clearest results is provided by the study of Meerwaldt and van Dongen (1988). Their subjects included six children, eight through fifteen years old, with unilateral right-hemisphere lesions and six children, seven through fifteen years old, with unilateral left-hemisphere lesions. On two tasks of spatial orientation (rod orientation and line orientation) and one of facial recognition, the right-lesion subjects were impaired and the left-lesion subjects were not. Unfortunately, the authors pro-vided no data on the age of onset of the lesions, although most were acquired lesions and it was noted that, in such cases, subjects were tested in the acute phase of their diseases. This would indicate that the age of lesion onset was close to the age at which the child was assessed, in many cases. The seven- to fifteen-year-old age range would fit the late-occurring lesion category in the comparable studies of left-hemisphere lesions and language impairment.

Stiles-Davis, Sugarman, and Nass (1985) found evidence of im-paired spatially based behavior in right hemisphere-lesioned children, two to three years old, all with lesion onset before three months of age. Four children with right-hemisphere lesions were compared to four children with left-hemisphere lesions; the children were of similar age and similar age at lesion onset, and they were also compared to normal controls. Deficits were apparent in the right-lesion group in terms of grouping objects by placing them side by side (as opposed to inside of or on top of). No general deficit in the ability to group objects was observed in the children with right-hemisphere lesions. Furthermore, left-lesion subjects and normal controls showed no evidence that side-by-side grouping was either weakly established or late in developing, indicating a genuine dissociation between this behavior and others in the right-lesion group, rather than an exaggeration of a normal devel-opmental pattern.

The study by Stiles-Davis, Sugarman, and Nass (1985) provides clear evidence of a spatial weakness in children with right- but not left-hemisphere lesions at a very early age. Generalizations from this study should be limited, however, for three reasons. First, the authors mentioned that preliminary data from the same children at older ages suggested that the observed deficits might not be permanent. Second, all of the subjects with right-hemisphere lesions were chosen because they had previously had difficulty with similar tasks, leaving open the question of whether their behavior was typical of children with right-hemisphere lesions. Finally, the authors' own interpretation of the problem encountered by the children with right-hemisphere lesions in grouping on a spatial ("next to") basis was that the use of side-by-side relations represented a more complex problem than did other types of grouping arrangement (e.g., "on" or "in") with regard to which there were no differences between lesion groups. Thus, they suggested that the problem may have lain in the need for integration of "more spatially relevant factors" in grouping side by side, rather than "in the construction of next-to relations per se" (1985, 407). If this is, in fact, the case, then to demonstrate a true spatial deficit it would be required to show that the complexity of the task was not the crucial variable.

Most surprising to us was the normal performance of the left-lesion children. As we will discuss further, visuospatial deficits are common among perinatally injured children with generalized lesions. Aram (1988) found that early left-hemisphere lesions were associated with lower Performance IQ than were late left-hemisphere lesions, suggesting that the transfer of language to the right hemisphere in children with early left-hemisphere lesions might interfere with the development of right hemisphere–based spatial skills. The result of Stiles-Davis, Sugarman, and Nass (1985), although provocative, is a trifle anomalous. Perhaps most important, Stiles-Davis et al. studied spontaneous grouping behavior rather than whether there was a limit to spatial ability. It is not clear that their subjects *could not have* used side-by-side grouping if instructed to do so. Spontaneous use of a behavior may, on the one hand, be a more subtle measure of a deficit and, on the other hand, fail to detect differences in the absolute limits of a skill.

Stiles-Davis et al. (1988) also contributed evidence that early right-hemisphere lesions may interfere with the development of spatial organization skills, whereas early left-hemisphere lesions do not have a similar effect. Their subjects were two five-year-old children with congenital right-hemisphere lesions and two five-year-old children with congenital left-hemisphere lesions. All children had a contralateral hemiparesis and evidence of unilateral injury on computed tomographic scan. Each child was asked to complete drawings of geometric shapes from the Beery Developmental Test of Visuo-Motor Integration, human figure drawings, and a picture of a house. Their drawings were compared to each others' as well as to those of a control group of neurologically normal children who were three and one-half to five years old.

The children with right-hemisphere lesions were markedly inferior to both those with left-hemisphere lesions and the normal controls. There were no differences between the latter two groups. The drawings of the two right hemisphere-lesion children were strikingly lacking in spatial organization. This was more apparent on "free drawings" of a house or a person than in simply copying geometric forms, although the latter was also impaired. In the case of the free drawings, it was clear that the children were aware of the elements that were to be included in the picture, but they simply didn't organize them in a way that had any physical resemblance to real houses or people. The authors remarked on the similarity between the drawing of the right hemisphere-lesion children and that of some adults with focal right hemisphere injury.

This study, like that of Stiles-Davis, Sugarman, and Nass (1985), is noteworthy in finding no obvious deficit in the performance of the two left-hemisphere-lesion children. Again, however, the sample size is small and we have no way of knowing how representative any of the children are of others with similar lesions. Still, both studies provide some tentative evidence for selective effects of early focal right-hemisphere lesions on spatial tasks.

In reviewing our own research and clinical findings, as well as those of others, what is most striking is the consistent finding of greater impairment of visuospatial abilities across a variety of types of early brain injury. This includes hydrocephalus, intraventricular hemorrhage, most infections and toxic disorders, complications associated with prematurity and perinatal injury in general, and most cases of cerebral palsy. The greater effect of early injury on visuomotor and visuospatial skills, rather than on language, has been a sufficiently pervasive phenomenon to prompt some writers to suggest that there is a bias toward preserving language at the expense of other skills in most cases of early injury (Witelson 1987).

Chapter 5 reviewed the large number of studies that found that visuospatial and visuomotor deficits were the most likely outcome of early brain injury resulting from complications of premature birth.

Table 7.1   Mean Scores on Developmental Assessments from Six to Twenty-four Months

Age (mo)	n	Bayley MDI		Bayley PDI	
		Mean	SD	Mean	SD
6	637	93.62	17.94	98.40	19.67
12	455	96.02	20.82	88.33	21.27
24	307	96.56	25.44	87.70	20.42

Note: MDI, Mental Development Index; PDI, Psychomotor Development Index.

Our own data on 307 to 637 prematurely born children, depending on the age of assessment, showed a similar pattern, as is shown in table 7.1.

A drop in psychomotor skills was evident at twelve months and persisted through twenty-four months. At six months the Bayley MDI and PDI were predicted by the same set of medical complications with correlations of approximately the same magnitude with each predictor variable for the two scores. For both the MDI and the PDI, the best predictors, in order of decreasing magnitude, were brain injury, the presence or absence of severe IVH, grade II IVH, grade III IVH, persisting neonatal illness, and being small for gestational age. In the case of both the MDI and the PDI, about one-third of the variability in scores was related to this set of predictors.

The two Bayley scores were correlated .84. By twelve months, however, those variables that continued to be predictors of the mental and motor scores began to diverge. Although the MDI and the PDI from the same age were still highly correlated, the size of the correlation decreased to .64 by twenty-four months. Furthermore, correlations from previous assessments were consistently higher between two mental scores or two motor scores than from one mental to one motor score and vice versa. Using multiple regression procedures, we found that the previous score on the same (mental or motor) scale was a much stronger predictor of current scores than was the alternative (mental or motor) scale. At twelve months, brain injury and persisting neonatal illness continued to be good predictors of both mental and motor scores, but by twenty-four months the only strong correlation between a medical factor and a developmental score was between brain injury and the motor scale.

Forty-eight of our subjects were administered the Beery Developmental Test of Visuo-Motor Integration at age five years. Since this test measures some combination of visuomotor and visuospatial skills, it should have been more highly related to early PDI scores than to MDI scores from the Bayley Scales. In fact, however, the pattern of correlations was just the opposite at six and twenty-four months. At twenty-four months the two Bayley scores were about equally correlated with Beery scores. However, using multiple regression and path analysis, we could show that the twenty-four-month Bayley PDI score was the best predictor of the five-year-old Beery score and that brain injury showed its effect by influencing early mental scale scores and the twenty-four-month PDI score. In fact, if taken by itself, the brain injury factor was nearly as good a predictor of Beery scores as was the twenty-four-month Bayley PDI.

Early brain injury clearly is a good predictor of the development of both overall intellectual ability and, specifically, visuomotor skills. In terms of simple correlations, brain injury is about equally predictive of IQ and visuomotor skill; the size of the correlation between the variables representing more severe IVH and visuomotor skills, however, was about twice that of the IQ. Possibly, IVH specifically lowers visuomotor ability because of its interference with motor pathways. As mentioned in chapter 5, IVH has consistently been associated with greater impairment of motor than mental development.

It is most interesting that even in the small sample of forty-eight children who we assessed at school age, visuomotor ability was considerably more impaired than IQ. WISC-R Full-Scale IQ was only 15 percent of one standard deviation below average, but Beery scores were 74 percent of one standard deviation below average in this group. This makes a great deal of sense in terms of the effects of brain injury and, especially, the hypothesized effects of IVH on visuomotor abilities, since the sample was biased toward a high incidence of IVH.

The data are not as neat as we would have liked them to be. In particular, the lowered Bayley PDI scores relative to MDI scores at twelve and twenty-four months, along with the lower Beery scores at five years, suggest more continuity in visuomotor impairment than is actually the case in our sample. Except at twenty-four months, the MDI scores are actually more highly correlated with Beery scores than are the PDI scores. Oddly enough, within our smaller sample of forty-eight children for whom we had five-year-old Beery scores, there was no discrepancy between Bayley MDI and PDI scores at the younger ages. Thus, the impression of continuity in visuomotor impairment is not borne out by the actual data.

Our sample included children with mild cerebral palsy, as have those of other investigators, although severe cases of cerebral palsy were excluded by us, as they usually have been by others. This raises the question of whether the typical finding of lower scores on visuo-motor tasks simply reflects motoric impairment in a substantial number of subjects in any sample of brain-injured children. Our own data as well as some other suggest that this is not so. In several studies that examined predictors of reading and spelling achievement in children and adolescents with cerebral palsy, we were able to use nonmotoric measures of visual perceptual ability. These proved to be the most impaired abilities in our subjects (Dorman 1987b; Dorman, Hurley, and Laatsch 1984; Dorman, Laatsch, and Hurley 1984).

In a fascinating article entitled "The Oblique Mystique," Rudel (1982) described the difficulty experienced by young children and older, brain-injured children and adolescents in dealing with oblique orientations. The problem occurs in discriminating opposite diagonals, in simply perceiving that a fine wire is present when in an oblique orientation, and in choosing oblique paths on motor tasks. It also occurs in adults with right-hemisphere brain damage. Rudel hypothesized that the accurate perception of oblique orientations may not be "built into" our nervous systems, although vertical and horizontal orientations are. She cited the case of a fifteen-year-old girl with neurological signs of right-hemisphere damage and an inability to dissociate eye movements from head movements (oculomotor apraxia). She was totally disinclined to pursue diagonal paths when walking map routes and was unable to do even simple block designs that involved diagonal patterns. Rudel speculated that her oculomotor disturbance did not allow her to build up the visual experiences that would support perceiving diagonal orientations as aspects of the environment to which she should respond.

Rudel pointed out that, although oblique orientations are not ubiquitous in the natural environment, they do occur in disproportionate numbers on psychological tests; the Raven Progressive Matrices, Block Design from the WISC-R, several designs from the Bender Gestalt, and many of the designs from the Beery Developmental Test of Visuo-Motor Integration are examples. Of course, these are the very tests on which brain-injured children often have difficulty. Whether this means that the deficit seen in brain-injured children is neurological or stems from experiential deprivation, or both, is difficult to say.

Visuomotor or visuospatial deficits may reflect deficits related to either common or different anatomical loci. On the other hand, visuospatial tasks may simply require greater overall brain functioning (whatever that may mean) than do most language tasks. Witelson (1987) suggested this possibility. If we can think of tasks that require more complex integration of more brain functions as those that emerge later in development, then it also fits in with Rudel's observations regarding the perception and orientation of oblique orientations, since these skills, which are required by a number of visuospatial tests, develop late in the normal child.

There are at least two ways to think of typical visuospatial tasks (those found on psychological tests) as being "harder" than language tasks. As Witelson described it, "Rather than language functions taking precedence over spatial functions, it may be that the apparent relative sparing of verbal ability compared to spatial ability following early left-sided lesions is a manifestation of the general effects of brain damage tapped by the visuo-spatial tasks of the Performance IQ" (1987, 177). An alternative explanation is that the same phenomenon is due to "some regions of the right hemisphere maturing later and therefore having greater plasticity to adopt new functions" (1987, 177). The new functions, in this case, would be language ones, which in the uninjured brain are represented in the left hemisphere. In other words, if the right hemisphere matures later than the left, as has been suggested by Yakovlev and Rakic (1966) and Goldman (1972), among others, then the right hemisphere is available to take over normally left-hemisphere functions, but the reverse is not true.

The available data seem to be more supportive of an argument based on visuospatial tasks requiring greater neurological integrity than of an argument based on a differential rate of maturation of the hemispheres. First, much of the evidence for greater impairment of visuospatial than language skills comes from disorders such as toxic influences, IVH, and hydrocephalus that are not usually lateralized to one hemisphere. Second, even in adults with generalized brain injury, Performance IQ is more vulnerable than Verbal IQ (Alexander 1987). Presumably, a maturational argument no longer applies in adulthood, especially since, when left-hemisphere language impairment occurs after adult injury, it tends not to resolve. Finally, even in children who have not shown impairment of Verbal IQ, more sophisticated assessment of language functions has often found deficits, particularly in syntactic comprehension (Kiessling, Denckla, and Carlton 1983; Vargha-Khadem, O'Gorman, and Watters 1985). In those cases of hemispherectomy after early unilateral brain lesions, when syntactic comprehension measures have been used, it would be difficult to say that language was less impaired by left hemispherectomy than visuospatial skills were by right hemispherectomy (Dennis and Whitaker 1976; Kohn and Dennis 1974).

All this is to say that it is not possible to conclude that the higher incidence of visuospatial impairment, as opposed to language impairment, after early brain injury actually reflects anything particularly revealing about brain development. The alternative explanation, which seems simpler to us, is that the tasks usually used to measure visuospatial abilities require more cognitive resources and, presumably, greater brain integrity than the tasks usually used to measure language abilities.

Language and visuospatial skills clearly do not require the same resources (whatever those might be). As we pointed out earlier in this chapter, each can be selectively impaired without equivalent impairment of the other. The likelihood remains, however, that visuospatial tasks often require *more* resources than language tasks. This probably has more to do with the selection of the tasks used to measure each domain than anything else. There is no obvious way to equate language and visuospatial tasks in terms of the resources required to perform them. Age-norming is an attempt to this, but there are many instances where this fails. Reading and spelling are good examples of this. Spelling seems to be more vulnerable to impairment than reading, since most poor readers are also poor spellers but a substantial number of poor spellers are good readers (Fletcher and Satz 1985; Van der Vlugt and Satz 1985). Because this dissociation shows up on tests that are age-normed on the same normative group, one could conclude that the tasks are equivalently difficult for the normal student but not for the impaired child.

It is puzzling that language, for which several innate or very early developing mechanisms for its perception have been identified, would be less vulnerable to perinatal injury. Put somewhat simplemindedly, if specific brain mechanisms for speech perception, for instance, are present at or soon after birth, why would it be so easy for other areas of the brain to assume this function in the case of early left-hemisphere lesions? We have no informed answer to this question (which may be a signal that it is a bad question). Furthermore, there is no reason to think that similar mechanisms do not exist for visuospatial perception. As researchers such as Gelman (1991) have demonstrated, the mechanisms that support the perception of objects, verticals and horizontals, expectations of continuity, inertia, and even primitive number concepts seem to be present very early in life and are possibly innate. These too may be relatively invulnerable to early brain lesions.

The vulnerability of visuospatial tasks to early brain lesions may be based on the selection of tasks that have little functional significance as well as that require widely dispersed brain resources. When language development is assessed, either we measure elementary abilities such as discrimination or articulation or we ask questions about *something*.

The *somethings* are relevant to day-to-day functioning in terms of the vocabulary used, the concepts employed, or the judgments made. If the basic mechanisms for language perception and comprehension survive, then most early childhood and school-age tests assess their products. (It is interesting that the highly sensitive tests of phonemic segmentation, found to be deficient in many reading-disabled children, may not fit this model. Phonemic segmentation seems to be a cognitive-perceptual skill that is not necessary for normal speech processing.)

On the other hand, the relationship of psychometric tests of figure-ground, spatial orientation, figure completion, and block construction to real-life accomplishments is rather suspect. Language-impaired children have trouble communicating, but what do visuospatially impaired children have trouble doing? We can't get too simpleminded here, for if we argue that these tasks are complex and are sensitive to just about any diminution in brain resources, then such children ought to be deficient in any areas that require the integration of a lot of brain functions. They may not be deficient on simple tasks that require visual or spatial perception and that are required for everyday functioning. Ratcliff (1982) pointed out that several "simple" tasks of spatial perception, such as spatial localization, as is involved in visually guided reaching, are probably not even cortically based and are rarely disrupted. Topographical orientation and locomotor route finding most often require bilateral lesions, although they may occur in unilateral right-hemisphere lesions. They may require skills that are different from those involved in spatial tasks in which the person has to deal with rearranging items in a fixed spatial array, like many of the visuospatial tasks on the Wechsler tests (Ratcliff 1982). The impairment in mathematics and social functioning, discussed extensively by Rourke (1987), that is often found in children with poor visuospatial as compared to verbal skills has not been convincingly linked to the visuospatial disturbance itself (see chapter 6). At any rate, it is not clear that the typical visuospatial task that appears on psychological tests is a measure of some sort of basic product that reflects the survival of underlying specific perceptual mechanisms.

We may have developed a technology for assessing difficult and relatively useless cognitive skills in the visuospatial realm. To the extent that this is the case, the basic mechanisms for visual perception and many types of spatial perception may survive just as well as those for language, but our assessment tasks require much more than these basic mechanisms for their accomplishment. This hypothesis receives some support from the studies of hemispherectomy patients who show impairment of higher level (later-developing) visuospatial abilities but not simpler ones, regardless of the hemisphere removed (Kohn and Dennis 1974). Similar conclusions should apply to the development of higher level thought processes in the language area, but these are often not assessed until late school age or adolescence.

As this argument has a high likelihood of being misunderstood, we will restate it a final time in a somewhat different form. Visuospatial tasks are peculiarly sensitive to brain injury. Recent, as yet unpublished, data by Hurley (personal communication) indicate that childhood impairment on visuospatial tasks, as seen in hydrocephalic subjects, is a better predictor of adult ability to master independent living skills than is impairment of verbal intelligence. We suggest that this is because visuospatial tasks are very sensitive to impaired brain functioning and that the type of impairment they measure may produce a deficit in any situation that requires the integration of skills in a complex environment. We also suggest that it is not because such tasks measure a specific perceptual skill that is also required of many real-life tasks that they can predict real-life impairment. Thus, individuals with low Performance IQ, for instance, who cannot learn mathematics or master independent living skills, have their difficulties because real-life tasks are, themselves, complex and require a reasonably intact brain, not because such tasks have a spatial perception component similar to that of those on the Performance section of the Wechsler tests or on measures of judgment of spatial orientation. This is, of course, a testable hypothesis for which we do not, at the moment, have very much convincing evidence.

8

Learning Disabilities after Early Brain Injury

The hypothesis of a "continuum of reproductive casualty" asserts that those types of perinatal brain injury that, in severe forms, result in death or major handicap will, in less severe forms, result in learning and behavior problems (Pasamanick and Knobloch 1961). It makes sense to extend this hypothesis to all types of early brain injury but for our purposes to restrict our attention to learning problems. In fact, we focus on academic learning problems, since motor coordination difficulties, visuospatial deficits, and language deficits have been discussed at length elsewhere. Although some authors tend to lump together attention problems, hyperactivity, and academic learning problems under the rubric "minimal brain dysfunction" (e.g., Nichols and Chen 1981), the data are clearest for academic learning problems and these seem the most "cognitive" of the categories of behavior, so we focus on them.

The data reviewed in the earlier chapters lead, straightforwardly, to several conclusions. If we define an academic learning disability as a level of skill in a generic academic subject (e.g., reading, spelling, or arithmetic) that is substantially lower than would be expected on the basis of one's Full-Scale IQ and in the presence of normal experience and motivation, then academic learning problems occur at above-average rates in subjects with some genetic disorders (e.g., Duchenne muscular dystrophy, sex chromosome abnormalities), congenital disorders (e.g., hydrocephalus), and perinatal brain injury. The type of disability is not the same in each type of disorder and, if all learning disabilities that are presumably caused by such disorders were counted together, they would account for only a fraction of all learning disabilities. Verified genetic, congenital, or perinatal brain disorders are simply too rare to account for the 10–15 percent of all children who have learning disabilities. This means either that the majority of learning-disabled children have a similar, unverified disorder (which seems unlikely) or that some combination of different types of genetic abnormality, inherent variability in the association between IQ and learning aptitude, and some types of later childhood experiences (e.g., head injury, social factors) produces the majority of learning-disabled students (which seems more likely).

Even though the disorders considered in this book may not account for the majority of learning-disordered children, a large proportion of the children with such disorders turn out to be learning disabled. For instance, in our own research with boys who had Duchenne muscular dystrophy, 46 percent had reading disabilities (Dorman, Hurley, and d'Avignon 1988). In our research with prematurely born children at high risk for brain injury, 52 percent were reading disabled and 46 percent were arithmetic disabled. Thirty-two percent of these subjects were disabled in both reading and arithmetic. In children with cerebral palsy, Seidel, Chadwick, and Rutter (1975) found that approximately 50 percent were reading disabled. As reported in chapter 3, mathematical disability is common among hydrocephalic children, but reading disability is not.

Although our own studies have indicated that either verified brain injury or a high risk for it increases the risk for learning disability, this has not been a uniform finding. As pointed out in chapter 5, some studies failed to find an increase in learning disabilities, especially reading disability, in prematurely born children.

We concluded in chapter 5 that, when learning disabilities occur in children at high risk for perinatal brain injury, they are more likely to be in arithmetic than reading and to be associated with other indications of neurological damage. Our own studies found that, although reading disability occurred slightly more often than arithmetic disability in our very high risk sample, arithmetic problems were more clearly predicted by neurological complications, whereas demographic variables such as gender, race, and socioeconomic status were more predictive of reading disability. Children who were disabled in reading only were less cognitively impaired, in terms of IQ scores, than either those disabled in just arithmetic or those disabled in both arithmetic and reading.

Our study of mathematical learning disabilities in prematurely born children confirmed the earlier findings of Klein, Hack, and Breslau (1989) that mathematical disability and visuomotor impairment often go together. Our conclusion, however, was that the association between visuomotor disability and mathematical disability was due to their both being sequelae of early brain injury, but not that visuomotor impairment was causal in producing mathematical disability. The study of reading disability by Gaines (1991) did not use the causal modeling procedures that would allow a similar analysis. However, relationships between reading and either perinatal medical complications or other cognitive variables were not so clear cut as in the case of arithmetic.

Reading Disabilities in Brain-injured Children

In a series of studies, we examined the cognitive variables associated with reading, spelling, and reading disability in neurologically handicapped children. Three of the studies involved children or adolescents with cerebral palsy. Dorman, Hurley, and Laatsch (1984) used nonmotoric cognitive tests, including the WISC-R and portions of the Luria-Nebraska Neuropsychological Battery, to predict reading recognition and spelling achievement in twenty-five adolescents with cerebral palsy. Measures of Verbal IQ and nonverbal auditory perception from the Luria-Nebraska (Rhythm Scale) were the best predictors of both reading and spelling.

   Dorman (1987a) replicated the above finding with another sample of thirty-one adolescents with different forms of moderate to severe cerebral palsy. Their mean Verbal IQ of 88 was in the low-average range. In this study, reading recognition (Wide Range Achievement Test) and reading comprehension (Peabody Individual Achievement Test) were the dependent variables. As a group, the sample was more impaired on both reading tests than on the intelligence measure. The mean standard score in reading recognition was 82 and that in reading comprehension was 67. Cognitive measures used to predict the reading scores included the WISC-R or WAIS-R Verbal IQ and factor scores from the Luria-Nebraska Battery that represented cognitive variables that were not only devoid of any motor component but also uncorrelated with motor measures from the Luria-Nebraska (Golden and Berg 1980a, 1980b) and required no reading. These included measures of verbal production and speech articulation (Word Repetition factor scale), speech sound discrimination (Phonemic Discrimination factor scale), nonverbal auditory perception (Rhythm and Pitch Perception factor scale), and visuospatial perception (Visual Organization factor scale).

The sample of thirty-one subjects was most impaired on the visuospatial measure (standard score of 69) and reading comprehension. They were least impaired on the measures of speech sound discrimination and speech production, both of which were average, except in the case of five athetoid subjects whose speech production scores were severely impaired. The degree of impairment, however, was not a good predictor of reading skill. For both reading recognition and reading comprehension, the best predictors were nonverbal auditory perception and Verbal IQ, in that order. With stepwise multiple linear regression, nonverbal auditory perception and Verbal IQ accounted for 40 percent of the variability in reading recognition scores. Nonverbal auditory perception by itself accounted for 33 percent of the variability in reading comprehension scores.

Although nonverbal auditory perception was not as impaired as visuospatial skills, the former was related to reading, whereas the latter was not. This is somewhat counterintuitive, since typical clinical assessment methods often explain academic difficulties in terms of whatever outstanding weaknesses appear in more basic cognitive skills. In this case, such an interpretation would be incorrect because the substantial weaknesses in visuospatial abilities shown by the students with cerebral palsy were not related to their reading skills. This is similar to our conclusions regarding visuomotor ability and arithmetical ability.

Our finding with regard to the high correlation between nonverbal auditory perception and reading is similar to that found by other researchers with dyslexic readers. Tallal reported deficits in the processing of nonverbal auditory stimuli in children with either language or reading impairment (Tallal 1980a, 1980b; Tallal and Piercy 1973). Byring and Pullianen (1984) used the same measure of nonverbal auditory perception as we used in our studies and found that it was related to dyslexia in adolescents, whereas measures of visuospatial perception were not.

Two studies examined cognitive differences between neurologically impaired poor readers and neurologically impaired good readers (Dorman 1987a; Dorman, Laatsch, and Hurley 1984). In the first study we examined differences on the Luria-Nebraska Neuropsychological Battery. The main differences between the two groups of students, who were mostly children with cerebral palsy, were on the verbal scales.

In a more ambitious study, Dorman (1987a) compared twenty-five neurologically impaired, reading-disabled students to twenty-five neurologically impaired good readers. In both groups, approximately 46 percent were diagnosed with cerebral palsy, 18 percent had spina bifida and hydrocephalus, 32 percent had neuromuscular disorders (mostly Duchenne muscular dystrophy), and 4 percent had incurred head injury. The mean age in both groups was 16.2 years. On the WRAT reading subtest, the reading-disabled group had a mean standard score of 71 and the non-reading-disabled group had a mean standard score of 103. The mean Verbal IQ of the reading-disabled group was 80 and that of the non-reading-disabled group was 92.

The study used three different methods for classifying students into subtypes of reading disability. All three methods, which included those used by Boder (1971, 1973), Doehring (Doehring and Hoshko 1977; Doehring, Hoshko, and Bryans 1979), and Mattis (1978; Mattis, French, and Rapin 1975), had been developed with dyslexic children. We applied them to both our reading-disabled and our non-reading-disabled groups with the aim of answering two questions: (1) Do the same subtypes that have been found in dyslexic children show up in neurologically impaired, reading-disabled children? (2) Do any of the subtypes also exist in neurologically impaired good readers? The answer to the latter question would tell us whether the subtypes were related to reading disability or to neurological impairment. We also hoped to find out whether there was any relationship between the type of neurological disorder and the subtype of reading disability.

The system developed by Boder used each subject's reading level and ability to spell words that he or she could read but were spelled irregularly in terms of phonetic rules or that he or she could not read but were phonetically regular in spelling to diagnose the subject as dysphonetic, dyseidetic, or a mixed dyslexic. Mattis's system utilized an extensive battery of cognitive tests in the areas of visual perceptual ability, auditory sequential information processing, auditory perception and analysis, receptive language, expressive language, and verbal knowledge. Using rules formulated by Mattis (1978), we classified subjects as falling into one or more subtypes based on having an anomic language disorder, articulatory-graphomotor dyscoordination disorder, or visuospatial perceptual disorder.

Doehring's subtype classification system was based on performance on a series of reading or reading-related tasks, some of which were presented on a computer console. Scores representing response latencies were computed for three activities: oral reading, auditory-visual matching, and visual-visual matching. Subtypes were generated using

Q-type factor analysis to classify subjects together who had similar profiles of scores across a total of twenty-two tasks in the three reading areas.

The design of the study was the same for all three subtyping systems. In each case, the reading-disabled subjects were classified into subtypes and then the non-reading-disabled subjects were similarly classified. Using Boder's system, 68 percent of the reading disabled subjects could be classified as either dysphonetic (28 percent), dyseidetic (12 percent), or mixed dyslexic type (28 percent). Eighty percent of the non-reading-disabled subjects fit none of the subtypes. There were no non-reading-disabled mixed types, 8 percent were dysphonetic, and 12 percent were dyseidetic. Since the same number of dyseidetic readers appeared in both the reading-disabled and the non-reading-disabled samples, it was concluded that this reading pattern was not related to having a reading disability.

Mattis's subtyping system was able to classify 84 percent of the reading-disabled subjects but also classified 64 percent of the non-reading-disabled subjects. Fifty-two percent of the non-reading-disabled subjects fell into the pure visuospatial perceptual disorder category. However, only 12 percent of the reading-disabled subjects fit this category. Reading-disabled subjects most often had a pure anomic-language disorder (36 percent) or a mixed anomic-language disorder and visuospatial perceptual disorder (28 percent). Sixty-eight percent of the reading-disabled subjects had an anomic-language disorder alone or in combination with another type of disorder, but this was true of only 8 percent of the non-reading-disabled subjects. Visuospatial perceptual disorder occurred alone or in combination with another type of disorder in 44 percent of reading-disabled subjects and 60 percent of non-reading-disabled subjects. It was clear that anomic-language disorder was related to having a reading disability, whereas visuospatial perceptual disorder was not. Interestingly, there was a fairly strong relationship between the type of neurological disorder and the subtype. Nearly all of the subjects with cerebral palsy had a visuospatial perceptual disorder, and most of the reading-disabled subjects with neuromuscular disorders had a pure anomic-language disorder. This latter finding was similar to that in our more in-depth analysis of cognitive abilities in subjects with Duchenne muscular dystrophy, among whom about half of the children had this disorder (Dorman, Hurley, and d'Avignon, 1988).

Using Doehring's system for subtyping subjects based on their oral reading and visual matching behavior, we were able to generate four subtypes in the reading-disabled sample, which included 64 percent of the subjects. Five subtypes were generated in the non-reading-disabled sample, encompassing 76 percent of the subjects. There were no similarities between the subtypes generated in the two samples, however. In the reading-disabled group, three of the subtypes were identical to those reported by Doehring et al. (1981) in dyslexic readers. These included a "sequencing deficit" subtype, an "oral reading deficit" subtype, and an "association deficit" subtype who were poor on auditory-visual matching. The fourth subtype in the reading disabled subjects was considered artifactual.

Only two of the subtypes in the non-reading-disabled sample could be interpreted as making any particular sense with regard to reading skills. One group was very good at reading nonsense syllables and at matching auditory and visual syllables and words. They were relatively poor at oral reading of real words and auditory-visual matching of letters. This subtype seemed to represent good phonetic but poor whole-word readers, a pattern of skills that evidently did not lower their overall level of reading achievement. The second interpretable subtype consisted of subjects who were quite adequate on all tasks except visual matching of complex mixed upper- and lower-case letter stimuli. This subtype was interpreted as representing a "visual-perceptual deficit" group. Since they were good readers, this type of deficit did not seem to impair their reading achievement. There was no obvious association between the type of neurological disorder and any of the subtypes.

Overall, we can say clearly that reading-disabled children with diagnosed neurological disorders show the same patterns of reading impairment as dyslexic children without obvious neurological disorders. Consistently, in this study and in our previous studies with children with cerebral palsy, we found that visuospatial impairment is a common outcome after perinatal brain injury but is not related to reading skill, at least by the time of adolescence (it could be more related to reading at younger ages).

One of our most interesting findings was evidence of visual-perceptual impairment on reading-related tasks themselves, as in matching visually complex letter sequences or in recalling irregular spelling patterns in familiar words (the dyseidetic pattern) in children who achieve normal reading levels on formal tests. This implies that visual perceptual deficits extend to the reading task itself but do not limit overall reading achievement. Word-finding problems (anomia), general language competence, and phonic skills seem to be crucial variables in determining reading achievement. This conclusion is no different from that reached by the majority of researchers in the area of dyslexia. Our results imply that there is no reason to invoke a different theory of reading impairment for dyslexic readers and neurologically impaired poor readers. Questions do remain, however, as to why the skills required for reading are so often impaired in neurologically abnormal children and why they are impaired in some but not others.

Of equal interest to us is that our studies of reading disability yielded a result provocatively similar to what we found in our study of mathematical learning disability in prematurely born children. In both instances we found a high incidence of visuospatial or visuomotor impairment along with academic learning disabilities. With regard to both reading and arithmetic, however, it appeared that both the visual perceptual disability and the academic learning disability were likely outcomes of perinatal injury, but we could find no evidence that the academic disability was related to the visual perceptual disability.

Subtypes of Neurologically Impaired and Nonneurologically Impaired Poor Readers

We attempted to extend our study of the similarities between neurologically impaired children with learning disabilities and more "garden variety" learning-disabled children by making a more direct comparison of the two groups. Our sample consisted of forty neurologically impaired children and forty children without neurological impairment. Within each group, half of the subjects had a reading disability, defined as having a WRAT reading standard score 10 or more points below the Verbal, Performance, or Full-Scale IQ on the WISC-R or WAIS-R. One-half of the subjects did not meet the criteria for a reading disability. None of the subjects was retarded.

Our neurologically impaired subjects all came from a school for handicapped children. In the reading-disabled group were six children with spina bifida and hydrocephalus, seven with Duchenne muscular dystrophy, six with cerebral palsy, and one with head injury. Their mean age was 15.5 years. In our non-reading-disabled group were ten children with spina bifida with hydrocephalus, four with Duchenne muscular dystrophy, four with cerebral palsy, one with a rare neuromuscular disorder, and one with a head injury. Their mean age was 14.7 years.

Our non–neurologically impaired subjects were all drawn from a private clinic for children with school problems. The reading-disabled group were all male and had a mean age of 12.8 years. The non-reading-disabled group were all academic underachievers. Sixteen were male and their mean age was 11 years.

We were interested in whether the subjects' cognitive abilities would be more related to their neurological status or their reading disability status. We chose to use the WISC-R or WAIS-R factor scores in verbal comprehension, spatial organization, and freedom from distractibility and the WRAT reading, spelling, and arithmetic scores to group the subjects based on similar patterns of cognitive and academic skills. The crucial question was whether those subjects with reading problems would show common patterns of cognitive and academic abilities, regardless of whether or not they had a neurological disorder. This was a broad question, and it was conceivable that we might find some types of neurological disorder in which reading-disabled subjects were similar to non–neurologically impaired reading-disabled subjects and some types of neurological disorder in which they were not. It also was possible that some non–neurologically impaired reading-disabled subjects would look like neurologically impaired reading-disabled children and some would not. The answers to these questions would give us a clue as to how many varieties of reading disability existed and therefore needed explanation. Our non-reading-disabled subjects were simply controls for the presence of a neurological disorder and for low academic achievement.

To establish subtypes, we used the method of cluster analysis. The Statistical Package for the Social Sciences (SPSS) was used to group subjects. Clustering was based on a similarity measure (cosine) because distance measures were more likely to reflect differences in profile elevations than profile patterns. To avoid exaggeration of the influence of any given measure on the clustering algorithm, we converted all scores to standard scores based on the mean and standard deviation of the sample as a whole. To ensure that the clustering solution was not an artifact of the clustering method being used, we conducted the analysis twice using two different methods: average and complete linkage. With both methods, we used a four-cluster solution to analyze the data. Because the clustering solution allows at least one cluster less than the number of variables used for computing the clusters and we used six test scores, we analyzed three-, four-, and five-cluster solutions. We decided that any solution that yielded a cluster with fewer than ten subjects was yielding too few subjects; using both methods, this resulted in a four-cluster solution.

The two clustering methods produced very similar results. Clusters 3 and 4 were essentially identical between the two methods, with only

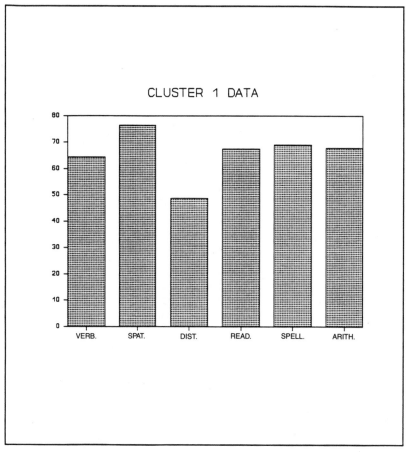

Figure 8.1   Profile of intellectual factor and academic achievement standard scores for cluster one (*n* = 24). *VERB.*, verbal comprehension; *SPAT.*, spatial organization; *DIST.*, freedom from distractibility; *READ.*, reading score; *SPELL.*, spelling score; *ARITH.*, arithmetic score.

one of forty-four subjects not being classified similarly using either method. Clusters 1 and 2 showed some overlap, particularly with subjects in cluster 2 often classified as belonging to cluster 1 using the alternative clustering method. This was the least reliable of the clusters using this criterion. We chose to analyze the composition of the clusters formed by using the average linkage method.

The profile of mean test scores for cluster 1 is shown in figure 8.1. All of the scores were below average, with somewhat higher scores on the spatial organization factor and lower scores on the freedom from distractibility factor. Of the twenty-four subjects who fell into this cluster, fifteen were from the neurologically impaired reading-disabled group, seven were from the non–neurologically impaired reading-disabled group, and two were neurologically impaired good readers. Among the neurologically impaired subjects, seven had spina bifida and hydrocephalus, seven had muscular dystrophy, two had cerebral palsy, and one had a rare neuromuscular disorder. This is a reading disability subtype that occurs more often in neurologically impaired subjects, especially those with either spina bifida and hydrocephalus or muscular dystrophy and less often those with cerebral palsy.

Cluster 2 contained eleven subjects. The profile of test scores for this cluster is shown in figure 8.2. These are clearly subjects with good verbal comprehension abilities and severely impaired spatial organization skills. All but two of the subjects, one reading disabled and one not, were neurologically impaired. Five of the neurologically impaired subjects were reading disabled, and four were not. Of the nine neurological cases, seven had cerebral palsy and one each had spina bifida and hydrocephalus or muscular dystrophy. This subtype was not particularly related to reading disability, since nearly one-half of the subjects were good readers. Primarily, it represented the type of severe visuospatial disability seen in many cases of cerebral palsy.

Cluster 3 contained fourteen subjects. The profile of scores for this cluster is shown in figure 8.3. They achieved high scores on the verbal comprehension factor and, especially, on spatial organization. They scored much lower on the freedom from distractibility factor and were impaired in all academic skills. Twelve of the fourteen subjects were from the non–neurologically impaired reading-disability group. Two subjects (one with muscular dystrophy and one with spina bifida and hydrocephalus) were from the non-reading-disabled neurologically impaired group. This cluster was nearly a pure reading-disability group. The children were generally very bright but significantly impaired in all academic subjects. This pattern does not seem to characterize neurologically impaired poor readers.

Cluster 4 contained thirty-one subjects. The profile of test scores for this cluster is shown in figure 8.4. Scores were average on all tests. None of the reading-disabled subjects fell into this group, which contained twelve neurologically impaired subjects and nineteen non–neurologically impaired subjects. The majority of neurologically impaired subjects (seven) had spina bifida and hydrocephalus. Two

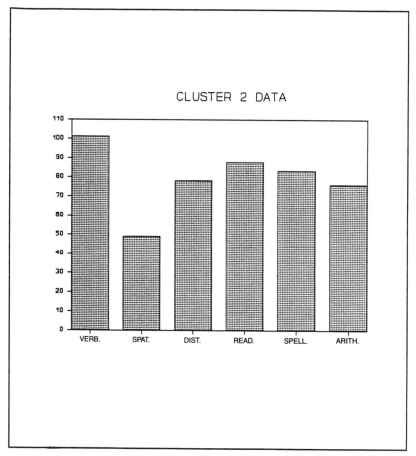

CLUSTER 2 DATA

Figure 8.2   Profile of intellectual factor and academic achievement standard scores for cluster 2 ($n = 11$).

had cerebral palsy, two had muscular dystrophy, and one had head injury.

We concluded from the results of this study that, using WISC-R or WAIS-R factor scores and WRAT achievement scores, reading-disabled subjects show any of three patterns of cognitive abilities. A pattern of scores that indicated mild overall cognitive impairment with the least impairment in visuospatial abilities and the greatest impairment in language and freedom from distractibility, with mild academic impairment relative to IQ, characterizes some reading-disabled children who have no other evidence of neurological disorder. This

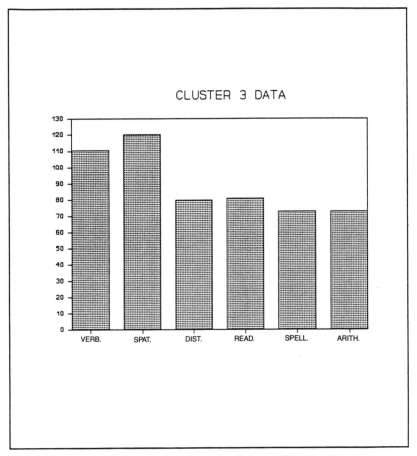

Figure 8.3   Profile of intellectual factor and academic achievement standard scores for cluster 3 (n = 14).

pattern is also found in neurologically impaired children with either spina bifida and hydrocephalus or Duchenne muscular dystrophy; it is rarely found in cerebral palsy. As we pointed out in chapter 3, severe reading disability is not a prominent finding in spina bifida and hydrocephalus, although mathematical skills are often impaired. Evidently, when it does occur, it reflects some reversal of the more typical pattern of impaired visuospatial abilities relative to language. The children with Duchenne muscular dystrophy showed a pattern of abilities that has been found in other studies. Our own research linked this pattern to reading problems and pointed out its similarity to some types of dyslexia (Dorman, Hurley, and d'Avignon 1988).

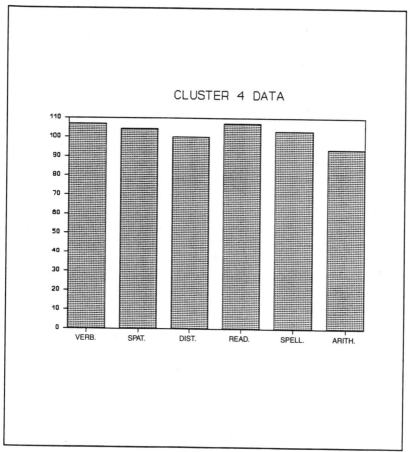

Figure 8.4 Profile of intellectual factor and academic achievement standard scores for cluster 4 ($n = 31$).

The impairment in reading, and in fact in all academic skills, shown by the children in this cluster seems hardly surprising, given their intellectual abilities. The discrepancy between their IQ and their achievement scores seems to be due to their strength on the spatial organization factor, which would have raised their Performance IQ high enough to meet our criterion for having a reading disability. This pattern characterized more than one-third of our non–neurologically impaired poor readers. It is similar to patterns identified by Mattis (1978) and Petrauskas and Rourke (1979). In discussing brain abnormalities in dyslexic subjects, Galaburda (1989) pointed out that left hemisphere-based language skills should be more impaired than right hemisphere-based visuospatial skills because of the evidence of more disorganized development of the left hemisphere.

It may be important that, in this study, our non–neurologically impaired poor readers resembled children with genetic or congenital neurological disorders but not those with perinatal injuries. It offers little support for the hypothesis that subtle perinatal brain injury is a source of learning disabilities in children without other evidence of neurological handicap. Genetic models might be a more fruitful source for theorizing.

Subjects with perinatal injury (i.e., those with cerebral palsy) clustered together, whether or not they had a reading problem. Their most outstanding cognitive characteristic was severe visuospatial impairment. This has been a repeated finding in our research. The majority of children with cerebral palsy are impaired in visuospatial abilities, but this does not differentiate those who read well from those who do not. Visuospatial impairment is strongly associated with perinatal injury, but its relevance to academic skill development remains to be demonstrated.

The majority of reading-disabled, non–neurologically impaired subjects formed a cluster nearly by themselves. We have some worry that this may partly reflect simply differences in general intellectual ability that characterized our groups to begin with. Nevertheless, the pattern of visuospatial skills being stronger than verbal skills, more extreme impairment in freedom from distractibility, and severe academic deficits is one that many researchers have reported for learning-disabled children (Kaufman 1979). The pattern is similar to that found in cluster 1, but the children are brighter and the discrepancy between their intelligence and their academic achievement is more dramatic. Of course, this is the subgroup of learning-disabled children for which no particular explanation of their disability is forthcoming.

In one sense, the fact that our non-reading-disabled subjects who fell into cluster 4 showed no cognitive or academic impairment whatsoever is hardly surprising. On the other hand, few neurologically impaired children other than those with spina bifida and hydrocephalus fit this pattern. Thus, especially in the case of cerebral palsy, no cognitive impairment may be unusual after a neurological disorder (however, our cerebral palsy subjects were all fairly severely handicapped and thus may have had more cognitive impairment than less severe cases).

The non–neurologically impaired good readers were all poor students. They were chosen as a control group because their academic difficulties might signal some other type of cognitive impairment (e.g., attention deficit disorder) that might or might not have something in common with the types of cognitive impairment found in the reading-disabled children. In fact, they were not cognitively impaired at all, so far as we could tell. If we favored diagnosis by default, we would say that they must be motivationally impaired. Of course, we really have no idea why they were not achieving well.

Our study had some serious limitations. The initial groups of subjects differed in terms of age, IQ, and gender. The numbers of subjects with different neurological disorders were not the same in the reading-disabled and non-reading-disabled groups. It is questionable whether subjects with spina bifida and hydrocephalus or with head injury should have been included at all. Especially the former group do not ordinarily have reading disabilities. Still, some of the relationships made sense in terms of our earlier findings, particularly in the case of subjects with cerebral palsy.

We must raise a note of caution regarding subtyping studies, in general. We have summarized the results of studies that used various methods for grouping subjects together. Some relied on reading behavior (Doehring's system), some on reading-spelling patterns (Boder's system), some on associated cognitive deficits (Mattis's system), and some, like the study reported above, on intelligence and achievement test patterns. Dorman (1988) examined the question of whether the subtypes produced by these various methods are related to one another. Using neurologically impaired poor readers and five different methods for subtyping the same sample, he asked whether subjects who were classified into a subtype using one method were any more likely to be classified into any particular subtype using another method. The answer, unfortunately, was generally no. When relationships between subtyping methods did exist, they tended to be between two methods that used similar behaviors as the basis for subtyping subjects. That is, some relationships existed between systems that were based on using associated cognitive abilities and some relationships existed between systems that were based on using reading behaviors, but nearly no relationships related a cognitive subtype to a reading behavior subtype.

This is not a healthy finding for the whole enterprise of trying to "explain" learning disabilities on the basis of patterns of cognitive deficits. On the other hand, it is conceivable that more relationships between cognitive abilities and academic deficits would be evident if the subjects being studied were less cognitively impaired (i.e., non–neurologically impaired dyslexic subjects). A difficulty with the subjects in our studies has been that, because of their neurological disorders, they may show all sorts of cognitive deficits, only some of which have anything to do with why they can't read or do math. The difficulty cannot be placed solely on the insensitivity of the cognitive measures being used. This may be true in the case of studies that use IQ tests as the primary measures of cognition. However, Dorman (1988) used sixteen neuropsychological tests in addition to the subtests from the WISC-R to establish cognitive subtypes.

At any rate, it is probably wiser to think of most subtyping research as a method for showing that some children are alike in either their cognitive abilities or their academic skills. The reason for their similarity will remain a mystery unless other extra test variables can be related to the subtypes. Our hypothesis that some children are alike because they have similar types of brain damage remains a hypothesis, but one that has some partial support.

Conclusions

We are able to draw a few, fairly simple-minded conclusions from the research cited in this chapter and elsewhere in this book. First, some types of neurological disorder in children are associated with a high incidence of academic learning problems. Mathematical disabilities are found in children with hydrocephalus and in children with perinatal brain injury. Reading disabilities occur at a high rate in subjects with Duchenne muscular dystrophy and in those with perinatal brain injury. It remains unclear whether, in the absence of any other evidence of neurological impairment, perinatal injuries can affect *only* academic learning. The most common cognitive deficit after perinatal injury is visuospatial impairment. Children with reading problems but no evidence of brain injury seldom are impaired in visuospatial abilities. In children with perinatal brain injuries, there is no evidence that their visuospatial impairment contributes to either their reading or their mathematical disabilities.

Children who have trouble learning to read and who have some type of brain impairment (e.g., hydrocephalus, perinatal injury, muscular dystrophy) are usually impaired in both auditory perception and overall language ability. Some non–neurologically impaired poor readers show this same pattern. Many non–neurologically poor readers do not show this pattern. Instead, they are not impaired in overall language abilities, at least as measured by the WISC-R. We do not know what their impairment is. They perform poorly, as a group, on the freedom from distractibility measure from the WISC-R, but it is not clear what abilities this factor measures. They may have difficulty with auditory perception, either in processing rapid acoustic stimuli, whether verbal or nonverbal, or in phonemic segmentation, since both of these skills have been found to be deficient in many poor readers (Bradley and Bryant 1978; Liberman et al. 1977). In our study of Duchenne muscular dystrophy (Dorman, Hurley, and d'Avignon 1988), we found a small number of subjects in whom phonemic segmentation and reading were both severely impaired but Verbal IQ was not. However, other language skills, most notably naming, were also impaired, which seems to be true of many poor readers (Mattis 1978; Wolf 1984).

Can early brain injury affect *only* the development of academic skills? The question probably makes no sense if we lump together all sorts of brain disorder. We can rephrase it. Do any known genetic disorders affect only academic skills? No . . . maybe. The question may ask for something that is unreasonable to expect. Since there is no reason to suppose that reading per se is old enough or important enough, in an evolutionary sense, to make it likely to be an innate module in Fodor's (1983) sense, it makes more sense to assume that this skill develops from some more basic cognitive/perceptual abilities. Therefore, some other abilities ought to be deficient in cases of reading disability. However, these other abilities may themselves be genetically determined in some specific way (i.e., in more than in the sense that everything is genetically determined). Here, now, there is some positive evidence. It comes from two sources. Genetic studies of reading disability by DeFries, Fulker, and LaBuda (1987) and Olson et al. (1989) found significant heritability for reading recognition, spelling, and WISC-R Digit Span in families of dyslexic readers. This is the same group of tests, among others, that show impairment in many reading-disabled children, including our own samples of non–neurologically impaired poor readers. Olson et al. (1989) found that phonological coding, measured by nonword reading, was strongly heritable and was the major factor contributing to the heritability of reading disability in the same sample of monozygotic and dizygotic twins used by DeFries, Fulker, and LaBuda (1987). Phonemic segmentation was the major cognitive contributor to nonword reading and was the primary heritable component underlying that skill. Interestingly, word reading by detecting orthographic similarities in the visual presentation of words was not inherited.

An inherited deficit in phonological coding may be common to more than one genetic type of reading disability. Pennington et al.

(1987) found that dyslexic subjects whose dyslexia seemed to be linked to chromosome 15 and dyslexic subjects who were not linked to this chromosome both showed similar deficits in phonological coding. This muddies the water somewhat. However, as Pennington and Smith (1988) pointed out, it may be that different genetic influences can lead to a cognitive phenotype that is common to most, if not all, genetically based dyslexic subjects.

About one-half of the subjects with Duchenne muscular dystrophy offer another avenue for viewing reading disability from a genetic basis. Duchenne muscular dystrophy is not a "clean" disorder in the sense of affecting only reading, but it is cleaner that most. Put simply, what is required in a genetic disorder is not that any or every cognitive ability be impaired, including academic skills, but rather that the cognitive and academic deficit be circumscribed, so it can be argued that specific deficit, not a generalized impairment, is inherited. This is more or less true of Duchenne muscular dystrophy. Overall IQ is usually low-average, with average Performance IQ and low-average Verbal IQ. This seems to represent two subgroups of cases: one with equal and unimpaired Verbal and Performance IQ and the other with impaired Verbal IQ. This is especially true of older children (Dorman, Hurley, and d'Avignon 1988).

About one-half of the subjects with Duchenne muscular dystrophy are reading disabled (Dorman, Hurley, and d'Avignon 1988; Liebowitz and Dubowitz 1981). Generally, but not always, these are the same children with low Verbal IQ. The reading-disabled subjects are also impaired in spelling and usually less so in arithmetic. Most striking, however, are their deficits in phonemic segmentation, phonetic reading, and naming. In fact, not only are their scores similar to each other on tests of these functions but also they make very similar errors, suggesting a common deficit (Dorman, Hurley, and d'Avignon 1988). Both their patterns of deficient scores and their error patterns are similar to those that have been identified in dyslexic subjects (Wolf 1984). It seems that Duchenne muscular dystrophy represents a disorder in which not only neuromuscular disease but also dyslexia is inherited. The main complication with this hypothesis is that half of the cases, with equivalent neuromuscular involvement, do not exhibit dyslexia. Thus far there has been one, not two genes identified as responsible for Duchenne muscular dystrophy. This is the gene at the p21 location on the X chromosome. The most likely explanation for this is that the muscular dystrophy gene is not the dyslexia gene, but that the two are close to each other on the X chromosome.

Alternatively, of course, it is possible that what looks like two groups of patients, in terms of their cognitive abilities, is just one group with differing degrees of impairment. If this is the case, then the sources of the neuromuscular impairment and the cognitive impairment are likely to be the same. This has always presented a puzzle in the case of Duchenne muscular dystrophy, for it was never clear what could commonly impair both neuromuscular and intellectual functioning. The discovery of dystrophin as the gene product that is deficient in Duchenne muscular dystrophy offers some suggestive possibilities, because dystrophin is also present in the brain, although its role is not known. Kakulas (1992) suggested that dystrophin might play a role in neuronal migration, leading to the migrational errors found in Duchenne patients by Rosman and Kakulas (1966). Whether or not this is the case, it seems clear that there is some genetic link between Duchenne muscular dystrophy and dyslexia.

Thus far we have discussed reading or, at most, reading and spelling. What about mathematics? There has been much less theorizing regarding the possible genetic basis for mathematical disabilities. We know of no genetic disorder in which mathematics is particularly affected in the absence of overall cognitive impairment. On the other hand, evidence from studies of very young infants by Gelman (1991) suggests that the tendency to respond to objects in terms of their number may be innate. This would suggest that we inherit a behavioral response tendency that may provide support for the later development of mathematical ability. How specific this tendency may be on a genetic or neurological basis is unclear, as is the extent to which later mathematical skills build on such early behavioral responses.

With regard to perinatal brain injury, we can ask a question similar to that we asked with regard to genetic disorders. Is there any evidence that perinatal brain injury affects the development of *only* academic skills? Again, we should not be unreasonable and expect virtually no evidence of cognitive impairment, since some cognitive skills ought to be related to academic ability. Still, it is conceivable that the development of academic skills requires such complex integration of more basic abilities or their precise application that very mild deficits do not show up on simpler cognitive tasks.

In fact, there is some evidence that academic skills can be impaired without overall cognitive abilities also being impaired. In our own studies of arithmetic and reading disabilities after premature birth, we found that about half of the sample had one or the other or both disabilities without equivalent impairment of intellectual ability. We must hasten to say that this does not mean that other cognitive abilities were unimpaired. A child with an IQ of 75, for instance, would be defined as disabled in an academic skill if his or her academic achievement level was below 60. However, it would be difficult to say that he or she was not cognitively impaired. In fact, we found that both arithmetic and reading disability were present in groups whose IQ scores did not differ from those of children without such disabilities. Especially with mathematical disability, our results must be considered tentative. There were, in fact, large differences in Performance and Full-Scale IQ between those children with mathematical disabilities and those without. However, the large amount of variability in the scores and the small sample size precluded these differences from being statistically significant. In the case of reading disability, however, there was no indication of differences in IQ between the reading-disabled and non-reading-disabled students.

Even in the case of mathematical disability, the results of our path analyses based on multiple regression indicated that early medical problems and developmental assessments were more highly related to the presence and type of arithmetic disability than were later IQ measures. Thus, with both reading and mathematics, specific disabilities may be present without overall intellectual impairment. Assessments of early development detect the precursors to these later academic disabilities by being more sensitive than some later IQ tests are to the effects of the brain injury associated with prematurity.

In terms of any real insight into either the brain or cognitive mechanisms that determine the development of academic skills, neither our own studies nor those done by others on groups of brain-injured children provide much evidence. As we conceptualize it, the first, most general question to be answered is whether some types of early brain impairment interfere with specific cognitive skills that later prove crucial for one or another type of academic skill or whether the interference is more generalized, perhaps in attentional factors or something equally non-domain specific, and the development of academic skills simply requires a higher development of this or these generalized abilities. The second question is whether whatever is impaired is more or less localized in the brain.

The evidence that, as in our own studies, both mathematics and reading were much more often impaired than only one or the other implies that some thing or things general are impaired and that they interfere with the development of academic skills more than with general cognitive development. The presence of some children with deficits in only one or the other skill, however, suggests that there also may be specific abilities related more to arithmetic or to reading that can be impaired more or less by themselves. After all, we did observe a double dissociation between reading and arithmetic. Furthermore, that we could predict such specific disabilities with reasonable accuracy from early childhood data adds more weight to the argument that such specific academic deficits are not just random occurrences or measurement error.

We have gone about as far as we can in either drawing conclusions or theorizing about cognitive development after early brain injury. The insights and information that the current knowledge in this field gives us are more clinically useful than theoretically illuminating. In the field of adult brain injury and cognitive neuropsychology, there is a rich interplay between the insights gained from clinical cases and that gained from studies of normal cognitive functioning. At some point we will achieve a similar state of affairs with regard to the development of cognitive skills. Cognitive mechanisms and brain-behavior relationships are a lot harder to pin down during the age of rapid development of both. Our own clinical approach to these issues has generally ignored most of the current work in either neuroscience or cognitive development. It is still very hard to link the subject matters of these two fields of study, even though both are perpetually exploding with new data and theories. We hope that we have provided an up-to-date assessment of the current findings in an area that may eventually contribute to a better understanding of neurocognitive development.

References

Abel, E. L. 1984. *Fetal Alcohol Syndrome and Fetal Alcohol Effects*. New York: Plenum Press.

Abercrombie, M. L., Lindon, R. L., and Tyson, M. C. 1964. Associated movements in normal and physically handicapped children. *Developmental Medicine and Child Neurology* 6:573–580.

Adams, M. M., Erickson, J. D., Layde, P. M., and Oakley, G. P. 1981. Down's syndrome: Recent trends in the United States. *Journal of the American Medical Association* 246:758–760.

Ahmann, P. A., Lazzara, A., Dykes, F., Brann, A. W., and Schwartz, J. F. 1978. IVH: Incidence and outcome. *Annals of Neurology* 4:186–189.

Alexander, D., Walker, H. T., and Money, J. 1964. Studies in direction sense: I. Turner's syndrome. *Archives of General Psychiatry* 10:337–339.

Alexander, M. P. 1987. The role of neurobehavioral syndromes in the rehabilitation and outcome of closed head injury. In H. S. Levin, J. Grafman, and H. M. Eisenberg (Eds.), *Neurobehavioral Recovery from Head Injury*, pp. 191–205. New York: Oxford University Press.

al-Qudah, A. A., Kobayashi, J., Chuang, S., Dennis, M., and Ray, P. 1990. Etiology of impairment in Duchenne muscular dystrophy. *Pediatric Neurology* 6:57–59.

Als, H., Duffy, F. H., and McAnulty, G. B. 1988. Behavioral differences between preterm and full-term newborns as measured with the APIB system scores: I. *Infant Behavior and Development* 11:305–318.

Amiel-Tison, C. 1973. Neurologic disorders in neonates associated with abnormalities of pregnancy and birth. *Current Problems in Pediatrics* 3:3–37.

Amin-Zaki, L., Elhassani, S., Majeed, M. A., Clarkson, T. W., Doherty, R. A., and Greenwood, M. 1974. Intrauterine methylmercury poisoning in Iraq. *Pediatrics* 54:587–595.

Anderson, E., and Spain, B. 1977. *The Child with Spina Bifida*. London: Methuen.

Annett, M. 1973. Laterality of childhood hemiplegia and the growth of speech and intelligence. *Cortex* 9:4–33.

Antonini, A., Berlucchi, G., and Lepore, F. 1983. Physiological organization of callosal connections of a visual lateral suprasylvian cortical area in the cat. *Journal of Neurophysiology* 49:902–921.

Apgar, V. 1953. A proposal for a new method of evaluation of the newborn infant. *Current Research in Anaesthesia and Analgesia* 32:260.

Aram, D. M. 1988. Language sequelae of unilateral brain lesions in children. In F. Plum (Ed.), *Language, Communication and the Brain*, pp. 171–197. New York: Raven Press.

Aram, D. M., and Ekelman, B. L. 1987. Unilateral brain lesions in childhood: Performance on the revised token test. *Brain and Language* 32:137–158.

Arnold, R., and Yule, W. 1985. The psychological characteristics of infantile hypercalcemia: A preliminary investigation. *Developmental Medicine and Child Neurology* 27:49–59.

Astbury, J., Orgill, A. A., Bajuk, B., and Yu, V. Y. H. 1986. Sequelae of growth failure in appropriate for gestational age, very low birthweight infants. *Developmental Medicine and Child Neurology* 28:472–479.

Aylward, G. P., Verhulst, S. J., and Bell, S. 1988. The early neuropsychologic optimality rating scale (ENORS-9): A new developmental follow-up technique. *Developmental and Behavioral Pediatrics* 9:140–146.

Babson, S. G. 1970. Growth of low-birthweight infants. *Journal of Pediatrics* 77:11–18.

Babson, S. G., Behrman, R. E., and Lessel, R. 1970. Fetal growth: Liveborn birth weights for 12 gestational age of white middle class infants. *Pediatrics* 45:937–944.

Badell-Ribera, H., Schulman, K., and Paddock, N. 1966. The relationship of non-progressive hydrocephalus to intellectual functioning in children with spina bifida cystica. *Pediatrics* 37:787–793.

Ball, M. J., and Nuttall, K. 1980. Neurofibrillary tangles, granulovacuolar degeneration, and neuron loss in Down syndrome: Quantitative comparison with Alzheimer dementia. *Annals of Neurology* 7:462–465.

Ball, M. J., Schapiro, M. B., and Rapoport, S. I. 1986. Neuropathological relationships between Down syndrome and senile dementia Alzheimer type. In J. Epstein (Ed.), *The Neurobiology of Down Syndrome*, pp. 45–58. New York: Raven Press.

Banker, G. A., and Cowan, W. M. 1979. Further observations on hippocampal neurons in dispersed cell culture. *Journal of Comparative Neurology* 187:469–494.

Bannister, C. M., Chapman, S. A., Cronley, J. J., Turnbull, I. W., and

Kulikowski, J. J. 1987. Occipital lobectomies in foetal lambs. *Zeitschrift fur Kinderchirurgie* 42 (Suppl.):5–9.

Baraitser, M. 1985. *The Genetics of Neurological Disorders.* Oxford: Oxford University Press.

Barlow, P. 1973. The influence of inactive chromosomes on human development. *Humangenetik* 17:105–136.

Barnes, M. A., and Dennis, M. 1992. Reading in children and adolescents after early onset hydrocephalus and in normally developing age peers: Phonological analysis, word recognition, word comprehension and passage comprehension skill. *Journal of Pediatric Psychology* 17:445–465.

Battaglia, F. C., and Lubchenko, L. O. 1967. A practical classification of newborn infants by weight and gestational age. *Journal of Pediatrics* 71:159–163.

Bavinck, J. N. B., Weaver, D. D., Ellis, F. O., and Ward, R. E. 1987. A syndrome of microcephaly, eye anomalies, short stature, and mental deficiency. *American Journal of Medical Genetics* 26:825–831.

Bayley, N. 1969. *Bayley Scales of Infant Development.* San Antonio: Psychological Corporation.

Bee, H. L. 1989. *The Developing Child.* New York: Harper & Row.

Beery, K. E. 1967. *Visual-Motor Integration.* Chicago: Follett Publishing co.

Bellinger, D., Leviton, A., Walternaux, C., Needleman, H., and Rabinowitz, M. 1987. Low-level lead exposure and child development assessment at age 5 of a cohort followed from birth. In S. E. Lindberg and T. C. Hutchinson (Eds.), *International Conference: Heavy Metals in the Environment,* Vol. 1. New Orleans: CEP Consultants.

Bellugi, U., Sabo, H., and Vaid, J. 1988. Spatial deficits in children with Williams syndrome. In J. Stiles-Davis, M. Kritchevsky, and U. Bellugi (Eds.), *Spatial Cognition: Brain Bases and Development,* pp. 273–298. Hillsdale, N.J.: Lawrence Erlbaum.

Belman, A. L., Diamond, G., Dickson, D., Horoupian, D., Llena, J., Lantos, G., and Rubinstein, A. 1988. Pediatric acquired immunodeficiency syndrome: Neurologic syndromes. *American Journal of Diseases of Children* 142:9–35.

Bender, B., Linden, M. G., and Robinson, A. 1989. Verbal and spatial processing efficiency in 32 children with sex chromosome abnormalities. *Pediatric Research* 25:577–579.

Bender, B., Puck, M., Salbenblatt, J., and Robinson, A. 1984. The development of four unselected 47,XYY boys. *Clinical Genetics* 25:435–445.

———. 1986. Cognitive development of children with sex chromosome abnormalities. In S. D. Smith (Ed.), *Genetics and Learning Disabilities,* pp. 175–201. San Diego: College-Hill Press.

Bennett, F. C., La Veck, B., and Sells, C. J. 1978. The Williams elfin facies syndrome: The psychological profile as an aid in syndrome identification. *Pediatrics* 61:303–306.

Bennett, F. C., Robinson, N. M., and Sells, C. J. 1983. Growth and development of infants weighing less than 800 grams at birth. *Pediatrics* 71:319–323.

Benson, P. F., and Fensom, A. H. 1985. *Genetic Biochemical Disorders*. Oxford: Oxford University Press.

Benton, A. L., Hamsher, D. deS., Varney, N. R., and Spreen, O. 1983. *Contributions to Neuropsychological Assessment: A Clinical Manual*. New York: Oxford University Press.

Berlucchi, G., Tassinari, G., and Antonini, A. 1986. The organization of the callosal connections according to Sperry's principle of supplementary complementary. In F. Lepore, M. Ptito, and H. H. Jaspers (Eds.), *Two Hemispheres—One Brain: Functions of the Corpus Callosum*, pp. 171–188. New York: Alan R. Liss.

Bickel, H., Gerrard, J., and Hickmans, E. M. 1954. The influence of phenylalanine intake on the chemistry and behavior of a phenylketonuric child. *Developmental Medicine and Child Neurology* 21:311–320.

Bigler, E. D., Rosenstein, L. D., Roman, M., and Nussbaum, N. L. 1988. The clinical significance of congenital agenesis of the corpus callosum. *Archives of Clinical Neuropsychology* 3:189–200.

Blomquist, H. K., Bohman, M., Edvinsson, S. O., Gillberg, C., Gustavson, K. H., Holmgren, G., and Wahlstrom, J. 1985. Frequency of the fragile X syndrome in infantile autism. *Clinical Genetics* 27:113–117.

Boder, E. 1971. Developmental dyslexia: A diagnostic screening procedure based on three characteristic patterns of reading and spelling. In B. Bateman (Ed.), *Learning Disorders*, Vol. 4. Seattle: Special Child Publications.

———. 1973. Developmental dyslexia: A diagnostic approach based on three atypical reading-spelling patterns. *Developmental Medicine and Child Neurology* 15:663–687.

Book, J. A., Schut, J. W., and Reed, S. C. 1953. A clinical and genetical study of microcephaly. *American Journal of Mental Deficiency* 57:637–660.

Bornstein, R. A., King, G., and Carroll, A. 1983. Neuropsychological abnormalities in Gilles de la Tourette syndrome. *Journal of Nervous and Mental Disorders* 171:497–502.

Bowman, R. E., Heironimus, M. P., and Allen, J. R. 1978. Correlation of PCB body burden with behavioral toxicology in monkeys. *Pharmacology, Biochemistry and Behavior* 9:49–56.

Bradley, L., and Bryant, P. 1978. Difficulties in auditory organization as a possible cause of reading backwardness. *Nature* 271:746–747.

Brandt, I. 1981. Brain growth, fetal malnutrition, and clinical consequences. *Journal of Perinatal Medicine* 3:1–26.

Brown, R. 1973. *A First Language: The Early Stages*. Cambridge: Harvard University Press.

Brown, W. T., Jenkins, E. C., Cohen, I. L., Fisch, G. S., Wolf-Schein, E. G., Gross, A., Waterhouse, L., Fein, D., Mason-Brothers, A., Ritvo, E., Rittenberg, B. A., Bentley, W., and Castells, S. 1986. Fragile X and autism: A multicenter survey. *American Journal of Medical Genetics* 23:341–352.

Brown, W. T., Jenkins, E. C., Friedman, E., Brooks, J., Wisniewski, K.,

Ragathu, S., and French, J. 1982. Autism is associated with the fragile X syndrome. *Journal of Autism and Developmental Disorders* 12:303–308.

Bryden, M. P., and Allard, F. 1978. Dichotic listening and the development of linguistic processes. In M. Kinsbourne (Ed.), *Asymmetrical Function of the Brain*, pp. 392–404. Cambridge: Cambridge University Press.

Buckley, S. 1985. Attaining basic educational skills: Reading, writing and number. In D. Lane and B. Stratford (Eds.), *Current Approaches to Down's Syndrome*, pp. 315–343. London: Holt, Rinehart & Winston.

Burbacher, T. M., Rodier, P. M., and Weiss, B. 1990. Methylmercury developmental toxicity: A comparison of effects in humans and animals. *Neurotoxicology and Teratology* 12:191–202.

Burd, L., Kauffman, D. W., and Kerbeshian, J. 1992. Tourette syndrome and learning disabilities. *Journal of Learning Disabilities* 25:598–604.

Burd, L., Kerbeshian, J., Wikenheiser, M., and Fisher, W. 1986. A Prevalence study of Gilles de la Tourette syndrome in North Dakota school-age children. *Journal of the American Academy of Child Psychiatry* 25:552–553.

Burton, B. K. 1981. Dominant inheritance of microcephaly with short stature. *Clinical Genetics* 20:25–27.

Butler, I. J., O'Flynn, M. E., Seifert, W. E., and Howell, R. R. 1981. Neurotransmitter defects and treatment of disorders of hyperphenylalaninemia. *Journal of Pediatrics* 98:729–733.

Byring, R., and Pullianen, V. 1984. Neurological and neuropsychological deficiencies in a group of older adolescents with dyslexia. *Developmental Medicine and Child Neurology* 26:765–773.

Caine, E. D., McBride, M. C., Chiverton, P., Bainford, K. A., Rediess, S., and Shiao, J. 1988. Tourette syndrome in Monroe County school children. *Neurology* 38:472–475.

Cajal, S. Ramon y. 1911. *Histologie du Systeme Nerveux de l'Homme et des Vertebres.* Paris: Moloine.

Cambridge, J., and Anderson, E. 1979. *The Handwriting of Spina Bifida Children: An Advisory Booklet for Teachers and Students.* London: Association for Spina Bifida and Hydrocephalus.

Carey, J. C., Lamb, J. M., and Hall, B. D. 1979. Penetrance and variability in neurofibromatosis: A genetic study of 60 families. *Birth Defects Original Articles Series* 15:271–281.

Carr, D. H., and Gedeon, M. 1977. Population cytogenetics of human abortuses. In E. B. Hook and I. H. Porter (Eds.), *Population Cytogenetics*, pp. 1–10. New York: Academic Press.

Carr, J. 1985. The development of intelligence. In D. Lane and B. Stratford (Eds.), *Current Approaches to Down's Syndrome*, pp. 167–186. London: Holt, Rinehart & Winston.

———. 1988. Six weeks to twenty-one years old: A longitudinal study of children with Down's syndrome and their families. *Journal of Child Psychology and Psychiatry* 29:407–431.

Carr, J., Halliwell, M., and Pearson, A. 1984. The relationship of disability and school type to everyday life. *Zeitschrift fur Kinderchirurgie* 39(Suppl.): 135–137.

Carr, J., and Hewett, S. 1982. Children with Down's syndrome growing up: A preliminary report. *Child Psychology and Psychiatry News* Spring:10–43.

Chiappelli, F., Taylor, A. N., Espinosa de los Monteras, A., and De Vellis, J. 1990. Fetal alcohol delays the developmental expression of myelin basic protein and transferrin in rat primary oligodendrocyte cultures. *International Journal of Developmental Neuroscience* 9:67–75.

Chiarello, C. 1980. A house divided? Cognitive functioning with callosal agenesis. *Brain and Language* 11:128–158.

Choo, K. H., Cotton, R. G. H., Jennings, I. G., and Danks, D. M. 1979. Observations indicating the nature of the mutation in phenylketonuria. *Journal of Inherited Metabolic Disease* 2:79–84.

Cianchetti, C., Filippi, G., Sannio-Fancello, G., Fratta, A. L., Marrosu, M. G., Dagna-Bricarelli, F., and Siniscalco, M. 1992. Permutation for the Martin-Bell syndrome analyzed in a large Sardinian family: II. Neuropsychological and behavioral data. *American Journal of Medical Genetics* 43:103–110.

Clark, E. V. 1973. Knowledge, context, and strategy in the acquisition of meaning. In D. P. Dato (Ed.), *Georgetown University Roundtable on Language and Linguistics*, pp. 77–98. Washington, D.C.: Georgetown University Press.

Clarren, S. K., Alvord, E. C., Sumi, S. M., Streissguth, A. P., and Smith, D. W. 1978. Brain malformations related to prenatal exposure to ethanol. *Journal of Pediatrics* 92:64–67.

Clarren, S. K., and Smith, D. W. 1978. The fetal alcohol syndrome. *New England Journal of Medicine* 298:1063–1067.

Cohen, D. J., Leckman, J. F., and Shaywitz, B. A. 1983. Tourette's syndrome and other tics. In D. Shaffer, A. A. Ehrhardt, and L. Greenhill (Eds.), *Diagnosis and Treatment in Pediatric Psychiatry*, pp. 3–28. New York: McMillan Free Press.

Cohen, S. E. 1983. The low-birthweight infant and learning disabilities. In M. Lewis (Ed.), *Learning Disabilities and Prenatal Risk*, pp. 153–193. Urbana, Ill.: University of Illinois Press.

Cohen, S. E., and Parmelee, A. 1983. Prediction of five year Stanford-Binet score in preterm infants. *Child Development* 54:1242–1253.

Coltheart, M. 1980. Reading, phonological recoding and deep dyslexia. In M. Coltheart, K. Patterson, and J. C. Marshall (Eds.), *Deep Dyslexia*, pp. 197–226. London: Routledge & Kegan Paul.

Comings, D. E. 1990. *Tourette Syndrome and Human Behavior*. Duarte, Calif.: Hope Press.

Comings, D. E., and Comings, B. G. 1987. A controlled study of Tourette syndrome. *American Journal of Human Genetics* 41:701–838.

Commey, J. O. O., and Fitzhardinge, P. M. 1979. Handicap in the preterm small-for-gestational age infant. *Journal of Pediatrics* 94:779–786.

Cory-Slechta, D. A. 1988. Chronic low-lead exposure: Behavioral consequences, biological exposure indices and reversibility. *Science and the Total Environmental* 71:433–440.

Cossu, G., Rossini, F., and Marshall, J. C. 1993. When reading is acquired but phonemic awareness is not: A study of literacy in Down's syndrome. *Cognition* 46:129–138.

Costello, A. M., Hamilton, P. A., Baudin, J., Townsend, J., Bradford, B. C., Stewart, A. L., and Reynolds, E. O. 1988. Prediction of neurodevelopmental impairment at four years from brain ultrasound appearance of very preterm infants. *Developmental Medicine and Child Neurology* 30:711–722.

Cotman, C. W., and Lynch, G. S. 1976. Reactive synaptogenesis in the adult nervous system: The effects of partial deafferentation on new synapse formation. In S. H. Barondes (Ed.), *Neuronal Recognition*, pp. 69–108 New York: Plenum Press.

Courville, C. B. 1971. *Birth and Brain Damage*. Pasadena, Calif.: M. F. Courville.

Cousens, P., Waters, B., Said, J., and Stevens, M. 1988. Cognitive effects of cranial irradiation in leukemia: A survey and meta-analysis. *Journal of Child Psychology and Psychiatry* 29:839–852.

Cowie, V. A. 1987. Microcephaly: A review of genetic implications in causation. *Journal of Mental Deficiency Research* 31:229–233.

Cox, C., Clarkson, T. W., Marsh, D. O., and Amin-Zaki, L. 1989. Dose-response analysis of infants prenatally exposed to methylmercury: An application of a single compartment model to single strand hair analysis. *Environmental Research* 49:318–332.

Cronister, A., Schreiner, R., Wittenberger, M., Amiri, K., Harris, K., and Hagerman, R. J. 1991. Heterozygous fragile X female: Historical, physical, cognitive and cytogenetic features. *American Journal of Medical Genetics* 43:111–115.

Crosson, B. 1985. Subcortical functions in language: A working model. *Brain and Language* 25:257–292.

Crowe, C. A., and Dickerman, L. H. 1986. A genetic association between microcephaly and lymphedema. *American Journal of Medical Genetics* 24:131–135.

Culler, F. L., Jones, K. L., and Deftos, L. J. 1985. Impaired calcitonin secretion in patients with Williams syndrome. *Journal of Pediatrics* 107:720–723.

Cusick, C. G., and Kaas, J. H. 1986. Interhemispheric connections of cortical sensory and motor representation in primates. In F. Lepore, M. Ptito, and H. H. Jaspers (Eds.), *Two Hemispheres—One Brain: Functions of the Corpus Callosum*, pp. 83–102. New York: Alan R. Liss.

Dameron, L. E. 1963. Development of intelligence of infants with mongolism. *Child Development* 34:733–738.

Davis, J. M., Otto, D. A., Weil, D. E., and Grant, L. D. 1990. The comparative developmental neurotoxicity of lead in humans and animals. *Neurotoxicity and Teratology* 12:215–229.

DeFries, J. C., Fulker, D. W., and LaBuda, M. C. 1987. Evidence for a genetic aetiology in reading disability of twins. *Nature* 329:536–539.

Delabar, J., Goldgaber, D., Lamour, Y., Nicole, A., Huret, J., deGrouchy, J., Brown, P., Gajdusek, D. C., and Sinet, P. 1987. Beta amyloid gene duplication in Alzheimer's disease and karyotypically normal Down syndrome. *Science* 235:1390–1392.

Dennis, M. 1976. Impaired sensory and motor differentiation with corpus callosum agenesis: A lack of callosal inhibition during ontogeny? *Neuropsychologia* 14:455–469.

———. 1980. Capacity and strategy for syntactic comprehension after early left or right hemidecortication. *Brain and Language* 10:287–317.

———. 1981. Language in a congenitally acallosal brain. *Brain and Language* 12:33–53.

———. 1985a. Intelligence after early brain injury: I. Predicting IQ scores from medical variables. *Journal of Clinical and Experimental Neuropsychology* 7:526–554.

———. 1985b. Intelligence after early brain injury: II. IQ scores of subjects classified on the basis of medical history variables. *Journal of Clinical and Experimental Neuropsychology* 7:555–576.

Dennis, M., Fitz, C. R., Netley, G. T., Sugar, J., Harwood-Nash, D. C. F., Hendrick, E. B., Hoffman, H. J., and Humphreys, R. P. 1981. The intelligence of hydrocephalic children. *Archives of Neurology* 38:607–617.

Dennis, M., Hendrick, E. B., Hoffman, H. J., and Humphrey, R. P. 1987. Language of hydrocephalic children and adolescents. *Journal of Clinical and Experimental Neuropsychology* 9:593–621.

Dennis, M., and Whitaker, H. A. 1976. Language acquisition following hemidecortication: Language superiority of the left over the right hemisphere. *Brain and Language* 3:404–433.

Denniston, J. C. 1963. Children of mothers with phenylketonuria. *Journal of Pediatrics* 63:461–463.

DeReuk, J. S., Chattha, A. S., and Richardson, E. P. 1972. Pathogenesis and evolution of periventricular leucomalacia in infancy. *Archives of Neurology* 27:229–236.

Dietrich, K. M., Krafft, K. M., Bornschein, R. L., Hammond, P. B., Berger, O., Succop, P. A., and Bier, M. 1987. Effects of low-level fetal lead exposure on neurobehavioral development in infancy. *Pediatrics* 80:721–730.

Dietrich, K. M., Krafft, K. M., Shukla, R., Sornschein, R. L., and Succop, P. A. 1989. The neurobehavioral effects of early lead exposure. In S. R. Schroeder (Ed.), *Toxic Substances and Mental Retardation: Neurobehavioral Toxicology and Teratology*, pp. 71–95. Washington, D.C.: American Association on Mental Deficiency.

Dietrich, K. M., Succop, P. A., Berger, O. G., Hammond, P. B., and Bornschein, R. L. 1991. Lead exposure and the cognitive development of urban preschool children: The Cincinnati lead study cohort at age 4 years. *Neurotoxicology and Teratology* 13:203–211.

Dobbing, J., and Sands, J. 1973. Quantitative growth and development of human brain. *Archives of Diseases in Childhood* 48:757–767.

Dodd, K. D. 1984. Where should spina bifida children go to school? *Zeitschrift fur Kinderchirurgie* 39(Suppl.):129–131.

Doehring, D. G., and Hoshko, I. M. 1977. Classification of reading problems by the Q-technique of factor analysis. *Cortex* 13:281–294.

Doehring, D. G., Hoshko, I. M., and Bryans, B. N. 1979. Statistical classification of children with reading problems. *Journal of Clinical Neuropsychology* 1:4–16.

Doehring, D. G., Trites, R. L., Patel, P. G., and Fiedorowicz, C. A. M. 1981. *Reading Disabilities*. New York: Academic Press.

Donders, J., Canady, A. I., and Rourke, B. P. 1990. Psychometric intelligence after infantile hydrocephalus. *Child's Nervous System* 6:118–151.

Donoso, A. D., and Santander, M. 1982. Hemialexia y afasia hemianoptica en agenesis del cuerpo calloso. *Revue Child Neuropsiquiatrica* 20:137–144.

Dooling, E. C., and Gilles, F. H. 1983. Intracranial hemorrhage: Topography. In A. Gilles, A. Leviton, and E. C. Dooling (Eds.), *The Developing Brain: Growth and Epidemiologic Neuropathology*. Boston: PSG.

Dorman, C. 1987a. Reading disability subtypes in neurologically impaired students. *Annals of Dyslexia* 37:166–188.

———. 1987b. Verbal, perceptual and intellectual factors associated with reading achievement in adolescents with cerebral palsy. *Perceptual and Motor Skills* 64:671–678.

———. 1988. Relationships between reading disability subtypes in neurologically impaired children. *International Journal of Clinical Neuropsychology* 10:165–177.

———. 1991a. Exceptional calendar calculation ability after early left hemispherectomy. *Brain and Cognition* 15:26–36.

———. 1991b. Microcephaly and intelligence. *Developmental Medicine and Child Neurology* 33:267–269.

———. 1992. Reply to Lynn. *Developmental Medicine and Child Neurology* 34:1024–1025.

Dorman, C., Hurley, A. D., and d'Avignon, J. 1988. Language and learning disorders in older boys with duchenne muscular dystrophy. *Developmental Medicine and Child Neurology* 30:316–327.

Dorman, C., Hurley, A. D., and Laatsch, L. K. 1984. Prediction of spelling and reading performance in cerebral palsied adolescents using neuropsychological tests. *International Journal of Clinical Neuropsychology* 6:142–144.

Dorman, C., Laatsch, L. K., and Hurley, A. D. 1984. A study of reading disability among neurologically impaired students using the Luria-Nebraska Neuropsychological Battery. *International Journal of Clinical Neuropsychology* 6:197–199.

Downey, J., Elkin, E. J., Erhardt, A. A., Meyer-Bahlburg, H. F., Bell, J. J., and Morishima, A. 1991. Cognitive ability and everyday functioning in women with Turner syndrome. *Journal of Learning Disabilities* 21:32–39.

Driscoll, C. D., Streissguth, A. P., and Riley, E. P. 1990. Prenatal alcohol exposure: Comparability of effects of human and animal models. *Neurotoxicity and Teratology* 12:231–237.

Dubowitz, L., Dubowitz, V., and Goldberg, C. 1970. Clinical assessment of gestational age in the newborn infant. *Journal of Pediatrics* 77:1–10.

Dubowitz, L. M. S., Bydder, G. M., and Mushin, J. 1985. Developmental sequence of periventricular leucomalacia. *Archives of Diseases in Childhood* 60:349–355.

Duckett, S. 1971. The establishment of internal vascularization in the human telencephalon. *Acta Anatomy* 80:107–113.

Duffen, L. 1976. Teaching reading to children with little or no language. *Remedial Education* 11:139–149.

Dunn, H. G. (Ed.). 1986. *Sequelae of Low Birthweight: The Vancouver Study.* Clinics in Developmental Medicine No. 95/96. Philadelphia: J. B. Lippincott.

Dunn, H. G., Hughes, C-J., and Schulzer, M. 1986. Physical growth. In H. G. Dunn (Ed.), *Sequelae of Low Birthweight: The Vancouver Study,* pp. 35–53. Clinics in Developmental Medicine No. 95/96. Philadelphia: J.B. Lippincott.

Dyer, N. C., Brill, A. B., Tsiantos, A. C., Sell, E., Victorin, L. H., and Stahlman, M. T. 1973. Timing of intracranial bleeding in newborn infants. *Journal of Nuclear Medicine* 14:807–811.

Edwards, D. R., Keppen, L. D., Rouells, J. D., and Gollin, S. M. 1988. Autism in association with fragile X syndrome in families: Implications for diagnosis and treatment in children. *Neurotoxicology* 9:359–365.

Einfield, S., Molony, H., and Hall, W. 1989. Autism is not associated with the fragile X syndrome. *American Journal of Medical Genetics* 34:187–193.

Eiser, C. 1980. Effects of chronic illness on intellectual development. *Archives of Diseases in Childhood* 55:766–770.

Elwood, J. M., and Elwood, J. H. 1980. *The Epidemiology of Anencephaly and Spina Bifida.* Oxford: Oxford University Press.

Emory, E. K., and Mapp, J. R. 1988. Effects of respiratory distress and prematurity on spontaneous startle activity in neonates. *Infant Behavior and Development* 11:71–81.

Emory, E. K., Tynan, W. D., and Davé, R. 1989. Neurobehavioral anomalies in neonates with seizures. *Journal of Clinical and Experimental Neuropsychology* 11:231–240.

Epstein, L. G., Sharer, L. R., Joshi, V. V., Fojas, M. M., Koenigsberger, M. R., and Oleske, J. M. 1985. Progressive encephalopathy in children with acquired immune deficiency syndrome. *Annals of Neurology* 17:488–496.

Epstein, L. G., Sharer, L. R., Oleske, J. M., Connor, E. M., Goudsmit, J., Bagdon, L., Robert-Guroff, M., and Koenigberger, M. R. 1986. Neurologic manifestations of human immunodeficiency virus infection in children. *Pediatrics* 78:678–687.

Ettlinger, G., Blakemore, C. B., Milner, A. D., and Wilson, J. 1972. Agenesis of the corpus callosum: A behavioral investigation. *Brain* 95:327–346.

———. 1974. Agenesis of the corpus callosum: A further behavioral investigation. *Brain* 97:225–234.

Fabregues, I., Ferrer, I., Gairi, J. M., Cahuana, A., and Giner, P. 1985. Effects of prenatal exposure to ethanol on the maturation of the pyramidal neurons in the cerebral cortex of the guinea-pig: A quantitative Golgi study. *Neuropathology and Applied Neurobiology* 11:291–298.

Fagan, J. F., and McGrath, S. K. 1981. Infant recognition memory and later intelligence. *Intelligence* 5:121–130.

Falloon, J., Eddy, J., Wiener, L., and Pizzo, P. A. 1989. Human immunodeficiency virus infection in children. *Journal of Pediatrics* 114:1–30.

Fanaroff, A. A., and Martin, R. J. 1983. *Behrman's Neonatal Perinatal Medicine: Diseases of the Fetus and Infant*, 3rd Edition. St. Louis: C. V. Mosby.

Fancourt, R., Campbell, S., Harvey, D., and Norman, A. P. 1976. Follow-up study of small-for-dates babies. *British Medical Journal* 1:1435–1437.

Fawer, C. L., Diebold, P., and Calame, A. 1987. Periventricular leukomalacia: A neurodevelopmental outcome in preterm infants. *Archives of Diseases in Childhood* 62:30–36.

Feldman, H. A. 1958. Toxoplasmosis. *Pediatrics* 22:559.

Fernell, E., Hagberg, B., Hagberg, G., and von Wendt, L. 1987. Epidemiology of infantile hydrocephalus in Sweden: III. Origin in preterm infants. *Acta Paediatrica Scandinavica* 76:418–423.

Ferrer, I., and Galofré, E. 1987. Dendritic spine anomalies in fetal alcohol syndrome. *Neuropediatrics* 18:161–163.

Ferris, G. S., and Dorsen, M. M. 1975. Agenesis of the corpus callosum: I. Neuropsychological studies. *Cortex* 11:95–122.

Fisch, G. S. 1992. Is autism associated with the fragile X syndrome? *American Journal of Medical Genetics* 43:47–55.

Fisch, G. S., Arinami, T., Froster-Iskenius, U., Fryns, J. P., Curfs, L. M., Borghgraef, M., Howard-Peebles, P. N., Schwartz, C. E., Simensen, R. J., and Shapiro, L. R. 1991. Relationship between age and IQ among fragile X males: A multicenter study. *American Journal of Medical Genetics* 38:481–487.

Fisch, G. S., Shapiro, L. R., Simensen, R., Schwartz, C. E., Fryns, J. P., Borghgraef, M., Curfs, L. M., Howard-Peebles, P. N., Arinami, T., and Mavrou, A. 1992. Longitudinal changes in IQ among fragile X males: Clinical evidence of more than one mutation? *American Journal of Medical Genetics* 43:28–34.

Fischer, K. W. 1987. Relations between brain and cognitive development. *Child Development* 58:623–632.

Fishler, K., Azen, C. G., Friedman, F. G., and Koch, R. 1989. School achievement in treated PKU children. *Journal of Mental Deficiency Research* 33:493–498.

Fitzhardinge, P. M., and Pape, K. E. 1977. Intrauterine growth retardation (IUGR): An added risk to the preterm infant. *Pediatric Research* 11:562 (abstr.).

Fitzhardinge, P. M., Pape, K., Aristikaitis, M., Boyle, M., Ashby, S., Rowley, A., Netley, C., and Sawyer, P. R. 1976. Mechanical ventilation in infants of less than 1501 grams birthweight: Health, growth, and neurologic sequelae. *Journal of Pediatrics* 88:531–541.

Fitzhardinge, P. M., and Steven, E. M. 1972. The small for date infant: I. Neurological and intellectual sequelae. *Pediatrics* 50:50–57.

Fleschig, P. 1920. *Anatomie des Menschlichen Gehirns und Ruckenmarks auf myelogenetischer Grundlage.* Leipzig: Georg Thieme.

Fletcher, J. M., Francis, D. J., Thompson, N. M., Brookshire, B. L., Bohan, T. P., Landry, S. H., Davidson, K. C., and Miner, M. E. 1992. Verbal and nonverbal skill discrepancies in hydrocephalic children. *Journal of Clinical and Experimental Neuropsychology* 14:593–609.

Fletcher, J. M., and Satz, P. 1985. Cluster analysis and the search for learning disability subtypes. In B. P. Rourke (Ed.), *Neuropsychology of Learning Disabilities: Essentials of Subtype Analysis,* pp. 40–64. New York: Guilford Press.

Fodor, J. A. 1983. *The Modularity of Mind.* Cambridge: Bradford/MIT Press.

Frankel, M., Cummings, J. L., Robertson, M. M., Trimble, M. R., Hill, M. A., and Benson, D. F. 1986. Obsessions and compulsions in Gilles de la Tourette's syndrome. *Neurology* 36:378–383.

Freeman, H. C., Shum, G., and Uthe, J. F. 1978. The selenium content in swordfish (*Xiphias giadius*) in relation to total mercury content. *Journal of Environmental Science and Health* 13:235–240.

Friede, R. L. 1975. *Developmental Neuropathology.* New York: Springer-Verlag.

Fujito, Y., Watanabe, S., Kobayashi, H., and Tsukahara, N. 1984. Lesion-induced sprouting in the red nucleus at the early developmental stage. In S. Finger and D. G. Stein (Eds.), *Early Brain Damage,* Vol. 2: *Neurobiology and Behavior,* pp. 35–47. New York: Academic Press.

Furshpan, E. J., MacLeish, P. R., O'Lague, P. H., and Potter, D. D. 1976. Chemical transmission between rat sympathetic neurons and cardiac myocytes developing in microcultures: Evidence for cholinergic, adrenergic and dual-function neurons. *Proceedings of the National Academy of Sciences of the United States of America* 73:4225–4229.

Gaines, K. A. 1991. Relationships among neonatal medical complications, demographics, developmental assessments and school age reading ability in prematurely born children. Ph.D. Diss., United States International University, San Diego.

Galaburda, A. M. 1989. Ordinary and extraordinary brain development: Anatomical variation in developmental dyslexia. *Annals of Dyslexia* 33:67–80.

Galaburda, A. M., Sherman, G. F., and Geschwind, N. 1983. Developmental dyslexia: Third consecutive case with cortical anomalies. *Society of Neuroscience Abstracts* 9:940 (abstr.).

Galin, D., Johnstone, J., Nakell, S., and Herron, J. 1979. Development of the capacity for information transfer between hemispheres in normal children. *Science* 204:1330–1332.

Garfinkel, E., Tejani, N., Boxer, H. S., Levinthal, C., Athern, V., Tuck, S., and Vidyasagar, S. 1988. Infancy and early childhood follow-up of neonates with periventricular or intraventricular hemorrhage or isolated ventricular dilation: A case controlled study. *American Journal of Perinatology* 5:214–219.

Gazzaniga, M. S., Bogen, J. E., and Sperry, R. W. 1962. Some functional effects of sectioning the cerebral hemispheres in man. *Brain* 88:221–236.

———. 1965. Observations on visual perception after disconnection of the cerebral commissures in man. *Proceedings of the National Academy of Sciences of the United States of America* 48:1765–1769.

Gazzaniga, M. S., and Sperry, R. W. 1967. Language after section of the cerebral commissures. *Brain* 90:131–148.

Gelman, R. 1991. Epigenetic foundations of knowledge structures: Initial and transcendent constructions. In S. Carey and R. Gelman (Eds.), *The Epigenesis of Mind: Essays on Biology and Cognition*. Hillsdale, N.J.: Lawrence Erlbaum.

Geoffroy, G., Lassonde, M., DeLisle, F., and DeCarie, M. 1983. Corpus callostomy for control of intractable epilepsy in children. *Neurology* 3:891–897.

Geschwind, N., and Behan, P. 1982. Left-handedness: Association with immune diseases, migraine and developmental learning disorder. *Proceedings of the National Academy of Sciences of the United States of America* 79:5097–6100.

Geschwind, N., and Galaburda, A. M. 1985. Cerebral lateralization: Biological mechanisms, association and pathology. I. A hypothesis and a programme for research. *Archives of Neurology* 42:428–459.

Gibson, D., and Harris, A. 1988. Aggregated early intervention effects for Down's syndrome persons: Patterning and longevity of benefits. *Journal of Mental Deficiency Research* 32:1–17.

Gilles, F. H., Shankle, W., and Dooling, E. C. 1983. Myelinated tracts: growth patterns. In F. H. Gilles, A. Leviton, and E. C. Dooling (Eds.), *The Developing Human Brain*, pp. 118–184. Boston: PSG.

Ginsburg, H. P., and Baroody, A. J. 1983. *Test of Early Mathematics Ability*. Austin: Pro-Ed.

Gladen, B. C., Rogan, W. J., Hardy, P., Thullen, J., Tingelstad, J., and Tully, M. R. 1988. Development after exposure to polychlorinated biphenyls and dichlorodiphenyl dichlorethene transplacentally and through breast milk. *Journal of Pediatrics* 113:991–995.

Goldberg, E., and Costa, L. D. 1981. Hemisphere differences in the acquisition and use of descriptive systems. *Brain and Language* 14:144–173.

Golden, C. J., and Berg, R. A. 1980a. Interpretation of the Luria-Nebraska Neuropsychological Battery by item intercorrelation: Items 1–24 of the Motor Scale. *Clinical Neuropsychology* 2:66–71.

———. 1980b. Interpretation of the Luria-Nebraska Neuropsychological Battery by item intercorrelation: Items 25–51 of the Motor Scale. *Clinical Neuropsychology* 3:105–108.

Golden, N. L., Sokol, R. J., Kuhnert, B. R., and Bottoms, S. 1982. Maternal alcohol use and infant development. *Journal of Pediatrics* 70:931–934.

Golding-Kushner, K., Weller, G., and Shprintzen, R. J. 1985. Velocardiofacial syndrome: Language and psychological profiles. *Journal of Craniofacial Genetics and Developmental Biology* 5:259–266.

Goldman, P. S. 1971. Functional development of the prefrontal cortex in early life and the problems of neuronal plasticity. *Experimental Neurology* 32:366–387.

———. 1972. Developmental determinants of cortical plasticity. *Acta Neurobiologica Experimentalis* 32:495–511.

———. 1974. An alternative to developmental plasticity: heterology of CNS structures in infants and adults. In D. G. Stein, J. J. Rosen, and N. Butters (Eds.), *Plasticity and Recovery of Function*, pp. 149–174. New York: Academic Press.

———. 1976. The role of experience in recovery of function following prefrontal lesions in infant monkeys. *Neuropsychologia* 14:401–412.

Goldman-Rakic, P. S. 1987. Development of cortical circuitry and cognitive function. *Child Development* 58:601–622.

Gott, P. S., and Saul, R. E. 1978. Agenesis of the corpus callosum: Limits of functional compensation. *Neurology* 28:1272–1279.

Graham, J. M., Bashir, A. S., Stark, R. E., Silbert, A., and Walzer, S. 1988. Oral and written language abilities of XXY boys: Implications for anticipatory guidance. *Pediatrics* 81:795–806.

Graham, M., Levene, M. I., and Trounce, J. Q. 1987. Prediction of cerebral palsy in very low birthweight infants: Prospective ultrasound study. *Lancet* 2:593–599.

Granroth, G. 1979. Defects of the central nervous system in Finland: IV. Associations with diagnostic X-ray examinations. *American Journal of Obstetrics and Gynecology* 133:191–194.

Grant, D. W., Goldberg, C., Guiney, E. J., and Fitzgerald, R. J. 1986. Should the tradition of right cerebral hemisphere shunting still prevail? *Zeitschrift fur Kinderchirurgie* 41(Suppl.):48–50.

Greene, T., and Ernhart, C. B. 1991. Prenatal and preschool age lead exposure: Relationship with size. *Neurotoxicology and Teratology* 13:417–427.

Grigsby, J., Kemper, M. B., and Hagerman, R. J. 1992. Verbal learning and memory among heterozygous fragile 27 X females. *American Journal of Medical Genetics* 43:111–115.

Grigsby, J. P., and Myers, C. S. 1987. Neuropsychological findings among heterozygous fragile X females. Paper presented at the First National Fragile X Conference, Denver, Colo.

Grimm, R. A. 1976. Hand function and tactile perception in a sample of children with myelomeningocele. *American Journal of Occupational Therapy* 30:234–240.

Gualtieri, C. T. 1987. Fetal antigenicity and maternal immunoreactivity: Factors in mental retardation. In S. R. Schroeder (Ed.), *Toxic Substances and Mental Retardation: Neurobehavioral Toxicology and Teratology*, pp. 33–69. Washington, D.C.: American Association on Mental Deficiency.

Hack, M., and Breslau, N. 1986. Very low birthweight infants: Effects of brain growth during infancy on intelligence quotients at 3 years of age. *Pediatrics* 77:196–202.

Hadenius, A. M., Hagberg, B., Hyttnes-Bensch, K., and Sjogren, I. 1962. The natural prognosis of infantile hydrocephalus. *Acta Paediatrica* 51:112.

Hagberg, B., Hagberg, G., and Olow, I. 1982. Gains and hazards of intensive neonatal care: An analysis from Swedish cerebral palsy epidemiology. *Developmental Medicine and Child Neurology* 24:13–19.

Hagberg, B., and Sjogren, I. 1966. The chronic brain syndrome of infantile hydrocephalus: A follow study of 13 spontaneously arrested cases. *American Journal of Diseases in Childhood* 112:189–196.

Hagerman, R. J. 1992. Annotation: Fragile X syndrome: Advances and controversy. *Journal of Child Psychology and Psychiatry* 33:1127–1139.

Hagerman, R. J., Schreiner, R. A., Kemper, M. B., Wittenberger, M. D., Zahn, B., and Habicht, K. 1989. Longitudinal IQ changes in fragile X males. *American Journal of Medical Genetics* 33:513–518.

Hagin, R. A., Beecher, R., Pagano, G., and Kreeger, H. 1982. Effects of Tourette syndrome on learning. In A. J. Friedhoff and T. N. Chase (Eds.), *Gilles de la Tourette Syndrome*, pp. 323–328. New York: Raven Press.

Hakim, S., and Adams, R. D. 1965. The special clinical problem of symptomatic hydrocephalus with normal cerebrospinal fluid pressure: Observations on cerebrospinal fluid dynamics. *Journal of Neurological Sciences* 2:307–327.

Halliwell, M., Carr, J., and Pearson, A. M. 1980. The intellectual and educational functioning of children with neural tube defects. *Zeitschrift fur Kinderchirurgie* 31:375–381.

Hambleton, G., and Wigglesworth, J. S. 1976. Origin of intraventricular hemorrhage in the preterm infant. *Archives of Diseases in Childhood* 51:651–659.

Hamburger, V. 1958. Regression versus peripheral control of differentiation in motor hypoplasia. *American Journal of Anatomy* 102:365–409.

———. 1975. Cell death in the development of the lateral motor column of the chick embryo. *Journal of Comparative Neurology* 160:535–546.

Hamburger, V., and Oppenheim, R. W. 1982. Naturally occurring neuronal death in vertebrates. *Neuroscience Commentary* 1:39–55.

Hammer, R. P., and Scheibel, A. B. 1981. Morphologic evidence for a delay of neuronal maturation in fetal alcohol exposure. *Experimental Neurology* 24:203–210.

Hammock, M. K., Milhorat, T. H., and Baron, I. S. 1976. Normal pressure hydrocephalus in patients with myelomeningocele. *Developmental Medicine and Child Neurology* 37:55–67.

Hankenson, L. G., Ozonoff, M. B., and Cassidy, S. B. 1989. Epiphyseal dysplasia with coxa vara, microcephaly and normal intelligence in sibs: Expanded spectrum of Lowry-Wood syndrome? *American Journal of Medical Genetics* 33:336–340.

Hansen, J. C. 1984. Selenium and its interrelationship with mercury in whole blood and hair in an East Greenlandic population. *Science of the Total Environment* 38:33–40.

Hansen, N. B., Kopechek, J., Miller, R. R., Menke, J. A., and Cordero, L. 1989. Prognostic significance of cystic intracranial lesions in neonates. *Developmental and Behavioral Pediatrics* 10:129–133.

Hanshaw, J. B. 1970. Developmental abnormalities associated with congenital cytomegalovirus infection. In D. H. M. Woollam (Ed.), *Advances in Teratology*, Vol. 4, pp. 64–94. New York: Academic Press.

Hanson, J. W., Streissguth, A. P., and Smith, D. W. 1978. The effects of moderate alcohol consumption during pregnancy on fetal growth and morphogenesis. *Journal of Pediatrics* 92:457–460.

Harada, Y. 1977. Congenital Minamata disease. In R. Tsubak and K. Irukayama (Eds.), *Minamata Disease: Methylmercury Poisoning in Minamata and Niigata, Japan*, pp. 209–239. Tokyo: Kodansha.

Haslam, R. H. A., and Smith, D. W. 1979. Autosomal dominant microcephaly. *Journal of Pediatrics* 95:701–705.

Havlicek, V., Childiaeva, R., and Chernick, V. 1977. EEG frequency spectrum characteristics of sleep states in infants of alcohol mothers. *Neuropaediatrie* 8:360–373.

Hier, D. B., Atkins, L., and Perlo, V. P. 1980. Learning disorders and sex chromosome aberrations. *Journal of Mental Deficiency Research* 24:17–26.

Hill, R. M. 1976. Fetal malformations and antepileptic drugs. *American Journal of Diseases of Children* 130:923–925.

Hingson, R., Alpert, J., Day, N., Dooling, E., Kayne, H., Morelock, S., and Zuckerman, B. 1982. Effects of maternal drinking and marijuana use on fetal growth and development. *Pediatrics* 70:539–546.

Hinton, V. J., Dobkin, C. S., Halperin, J. M., Jenkins, E. C., Brown, W. T., Ding, X. H., Cohen, I. L., Rousseau, F., and Miezejeski, C. M. 1992. Mode of inheritance influences behavioral expression and molecular control of cognitive deficits in female carriers of the fragile X syndrome. *American Journal of Medical Genetics* 43:87–95.

Hirata, T., Epcar, J. T., Walsh, A., Mednick, J., Harris, M., McGinnis, M. S., Sehring, S., and Papedo, G. 1983. Survival and outcome of infants 501–750 gm: A six year experience. *Journal of Pediatrics* 102:741–748.

Hollingshead, A. B., and Redlich, F. C. 1958. *Social Class and Mental Illness*. New York: John Wiley & Sons.

Hollyday, M., and Hamburger, V. 1976. Reduction of the naturally occurring motor neuron loss by enlargement of the periphery. *Journal of Comparative Neurology* 170:311–320.

Hope, P. L., Cady, E. B., Tofts, P. S., Hamilton, P. A., Costello, A. M. L., Dalpy, D. T., Chu, A., Reynolds, E. O. R., and Wilkie, D. R. 1984. Cerebral energy metabolism studied with phosphorous NMR spectroscopy in normal and birth-asphyxiated infants. *Lancet* 2:366–369.

Horwood, S. P., Boyle, M. H., Torrance, G. W., and Sinclair, J. C. 1982.

Mortality and morbidity of 500 to 1499 gram birthweight infants live-born to residents of defined geographic region before and after neonatal intensive care. *Pediatrics* 69:613–620.

Hubel, D. H., and Wiesel, T. N. 1963. Receptive fields of cells in striate cortex of very young, visually inexperienced kittens. *Journal of Neurophysiology* 26:994–1002.

———. 1965. Binocular interaction in striate cortex of kittens reared with artificial squint. *Journal of Neurophysiology* 28:1041–1059.

———. 1970. The period of susceptibility to the physiological effects of unilateral eye closure in kittens. *Journal of Physiology (London)* 206:419–436.

Hubel, D. H., Wiesel, T. N., and LeVay, S. 1977. Plasticity of ocular dominance columns in the monkey striate cortex. *Philosophical Transactions of the Royal Society of London (Biology)* 278:377–409.

Hunt, G. M., and Holmes, A. E. 1975. Some factors relating to intelligence in treated children with spina bifida cystica. *Developmental Medicine and Child Neurology* 17(Suppl.):65–70.

Hunt, J. V., Cooper, B. A. B., and Tooley, W. H. 1988. Very low birthweight infants at 8 and 11 years of age: Role of neonatal illness and family status. *Pediatrics* 82:596–603.

Hunt, N. 1966. *The World of Nigel Hunt*. London: Darwen Finlayson.

Hurley, A. D., Dorman, C., Laatsch, L. K., Bell, S., and d'Avignon, J. 1990. Cognitive functioning in patients with spina bifida and hydrocephalus and the "cocktail party" syndrome. *Developmental Neuropsychology* 6:151–172.

Hurley, A. D., Laatsch, L. K., and Dorman, C. 1983. Comparison of spina bifida patients and matched controls on neuropsychological tests. *Zeitschrift fur Kinderchirurgie* 38(Suppl. 11):116–118.

Huttenlocher, P. R. 1974. Dendritic development in neocortex of children with mental defect and infantile spasms. *Neurology* :203–210.

Ingram, T. T. S., and Naughton, J. A. 1962. Pediatric and psychological aspects of cerebral palsy associated with hydrocephalus. *Developmental Medicine and Child Neurology* 4:287–292.

Innocenti, G. M. 1981. Growth and reshaping of axons in the establishment of visual callosal connections. *Science* 212:824–827.

———. 1986. What is so special about callosal connections? In F. Lepore, M. Ptito, and H. H. Jasper (Eds.), *Two Hemispheres—One Brain: Functions of the Corpus Callosum*, pp. 75–81. New York: Alan R. Liss.

Ivey, G. O., and Killackey, H. P. 1982. Ontogenetic changes in the projections of neocortical neurons. *Journal of Neuroscience* 6:735–743.

Jacobson, J. L., Jacobson, S. W., Fein, G. G., Schwartz, P. M., and Dowler, J. K. 1984. Prenatal exposure to an environmental toxin: A test of the multiple effects model. *Developmental Psychology* 20:523–532.

Jacobson, M. 1978. *Developmental Neurobiology*, 2nd Edition. New York: Plenum Press.

Jacobson, S. W., Fein, G. G., Jacobson, J. L., Schwartz, P. M., and Dowler, J. K.

1985. The effect of intrauterine exposure on visual recognition memory. *Child Development* 56:853–860.

Jagadha, V., and Becker, L. E. 1988. Brain morphology in muscular dystrophy: A Golgi study. *Pediatric Neurology* 1:87–92.

Jammes, J. L., and Gilles, F. H. 1983. Telencephalic development: Matrix volume and isocortex and allocortex surface areas. In F. H. Gilles, A. Leviton, and E. C. Dooling (Eds.), *The Developing Human Brain*, pp. 87–93. Boston: PSG.

Janowsky, J. S., and Finlay, B. L. 1986. The consequences of early brain damage: The role of normal neuron loss and axon retraction. *Developmental Medicine and Child Neurology* 28:375–389.

Jeeves, M. A. 1979. Some limits to interhemispheric integration in cases of callosal agenesis and partial commissurotomy. In I. S. Russell, M. W. Van Hof, and G. Berlucchi (Eds.), *Structure and Function of the Callosal Commissures*. London: Macmillan.

———. 1986. Callosal agenesis: Neuronal and developmental adaptations. In F. Lepore, M. Ptito, and H. H. Jasper (Eds.), *Two Hemispheres—One Brain: Functions of the Corpus Callosum*, pp. 403–421. New York: Alan R. Liss.

Johnson, F. W. 1991. Biological factors and psychometric intelligence: A review. *Genetic, Social and General Psychology Monographs* 117:313–357.

Johnson, J. D., Malachowshi, N. C., Grebstein, R., Welsh, J. D., Daily, W. I. R., and Sunshine, P. 1974. Prognosis of children surviving with the aid of mechanical ventilation in the newborn period. *Journal of Pediatrics* 84:272–276.

Jones, K. L., and Smith, D. W. 1973. Recognition of the fetal alcohol syndrome in early infancy. *Lancet* 2:999–1001.

———. 1975a. The fetal alcohol syndrome. *Teratology* 12:1–10.

———. 1975b. The Williams elfin facies syndrome: A new perspective. *Journal of Pediatrics* 86:718–723.

Jones, K. L., Smith, D. W., Streissguth, A. P., and Myrianthopolous, N. C. 1974. Pattern of malformation in offspring of chronic alcoholic women. *Lancet* 1:1076–1078.

Jones, K. L., Smith, D. W., Ulleland, C. N., and Streissguth, A. P. 1973. Pattern of malformation in offspring of chronic alcoholic mothers. *Lancet* 1:1267–1271.

Jones, R. A. K., Cummins, M., and Davies, P. A. 1979. Infants of very low birthweight: A 15 year analysis. *Lancet* 1:1332–1335.

Jovaisas, E., Koch, M. A., Schafer, A., Stauber, M., and Lowenthal, D. 1985. LAV/HTLV-III in 20-week fetus. *Lancet* 2:1129–1130.

Kaiser, G. 1985. Hydrocephalus following toxoplasmosis. *Zeitschrift fur Kinderchirurgie* 40 (Suppl.):129–131.

Kakulas, B. A. 1992. Pathological features of Duchenne and Becker muscular dystrophy. In B. A. Kakulas, J. M. Howell, and A. D. Roses (Eds.), *Duchenne Muscular Dystrophy: Animal Models and Genetic Manipulation*, pp. 11–18. New York: Raven Press.

Kaplan, I. C., Osborne, P., and Elias, E. 1986. The diagnosis of muscular dystrophy in patients referred for language delay. *Journal of Child Psychology and Psychiatry* 27:545–549.

Karagan, N. J. 1979. Intellectual functioning in Duchenne muscular dystrophy: A review. *Psychological Bulletin* 86:250–259.

Karagan, N. J., and Zellweger, H. U. 1978. Early verbal disability in children with Duchenne muscular dystrophy. *Developmental Medicine and Child Neurology* 20:435–441.

Katzir, B. 1992. A Follow-up Study of Mathematical Learning Disabilities in Children Born Prematurely. Ann Arbor: University Microfilms.

Kaufman, A. S. 1979. *Intelligent Testing with the WISC-R.* New York: John Wiley & Sons.

Kawashima, H., and Tsuji, N. 1987. Syndrome of microcephaly, deafness/malformed ears, mental retardation and peculiar facies in a mother and son. *Clinical Genetics* 31:303–307.

Kemper, M. B., Hagerman, R. J., Ahamad, R. S., and Mariner, R. C. 1986. Cognitive profiles and the spectrum of clinical manifestation in heterozygous fragile X females. *American Journal of Medical Genetics* 23:139–156.

Kemper, M. B., Hagerman, R. J., and Altshul-Stark, D. 1988. Cognitive profiles of boys with fragile X 34 syndrome. *American Journal of Medical Genetics* 30:191–200.

Kemper, T. L. 1984. Asymmetrical lesions in dyslexia. In N. Geschwind and A. M. Galaburda (Eds.), *Cerebral Dominance: The Biological Foundations*, pp. 75–92. Cambridge: Harvard University Press.

Kennan, K. E. 1984. Time in her life: A Down's woman's personal account. *Dissertation Abstracts International* 45:1806 (abstr.).

Kennard, M. A. 1936. Age and other factors in motor recovery from precentral lesions in monkeys. *American Journal of Physiology* 115:138–146.

———— 1938. Reorganization of motor function in the cerebral cortex of monkeys deprived of motor and premotor areas in infancy. *Journal of Neurophysiology* 1:477–496.

———— 1942. Cortical reorganization of motor function. *Archives of Neurology and Psychiatry* 48:227–240.

Kier, E. L. 1974. Fetal cerebral arteries: A phylogenetic and ontogenetic study. In T. H. Newton and D. G. Potts (Eds.), *Radiology of the Skull and Brain*, Vol. 2, Book 1, pp. 1089–1130. St. Louis: C. V. Mosby.

Kiessling, L. S., Denckla, M. B., and Carlton, M. 1983. Evidence for differential hemispheric function in children with cerebral palsy. *Developmental Medicine and Child Neurology* 25:727–734.

Kinsbourne, M., and Warrington, E. K. 1963. The development of finger differentiation. *Quarterly Journal of Experimental Psychology* 15:132–137.

Kjellstrom, T., Kennedy, P., Wallis, S., and Mantell, C. 1986. Physical and mental development of children with prenatal exposure to mercury from fish. Stage 1: Preliminary tests at age 4. Report 3080. Solna, Sweden: National Swedish Environmental Protection Board.

Kleczkowska, A., Kubien, E., Dmoch, E., Fryns, J. P., and Van den Berghe, H. 1990. Turner syndrome II. Associated anomalies, mental performance and psychological problems in 218 patients diagnosed in Leuven in the period 1965–1989. *Genetic Counseling* 1:241–249.

Klein, N. K. 1988. Children who were very low birthweight: Cognitive abilities and classroom behavior at five years of age. *Journal of Special Education* 22:41–54.

Klein, N. K., Hack, M., and Breslau, N. 1989. Children who were very low birthweight: Developmental and academic achievement at nine years of age. *Developmental and Behavioral Pediatrics* 10:32–37.

Klein, N. K., Hack, M., Gallagher, J., and Fanaroff, A. A. 1985. Preschool performance of children with normal intelligence who were very low birthweight infants. *Pediatrics* 75:531–537.

Kloepfer, H. W., Platou, R. V., and Handshe, W. J. 1964. Manifestations of a recessive gene for microcephaly in a population isolate. *Journal de Genetique Humaine* 13:52–59.

Knobloch, H., Malone, A., Ellison, P. H., Stevens, F., and Zdeb, M. 1982. Considerations in evaluating changes in outcome for infants weighing less than 1501 grams. *Pediatrics* 69:285–295.

Knobloch, H., and Pasamanick, B. 1960. Complications of pregnancy and mental deficiency. Presented at the 1st International Congress on Mental Retardation (pp. 182–193) (abstr.).

Koch, R., Azen, C., Friedman, E. G., and Williamson, M. L. 1984. Paired comparisons between early treated PKU children and their matched sibling controls on intelligence and school achievement test results at eight years of age. *Journal of Inherited Metabolic Disease* 7:86–90.

Koeda, T., and Takeshita, K. 1993. Tactile naming disorder of the left hand in two cases with corpus callosum agenesis. *Developmental Medicine and Child Neurology* 35:65–78.

Kohn, B., and Dennis, M. 1974. Patterns of hemispheric specialization after hemidecortication for infantile hemiplegia. In M. Kinsbourne and W. L. Smith (Eds.), *Hemispheric Disconnection and Cerebral Function*, pp. 34–47. Springfield, Ill.: Charles C Thomas.

Konermann, G. 1986. Brain development in mice after prenatal irradiation: Modes of effect manifestation. Dose-response relationships and the RBE of neutrons. In H. Kriegel, W. Schmahl, G. B. Gerber, and F. E. Stieve (Eds.), *Radiation Risks to the Developing Nervous System*, pp. 93–116. Stuttgart: Gustav Fischer.

Kopp, C. B., and Vaughn, B. E. 1982. Sustained attention during exploratory manipulation as a predictor of cognitive competence in preterm infants. *Child Development* 53:174–182.

Kostrzewski, J. 1965. The dynamics of intellectual and social development in Down's syndrome: Results of experimental investigation. *Roczniki: Filozoficzne* 13:5–32.

Kovelman, J. A., and Scheibel, A. B. 1983. A neuroanatomical study of schizophrenia. *Society of Neuroscience Abstracts* 9:850 (abstr.).

Lachiewicz, A. M., Gullion, C. M., Spiridigliozzi, G. A., and Aylsworth, A. S. 1987. Declining IQs of young males with fragile X syndrome. *American Journal of Mental Retardation* 92:272–278.

Land, P. W., and Lund, R. D. 1979. Development of the rat's uncrossed retinotectal pathway and its relation to plasticity studies. *Science* 205:698–700.

Landesman-Dwyer, S., Keller, L. S., and Streissguth, A. P. 1978. Naturalistic observations of newborns: Effects of maternal alcohol intake. *Alcohol: Clinical and Experimental Research* 2:171–177.

Landman, G. B., Levine, M. D., Fenton, T., and Solomon, B. 1986. Minor neurological indicators and developmental function in preschool children. *Developmental and Behavioral Pediatrics* 7:97–101.

Landry, S. H., and Chapieski, M. L. 1988. Visual attention during toy exploration in preterm infants: Effects of medical risk and maternal interactions. *Infant Behavior and Development* 11:187–204.

Landry, S. H., Fletcher, J. M., Zarling, C. L., Chapieski, L., Francis, D. J., and Denson, S. 1984. Differential outcomes associated with early medical complications in premature infants. *Journal of Pediatric Psychology* 9:384–401.

Landry, S. H., Leslie, N. A., Fletcher, J. M., and Francis, D. J. 1985. Visual attention skills of premature infants with and without intraventricular hemorrhage. *Infant Behavior and Development* 8:309–321.

Landry, S. H., Schmidt, M., and Richardson, M. A. 1989. The effects of intraventricular hemorrhage on functional communication skills in preterm toddlers. *Developmental and Behavioral Pediatrics* 10:299–306.

Lapointe, N., Michaud, J., Pekovic, D., Chausseau, J. P., and Dupuy, J. M. 1985. Transplacental transmission of HTLV-III virus. *New England Journal of Medicine* 312:1325–1326.

Largo, R. H., Molinari, L., Commenale-Pinto, L., Weber, M., and Duc, G. 1986. Language development of term and preterm children during the first five years of life. *Developmental Medicine and Child Neurology* 28:333–350.

Largo, R. H., Pfister, D., Molinari, L., Kundu, S., Lopp, A., and Duc, G. 1989. Significance of prenatal, perinatal and postnatal factors in the development of AGA preterm infants at five to seven years. *Developmental Medicine and Child Neurology* 31:440–456.

Larroche, J. 1977. *Developmental Pathology of the Neonate.* Amsterdam: Excerpta Medica.

Lashley, K. S. 1929. *Brain Mechanisms and Intelligence: A Quantitative Study of Injuries to the Brain.* Chicago: University of Chicago Press.

Lassen, N. A. 1959. Cerebral blood flow and oxygen consumption in man. *Physiological Reviews* 39:183–238.

———. 1974. Control of cerebral circulation in health and disease. *Circulation Research* 34:749–760.

Lassonde, M. 1986. The facilitory influence of the corpus callosum on intra-hemispheric processing. In F. Lepore, M. Ptito, and H. H. Jasper (Eds.), *Two Hemispheres—One Brain: Functions of the Corpus Callosum*, pp. 361–368. New York: Alan R. Liss.

Lassonde, M., Sauerwein, H., McCabe, N., Laurencelle, L., and Geoffroy, G. 1988. Extent and limits of cerebral adjustment to early section of congenital absence of the corpus callosum. *Behavioral Brain Research* 30:165–181.

Laurence, K. M. 1958. The natural history of hydrocephalus. *Lancet* 2:1152.

———. 1964. The natural history of spina bifida cystica. *Archives of Diseases in Childhood* 39:41–57.

———. 1969. Neurological and intellectual sequelae of hydrocephalus. *Archives of Neurology* 20:73–81.

———. 1985. The apparently declining prevalence of neural tube defect in two countries in South Wales over three decades illustrating the need for continuing action and vigilance. *Zeitschrift fur Kinderchirurgie* 40(Suppl.):58–60.

Laurence, K. M., Campbell, H., and James, N. E. 1983. Double blind randomized controlled trial of preconceptional folic acid supplementation in the prevention of neural tube defects. In J. Dobbing (Ed.), *Prevention of Spina Bifida and Other Neural Tube Defects*, pp. 127–154. London: Academic Press.

Laurence, K. M., and Cavanaugh, J. B. 1968. Progressive degeneration of the cerebral cortex in infancy. *Brain* 91:261.

Laurence, K. M., Miller, J. N., and Campbell, H. 1980. The increased risk of recurrence of pregnancies complicated by fetal neural tube defects in mothers on poor diets and the possible benefits of dietary counseling. *British Medical Journal* 280:1592–1594.

Laurence, K. M., Miller, J. N., Tennant, G. B., and Campbell, H. 1981. Double-blind randomised controlled trial of folate treatment before conception to prevent recurrence of neural tube defects. *British Medical Journal* 282:1509–1511.

Lee, K. S., Paneth, N., Gartner, L. M., Pearlman, M. A., and Gruss, L. 1980. Neonatal mortality: An analysis of the recent improvements in the United States. *American Journal of Public Health* 70:15–21.

Leech, R. W., and Kohnen, P. 1974. Subependymal and intraventricular hemorrhages in the newborn. *American Journal of Pathology* 77:465–475.

Lemire, R. J., Loesser, J. D., Leech, R. W., and Alvord, E. C. 1975. *Normal and Abnormal Development of the Nervous System*. Hagerstown, Md.: Harper & Row.

Lemoine, P., Harousseau, H., Borteyru, J. P., and Menuet, J. C. 1968. Les enfants de parents alcoholiques: Anomalies observee a propos 127 cas. *Paris Ouest Medical* 21:476–482.

Lepore, F., Ptito, M., and Guillemot, J. P. 1986. The role of the corpus callosum in midline fusion. In F. Lepore, M. Ptito, and H. H. Jasper (Eds.), *Two Hemispheres—One Brain: Functions of the Corpus Callosum*, pp. 211–229. New York: Alan R. Liss.

Le Provost, P. A. 1983. Using the Makaton vocabulary in early language training. *Mental Handicap* 11:29–30.

Leung, A. K. C. 1985. Dominantly inherited syndrome of microcephaly and congenital lymphedema. *Clinical Genetics* 27:611–612.

Levin, E. D., Schantz, S. L., and Bowman, R. E. 1988. Delayed spatial alternation deficits resulting from perinatal PCB exposure of monkeys. *Archives of Toxicology* 62:267–273.

Levine, S. C., Huttenlocher, P., Banich, M. T., and Duda, E. 1987. Factors affecting cognitive functioning of hemiplegic children. *Developmental Medicine and Child Neurology* 29:27–35.

Leviton, A., Gilles, F. H., and Dooling, E. C. 1983. The epidemiology of delayed myelination. In F. H. Gilles, A. Leviton, and E. C. Dooling (Eds.), *The Developing Human Brain*, pp. 185–192. Boston: PSG.

Levitt, P., and Rakic, P. 1980. Immunoperoxidase localization of glial fibrillary acidic protein in radial glial-cells and astrocytes of the developing rhesus-monkey brain. *Journal of Comparative Neurology* 193:815–840.

Lewis, M., and Brooks-Gunn, J. 1981. Visual attention at three months as a predictor of cognitive functioning at two years of age. *Intelligence* 5:131–140.

Liberman, I. Y., Shankweiler, D., Liberman, A. M., Fowler, C., and Fisher, F. W. 1977. Phonetic segmentation and recoding in the beginning reader. In A. S. Reber and D. L. Scarborough (Eds.), *Toward a Psychology of Reading*, pp. 207–226. New York: Halstead Press.

Liebowitz, D., and Dubowitz, V. 1981. Intellect and behavior in Duchenne muscular dystrophy. *Developmental Medicine and Child Neurology* 23:577–590.

Lindsley, O. R. 1965. Can deficiency produce superiority? The challenge of the idiot savant. *Exceptional Children* 31:225–232.

Lipson, A. H., Yu, J. S., O'Halloran, M. T., and Williams, R. 1981. Alcohol and phenylketonuria. *Lancet* 1:717–718.

Loesser, J. D., and Alvord, E. C. 1968. Agenesis of the corpus callosum. *Brain* 91:553–570.

Lonton, A. P. 1976. Hand preference in children with myelomeningocele and hydrocephalus. *Developmental Medicine and Child Neurology* 18(Suppl.): 143–149.

———. 1979. Prediction of intelligence in spina bifida neonates. *Zeitschrift fur Kinderchirurgie* 37:172.

Lopez-tejero, D., Ferrer, M., Llobera, M., and Herrera, E. 1986. Effects of prenatal ethanol exposure on physical growth, sensory reflex maturation and brain development in the rat. *Neuropathology and Applied Neurobiology* 12:251–260.

Lorber, J. 1961. Systematic ventriculographic studies in infants born with meningomyelocele and encephalocele: The incidence and development of hydrocephalus. *Archives of Diseases in Childhood* 36:381–389.

———. 1965. The family history of spina bifida cystica. *Pediatrics* 35:589–595.

———. 1983. Is your brain really necessary? In D. Voth (Ed.), *Hydrocephalus im Fruhen Kindesalter*. Stuttgart: Ferdinand Enke.

Lorber, J., and Ward, A. M. 1985. Spina bifida: A vanishing nightmare? *Archives of Diseases of Childhood* 60:1086–1091.

Lott, I. T. 1986. The neurology of Down syndrome. In C. J. Epstein (Ed.), *The Neurobiology of Down Syndrome*, pp. 17–28. New York: Raven Press.

Lou, H. C., Griesen, G., and Tweed, A. 1988. Hypoxia, loss of autoregulation and intracranial hemorrhage. In F. Kubli, N. Patel, W. Schmidt, and O. Lindercamp (Eds.), *Perinatal Events and Brain Damage in Surviving Children*, pp. 211–215. New York: Springer-Verlag.

Lou, H. C., Lassen, N. A., and Friis-Hansen, B. 1977. Low cerebral blood flow in hypotensive perinatal distress. *Acta Neurologica Scandinavica* 56:343–352.

———. 1979. Impaired autoregulation of cerebral blood flow in the distressed newborn infant. *Journal of Pediatrics* 94:118–121.

Low, J. A., Galbraith, R. W., Muir, D. W., Broekhoven, L. H., Wilkinson, J. W., and Karchmar, E. J. 1985. The contributions of fetal-newborn complications to motor and cognitive deficits. *Developmental Medicine and Child Neurology* 27:578–587.

Luria, A. R. 1980. *Higher Cortical Functions in Man.* New York: Basic Books.

Lynn, R. 1992. Microcephaly and intelligence re-examined. *Developmental Medicine and Child Neurology* 34:1023–1024.

Lynn, R. B., Buchanan, D. C., Fenichel, G. M., and Freeman, F. R. 1980. Agenesis of the corpus callosum. *Archives of Neurology* 37:444–445.

Lyon, M. F. 1962. Sex chromatin and gene action in the mammalian X-chromosome. *American Journal of Human Genetics* 14:135–148.

MacDonald, G. W., and Roy, D. L. 1988. Williams syndrome: A neuropsychological profile. *Journal of Clinical and Experimental Psychology* 10:125–131.

Mahaffey, K. R., Annest, J. L., Roberts, J., and Murphy, R. S. 1982. National estimates of blood lead levels, United States, 1976–1980: Association with selected demographic and socioeconomic factors. *New England Journal of Medicine* 307:573–579.

Majewski, F. 1978. Uber schadigende Einflusse des Alkohols auf die Nachkommen. *Nervenartz* 49:410–414.

Mannino, F. L., and Merritt, T. A. 1986. The management of respiratory distress syndrome. In D. W. Thibeault and G. A. Gregory (Eds.), *Neonatal Pulmonary Care*, pp. 427–459. East Norwalk, Conn.: Appleton-Century-Crofts.

Marcell, M. M., and Armstrong, V. 1982. Auditory and visual sequential memory of Down syndrome and non-retarded children. *American Journal of Mental Deficiency* 87:86–95.

Marcell, M. M., and Weeks, S. L. 1988. Short-term memory difficulties and Down's syndrome. *Journal of Mental Deficiency Research* 32:153–162.

Marino, R. V., Scholl, T. O., Karp, R. J., Yanoff, J. M., and Therington, J. 1987. Minor physical anomalies and learning disability: What is the prenatal component? *Journal of the National Medical Association* 79:7–39.

Marin-Padilla, M. 1972. Structural abnormalities of the cerebral cortex in human chromosomal aberrations: A Golgi study. *Brain Research* 44:625–629.

Marsh, D. O. 1987. Dose-response relationships in humans: Methyl mercury epidemics in Japan and Iraq. In C. U. Eccles and Z. Annau (Eds.), *The Toxicity of Methyl Mercury.* Baltimore: Johns Hopkins University Press.

Marsh, G. G., and Munsat, T. L. 1974. Evidence for early impairment of verbal intelligence in Duchenne muscular dystrophy. *Archives of Diseases in Childhood* 49:118–122.

Marshall, J. C. 1985. On some relationships between acquired and developmental dyslexics. In F. H. Duffy and N. Geschwind (Eds.), *Dyslexia: A Neuroscientific Approach to Clinical Evaluation,* pp. 55–66. Boston: Little, Brown & Co.

Martin, J. C., Martin, D. C., Lund, C. A., and Streissguth, A. P. 1977. Maternal alcohol ingestion and cigarette smoking and their effects on newborn conditioning. *Alcoholism* 1:243–247.

Matilainen, R., Heinonen, K., and Siren-Tiusanen, H. 1988. Effect of intrauterine growth retardation (IUGR) on the psychological performance of preterm children at preschool age. *Journal of Child Psychology and Psychiatry* 29:601–609.

Matsumoto, H., Koya, G., and Takeuchi, T. 1965. Fetal Minamata disease: A neuropathological study of two cases of intrauterine intoxication by a methylmercury compound. *Journal of Neuropathology and Experimental Neurology* 24:563–574.

Mattis, S. 1978. Dyslexia syndromes: A working hypothesis that works. In A. L. Benton and D. Pearl (Eds.), *Dyslexia: An Appraisal of Current Knowledge,* pp. 43–66. New York: Oxford University Press.

Mattis, S., French, J. H., and Rapin, I. 1975. Dyslexia in children and young adults: Three independent neuropsychological syndromes. *Developmental Medicine and Child Neurology* 17:150–163.

Mayr, U., Aichner, F., Menardi, G., and Hager, J. 1986. Computer-tomographical appearances of the chiari malformation of the posterior fossa. *Zeitschrift fur Kinderchirurgie* 41 (Suppl.):33–35.

Mazzocco, M. M. M., Hagerman, R. J., Cronister-Silverman, A., and Pennington, B. F. 1992. Specific frontal lobe deficits among women with the fragile X gene. *Journal of the American Academy of Child and Adolescent Psychiatry* 31:1141–1148.

Mazzocco, M. M. M., Hagerman, R. J., and Pennington, B. F. 1992. Problem solving limitations among cytogenetically expressing fragile X women. *American Journal of Medical Genetics* 43:78–86.

McBurney, A. K., and Eaves, L. C. 1986. Evolution of developmental and psychological test scores. In H. G. Dunn (Ed.), *Sequelae of Low Birthweight: The Vancouver Study,* pp. 54–67. Clinics in Developmental Medicine No. 95/96. Philadelphia: J. B. Lippincott Co.

McDade, H. L., and Adler, S. 1980. Down syndrome and short-term memory impairment: A storage or retrieval deficit? *American Journal of Mental Deficiency* 84:561–567.

McDonald, A. D. 1981. Survival and handicap in infants of very low birthweight. *Lancet* 2:194.

McKean, C. M. 1971. Effect of totally synthetic low phenylalanine diet on adolescent phenylketonuric patients. *Archives of Diseases in Childhood* 46:606–615.

McLone, D. G., Czewski, D., Raimondi, A. J., and Sommers, R. C. 1982. Central nervous system infections as a limiting factor in the intelligence of children with myelomeningocele. *Pediatrics* 70:338–342.

McLone, D. G., and Naidich, T. P. 1989. Embryology of the cerebral vascular system. In M. S. B. Edwards and H. J. Hoffman (Eds.), *Cerebral Vascular Disease in Children and Adolescents*, pp.1–16. Baltimore: Williams & Wilkins.

Meadows, A. T., Massari, D. J., Fergiusson, J., Gordon, J., Littman, P., and Moss, K. 1981. Declines in IQ scores and cognitive dysfunctions in children with acute lymphocytic leukaemia treated with cranial irradiation. *Lancet* 2:1015–1018.

Mearig, J. S. 1979. The assessment of intelligence in boys with Duchenne muscular dystrophy. *Rehabilitation Literature* 40:262–274.

Meerwaldt, J. D., and van Dongen, H. R. 1988. Disturbances of spatial perception in children. *Behavioral Brain Research* 31:131–134.

Meyer, M. B., Tonascia, J. A., and Merz, T. 1976. Long-term effects of prenatal X-ray on development and fertility of human females. In(Ed.), *Biological and Environmental Effects of Low-level Radiation*, Vol.2, pp. 273–277. Vienna: IAEA.

Michejda, M. 1984. Intrauterine treatment of spina bifida: Primate models. *Zeitschrift fur Kinderchirurgie* 39:259–261.

Michejda, M., and McCollough, D. 1987. New animal model for the study of neural tube defects. *Zeitschrift fur Kinderchirurgie* 42(Suppl.):32–35.

Michel, V., Schmidt, F., and Ratzler, V. 1990. Results of psychological testing of patients age 3–6 years. *European Journal of Pediatrics* 149(Suppl.): 534–538.

Miezejeski, C. M., Jenkins, E. C., Hill, A. L., Wisniewski, K., French, J. H., and Brown, W. T. 1986. A profile of cognitive deficit in females from fragile X families. *Neuropsychologia* 24:405–410.

Milhorat, T. H., and Hammock, M. K. 1972. Arrested versus normal pressure hydrocephalus in children. *Clinical Proceedings of the Childrens Hospital National Medical Center* 28:168 (abstr.).

Miller, E., and Sethi, L. 1971a. The effect of hydrocephalus on perception. *Developmental Medicine and Child Neurology* 13(Suppl.):77–81.

———. 1971b. Tactile matching in children with hydrocephalus. *Neuropediatrics* 3:191–194.

Miller, M. W. 1985. Cogeneration of retrogradely labeled corticocortical projection and GABA-immunoreactive local circuit neurons in cerebral cortex. *Developmental Brain Research* 23:187–192.

Molfese, D. L. 1978. Left and right hemisphere involvement in speech perception: Electrophysiological involvement. *Perception and Psychophysics* 23:237–243.

Molfese, D. L., Burhke, R. A., and Wang, S. L. 1985. The right hemisphere and temporal processing of consonant durations: Electrophysiological correlates. *Brain and Language* 26:49–62.

Money, J. 1973. Turner's syndrome and parietal lobe functions. *Cortex* 9:385–393.

Money, J., and Alexander, D. 1966. Turner's syndrome: Further demonstration of the presence of specific cognitional deficiencies. *Journal of Medical Genetics* 3:47–48.

Money, J., and Erhardt, A. A. 1972. *Man and Woman, Boy and Girl*. Baltimore: Johns Hopkins University Press.

Moses, K. 1981. Declines in IQ scores and cognitive dysfunctions in children with acute lymphocytic leukaemia treated with cranial irradiation. *Lancet* 2:1015–1018.

Nadel, L. 1986. Down syndrome in neurobiological perspective. In J. Epstein (Ed.), *The Neurobiology of Down Syndrome*, pp. 239–251. New York: Raven Press.

Naeye, R. L., and Peters, E. C. 1988. Antepartum events and cerebral handicap. In N. Kubli, N. Patel, W. Schmidt, and O. Lindercamp (Eds.), *Perinatal Events and Brain Damage in Surviving Children*, pp. 83–91. New York: Springer-Verlag.

Needleman, H. L., Rabinowitz, M., Leviton, A., Linn, S., and Schoenbaum, S. 1984. The relationship between prenatal exposure to lead and congenital anomalies. *Journal of the American Medical Association* 251:2956–2959.

Neligan, G. A., Kolvin, I., Scott, D. M., and Garside, R. F. 1976. *Born Too Soon or Born Too Small: A Follow-up Study to Seven Years of Age*. London: Spastics International Medical Publications.

Nelson, K. B., and Ellenberg, J. H. 1982. Children who "outgrew" cerebral palsy. *Pediatrics* 69:529–536.

Netley, C. 1988. Relationships between hemispheric lateralization, sex hormones, quality of parenting and adjustment in 47,XXY males prior to puberty. *Journal of Child Psychology and Psychiatry* 29:281–287.

———. 1992. Time of pubertal onset, testosterone levels and intelligence in 47,XXY males. *Clinical Genetics* 42:31–34.

Netley, C., and Rovet, J. 1982. Handedness in 47,XXY males. *Lancet* 2:267.

———. 1983. Relationships among brain organization, maturation rate and development of verbal and nonverbal ability. In S. Segalowitz (Ed.), *Language Functions and Brain Organization*, pp. 246–266. New York: Academic Press.

Neumeister, K. 1978. Findings in children after radiation exposure in utero from X-ray examination of mothers. In *Late Biological Effects of Ionizing Radiation*, Vol. 1, pp. 119–134. Vienna: IAEA.

Neville, H. 1988. Cerebral organization for spatial attention. In J. Stiles-Davis,

M. Kritchevsky, and U. Bellugi (Eds.), *Spatial Cognition: Brain Bases and Development.* Hillsdale, N.J.: Lawrence Erlbaum.

Nichols, P. L., and Chen, T. C. 1981. *Minimal Brain Dysfunction: A Prospective Study.* Hillsdale, N.J.: Lawrence Erlbaum.

Nielsen, J., Silbeson, I., Sorensen, A. M., and Sorensen, K. 1979. Follow-up until age 4 to 8 of 25 unselected children with sex chromosome abnormalities compared with sibs and controls. *Birth Defects Original Article Series* 15:15–73.

Nielsen, J., and Sorensen, K. 1984. The importance of early diagnosis of Klinefelter's syndrome. In H. J. Bandmann and R. Breit (Eds.), *Klinefelter's Syndrome,* pp. 170–187. New York: Springer-Verlag.

Nielsen, J., and Wohlert, M. 1990. Sex chromosome abnormalities found among 34,910 newborn children: Results from a 13-year incidence study in Arhus, Denmark. *Birth Defects Original Article Series* 26:209–223.

Nonneman, A. J., Corwin, J. V., Sahley, C. L., and Vicedomini, J. P. 1984. Functional development of the prefrontal system. In S. Finger and D. G. Stein (Eds.), *Early Brain Damage,* Vol. 2: *Neurobiology and Behavior,* pp. 139–153. New York: Academic Press.

Novotny, E. J. 1989. Hypoxic-ischemic encephalopathy. In D. K. Stevenson and P. Sunshine (Eds.), *Fetal and Neonatal Brain Injury,* pp. 113–122. Philadelphia: B. C. Decker.

Nowakowski, R. S. 1987. Basic concepts of CNS development. *Child Development* 58:568–595.

Nowakowski, R. S., and Davis, T. L. 1985. Dendritic arbors and dendritic excrescences of abnormally positioned neurons in area CA3c of mice carrying the mutation "hippocampal lamination defect." *Journal of Comparative Neurology* 239:267–275.

Nowakowski, R. S., and Rakic, P. 1981. The site of origin and route and rate of migration of neurons to the hippocampal region of the rhesus monkey. *Journal of Comparative Neurology* 196:129–154.

Nudel, U., Zuk, D., Einat, P., Zeelon, E., Levy, Z., Neuman, S., and Yaffe, D. 1989. The Duchenne muscular dystrophy product is not identical in muscle and brain. *Nature* 337:76–77.

Oberle, I., Rousseau, F., Heitz, D., Kretz, C., Devys, D., Hanauer, A., Boue, J., Bertheas, M. F., and Mandel, J. L. 1991. Instability of a 550-base pair DNA segment, and abnormal methylation in fragile X syndrome. *Science* 252:1097–1102.

O'Connell, E. J., Feldt, R. H., and Stickler, G. B. 1965. Head circumference, mental retardation and growth failure. *Pediatrics* 36:62–66.

Oleson, J. 1973. Quantitative evaluation of normal and pathologic cerebral blood flow regulation to perfusion pressure changes in man. *Archives of Neurology* 28:143–149.

Olson, R. K., Wise, B., Conners, F., Rack, J., and Fulker, D. 1989. Specific deficits in component reading and language skills: Genetic and environmental influences. *Journal of Learning Disabilities* 22:339–348.

Otake, M., and Schull, W. J. 1984. In utero exposure to A-bomb radiation and mental retardation: A reassessment. *British Journal of Radiology* 57:409–414.

Otake, M., Schull, W. J., Fujikoshi, Y., and Yoshimaru, H. 1988. Effect on school performance of prenatal exposure to ionizing radiation in Hiroshima: A comparison of the T65DR and DS86 dosimetry systems. Radiation Effects Research Foundation Technical Report 2-88.

Otake, M., Yoshimaru, H., and Schull, W. J. 1987. Severe mental retardation among the prenatally exposed survivors of the atomic bombing of Hiroshima and Nagasaki: A comparison of the T%DR and DS dosimetry systems. Radiation Effects Research Foundation Technical Report 16-87.

Oulette, E. M., Rosett, H. L., Rosman, N. P., and Weiner, L. 1977. Adverse effects on offspring of maternal alcohol abuse during pregnancy. *New England Journal of Medicine* 297:528–530.

Ozanna, A. F., Krimmer, H., and Murdoch, B. F. 1990. Speech and language skills in children with early treated phenylketonuria. *American Journal of Mental Retardation* 94:625–632.

Padgett, D. H. 1948. The development of the cranial arteries in the human embryo. Carnegie Institute of Washington Publication 575. *Contributions to Embryology* 32:205–261.

———. 1956. The cranial venous system in man in reference to development, adult configuration, and relation to arteries. *American Journal of Anatomy* 98:307–356.

Paine, R. S. 1957. The variability in manifestations of untreated patients with phenylketonuria (phenylpyruvic aciduria). *Pediatrics* 20:290–302.

Paludetto, R., Maansi, G., Rinaldi, P., DeLuca, T., Corchia, G., DeCurtis, M., and Andolfi, M. 1982. Behavior of preterm newborns reaching term without any serious disorder. *Human Development* 6:357–363.

Pandya, D. N., and Seltzer, B. 1986. The topography of the commissural fibers. In F. Lepore, M. Ptito, and H. H. Jasper (Eds.), *Two Hemispheres—One Brain: Functions of the Corpus Callosum*, pp. 47—73. New York: Alan R. Liss.

Pape, K. E., Armstrong, D. L., and Fitzhardinge, P. M. 1977. A reply to the commentary of Drs. Shuman and Oliver. *Pediatrics* 60:787–788.

Pape, K. E., and Wigglesworth, J. S. 1979. *Hemorrhage, Ischaemia and the Perinatal Brain*. London: William Heineman Medical Books.

Papile, L. A., Burstein, J., Burstein, R., and Koffler, H. 1978. Incidence and evolution of subependymal and intraventricular hemorrhage: A study of infants with birthweight less than 1500 grams. *Journal of Pediatrics* 92:529 (abstr.).

Papile, L. A., Munsick-Bruno, G., and Lòwe, J. 1988. Grade III and IV periventricular-intraventricular hemorrhage (PIVH): Longitudinal neurodevelopmental outcome. *Pediatric Research* 23:453 (abstr.).

Papile, L. A., Munsick-Bruno, G., and Schaefer, A. 1983. Relationship of cerebral intraventricular hemorrhage and early childhood handicaps. *Pediatrics* 103:273–277.

Pasamanick, B., and Knobloch, H. 1961. Epidemiologic studies on the complications of pregnancy and the birth process. In G. Caplan (Ed.), *Prevention of Mental Disorders in Childhood*, pp. 74–94. New York: Basic Books.

———. 1966. Retrospective studies on the epidemiology of reproductive casualty: Old and new. *Merrill Palmer Quarterly* 12:7–26.

Paul, R., Cohen, D. J., Breg, W. R., Watson, M., and Herman, S. 1984. Fragile X syndrome: Its relation to speech and language disorders. *Journal of Speech and Hearing Disorders* 49:328–332.

Pederson, D. R., Evans, B., Chance, G. W., Bento, S., and Fox, A. M. 1988. Predictors of one-year developmental status in low birthweight infants. *Developmental and Behavioral Pediatrics* 9:287–292.

Pennington, B., Bender, B., Puck, M., Saltenblatt, J., and Robinson, A. 1982. Learning disabilities in children with sex chromosome abnormalities. *Child Development* 53:1182–1192.

Pennington, B., Heaton, R., Karzmark, P., Pendleton, M. G., Lehman, R., and Shucard, D. W. 1985. The neuropsychological phenotype in Turner syndrome. *Cortex* 21:391–404.

Pennington, B. F., Lefly, D. L., Van Orden, G. C., Bookman, M. O., and Smith, S. D. 1987. Is phonology bypassed in normal or dyslexic development? *Annals of Dyslexia* 37:62–89.

Pennington, B. F., and Smith, S. D. 1988. Genetic influences on learning disabilities: An update. *Journal of Consulting and Clinical Psychology* 56:817–823.

Penrose, L. S. 1963. *Biology of Mental Defect*. London: Sidgwick & Jackson.

Petrauskas, R., and Rourke, B. P. 1979. Identification of subgroups of retarded readers: A neuropsychological, multivariate approach. *Journal of Clinical Neuropsychology* 1:17–37.

Pharoah, P. O. D., and Alberman, E. O. 1981. Mortality of low birthweight infants in England and Wales, 1953–1979. *Archives of Diseases in Childhood* 56:86–89.

Pilar, G. L., Landmesser, L., and Burstein, L. 1980. Competition for survival among developing ciliary ganglion cells. *Journal of Neurophysiology* 43:233–254.

Piper, M. C., Kunos, I., Willis, D. M., and Mazer, B. 1985. Effects of gestational age on neurological functioning of the very low-birthweight infant at 40 weeks. *Developmental Medicine and Child Neurology* 27:596–605.

Pizzo, P. A., Eddy, J., Falloon, J., Balis, F. M., Murphy, R. F., Moss, H., Wolters, P., Brouwers, P., Jarosinski, P., Rubin, M., Broder, S., Yarchoan, R., Brunetti, A., Haha, M., Nusinoff-Lehrman, S., and Poplack, D. G. 1988. Effect of continuous intravenous infusion of zidovudine (AZT) in children with symptomatic HIV infection. *New England Journal of Medicine* 319:889–896.

Plant, M. L. 1985. *Women, Drinking and Pregnancy*. London: Tavistock.

Plant, M. L., and Plant, M. A. 1988. Maternal use of alcohol and other drugs during pregnancy and birth abnormalities: Further results from a prospective study. *Alcohol and Alcoholism* 23:229–233.

Polani, P. E. 1977. Abnormal sex chromosomes, behavior and mental disorder. In J. M. Tanner (Ed.), *Developments in Psychiatric Research*. London: Hodder & Stoughton.

Potolsky, C., and Grigg, A. E. 1942. A revision of the prognosis in mongolism. *American Journal of Orthopsychiatry* 12:503.

Potter, D. D., Landis, S. C., and Furshpan, E. J. 1980. Dual function during development of rat sympathetic neurons in culture. *Journal of Experimental Biology* 89:57–71.

Poundstone, W. 1992. *Prisoner's Dilemma*. New York: Doubleday.

Pryor, H. B., and Thelander, H. 1968. Abnormally small head size and intellect in children. *Journal of Pediatrics* 73:593–598.

Puri, P., Malone, M., and Guiney, E. J. 1977. Primary hydrocephalus: The effect of timing of first valve insertion, valve revisions and the nature of the revisions on intelligence. *Zeitschrift fur Kinderchirurgie* 22:506–509.

Purpura, D. P. 1975. Dendritic differentiation in human cerebral cortex: Normal and aberrant developmental patterns. *Advances in Neurology* 12:91–134.

Purves, D., and Lichtman, J. W. 1980. Elimination of synapses in the developing nervous system. *Science* 210:153–157.

———. 1985. *Principles of Neural Development*. Sunderland, Mass.: Sinauer Associates.

Quazi, Q. H., and Reed, T. E. 1975. A possible major contribution to mental retardation in the general population by the gene for microcephaly. *Clinical Genetics* 7:85–90.

Rakic, P. 1975. Synaptic specificity in the cerebellar cortex: Study of anomalous circuits induced by single gene mutations in mice. *Cold Spring Harbor Symposium in Quantitative Biology* 40:333–346.

———. 1976. Prenatal genesis of connections subserving ocular dominance in the rhesus monkey. *Nature* 261:467–471.

———. 1990. Principles of neural cell migration. *Experientia* 46:882–891.

Rakic, P., and Sidman, R. L. 1973. Sequence of developmental abnormalities leading to granule cell deficit in cerebellar cortex of Weaver mutant mice. *Journal of Comparative Neurology* 152:103–132.

Rakic, P., Stensaas, L. J., Sayre, E. P., and Sidman, R. L. 1974. Computer aided three-dimensional reconstruction and quantitative analysis of cells from serial electron microscopic montages of foetal monkey brain. *Nature* 250:31–34.

Rakic, P., and Yakovlev, P. I. 1968. Development of the corpus callosum and the cavum septi in man. *Journal of Comparative Neurology* 132:14–72.

Ramirez, M. L., Rivas, F., and Cantu, J. M. 1983. Silent microcephaly. A distinct autosomal dominant trait. *Clinical Genetics* 23:281–286.

Ramsay, M., and Piper, M. C. 1980. A comparison of two developmental scales in evaluating infants with Down syndrome. *Early Human Development* 4:89–95.

292   References

Ratcliff, G. 1982. Disturbances of spatial cognition associated with cerebral lesions. In M. Potegal (Ed.), *Spatial Abilities: Development and Physiological Foundations*, pp. 301-334. New York: Academic Press.

Ratcliffe, S. G. 1984. Klinefelter's syndrome in children: A longitudinal study of 47,XXY boys identified by population screening. In H. J. Bandmann and R. Breit (Eds.), *Klinefelter's Syndrome*, pp. 38–47. New York: Springer-Verlag.

Ratcliffe, S. G., Tierney, I., Nshaho, J., Smith, L., Springbett, A., and Callan, S. 1982. The Edinburgh study of growth and development of children with sex chromosomal abnormalities. *Birth Defects Original Article Series* 18:41–60.

Reinisch, J., Gandelman, R., and Spiegel, F. 1979. Prenatal influences on cognitive abilities. In M. Wittig and A. Petersen (Eds.), *Sex-related Differences in Cognitive Functioning*, pp. 215–240. New York: Academic Press.

Reinisch, J. M. 1976. Effects of prenatal hormone exposure on physical and psychological development in humans and animals, with a note on the state of the field. In E. J. Sachar (Ed.), *Hormones, Behavior and Psychopathology*. New York: Raven Press.

Reiss, A. L., and Freund, L. 1992. Behavioral phenotype of fragile X syndrome: DSM-III-R autistic behavior in male children. *American Journal of Medical Genetics* 43:35–46.

Reiss, A. L., Freund, L., Vinogradov, S., Hagerman, R. J., and Cronister, A. 1989. Parental inheritance and psychological disability in fragile X females. *American Journal of Human Genetics* 45:697–703.

Reyes, E., Rivera, J. M., Saland, L. C., and Murray, H. M. 1983. Effects of maternal administration of alcohol on fetal brain development. *Neurobehavioral Toxicology and Teratology* 5:263–267.

Reynolds, E. O. R., and Hamilton, P. S. 1988. Magnetic resonance spectroscopy of the brain and early neurodevelopmental outcome. In F. Kubli, N. Patel, W. Schmidt, and O. Lindercamp (Eds.), *Perinatal Events and Brain Damage in Surviving Children*, pp. 245–256. New York: Springer-Verlag.

Robinson, G. C., Conry, J. L., and Conry, R. F. 1987. Clinical profile and prevalence of fetal alcohol syndrome in an isolated community in British Columbia. *Canadian Medical Association Journal* 137:203–208.

Rogan, W. J., Gladen, B. C., Hung, K. L., Koong, S. L., Shia, L. Y., Taylor, J. S., Wu, Y. C., Yang, D., Ragan, N. B., and Hsu, C. C. 1988. Congenital poisoning by polychlorinated biphenyls and their contaminants in Taiwan. *Science* 241:334–336.

Rogers, M. F., Thomas, P. A., Starcher, E. T., Noa, M. C., Bush, T. J., and Jaffe, H. W. 1987. Acquired immunodeficiency syndrome in children: Report of the Centers for Disease Control National Surveillance, 1982 to 1985.

Rogers, S. C. 1976. Congenital malformations in Europe in war and at peace. *Health Trends* 8:20–21.

Rose, S. A. 1983. Differential rates of visual information processing in full-term and preterm infants. *Child Development* 54:1189–1198.

Rosett, H. L. 1980. A clinical perspective on the fetal alcohol syndrome. *Alcoholism* 4:119–122.

Rosett, H. L., and Weiner, L. 1984. *Alcohol and the Fetus: A Clinical Perspective.* New York: Oxford University Press.

Rosett, H. L., Weiner, L., Lee, A., Zuckerman, B., Dooling, E., and Oppenheimer, E. 1983. Patterns of alcohol consumption and fetal development. *Obstetrics and Gynecology* 61:539–546.

Rosman, N. P., and Kakulas, B. A. 1966. Mental deficiency associated with muscular dystrophy: A neuropathological study. *Brain* 89:769–788.

Ross, J. J., and Frias, J. L. 1977. Microcephaly. In P. J. Vinken and A. W. Bruyn (Eds.), *Handbook of Clinical Neurology,* vol. 30: *Congenital Malformations of the Brain and Skull.* Amsterdam: North Holland Publishing.

Rossi, L. N., Candini, G., Scarlotti, G., Rossi, G., Prins, E., and Alberti, S. 1987. Autosomal dominant microcephaly without mental retardation. *American Journal of Diseases of Children* 141:655–659.

Rourke, B. P. 1989. *Non-verbal Learning Disability Syndrome.* New York: Guilford Press.

Rourke, B. P., and Finlayson, M. A. J. 1978. Neuropsychological significance of variations in patterns of academic performance: Verbal and visual-spatial abilities. *Journal of Abnormal Child Psychology* 6:121–123.

Rourke, B. P., and Strang, J. D. 1978. Neuropsychological significance of variation in patterns of academic performance: Motor, psychomotor and tactile perceptual abilities. *Journal of Pediatric Psychology* 3:62–66.

———. 1983. Subtypes of reading and arithmetic disabilities: A neuropsychological analysis. In M. Rutter (Ed.), *Developmental Neuropsychiatry,* pp. 473–488. New York: Guilford Press.

Rousseau, F., Heitz, D., Biancalana, V., Blumenfeld, S., Kretz, C., Boue, J., Tommerup, N., Van der Hagen, C., De Lozin-Blanchet, C., Croquette, M. F., Gilgenkrantz, S., Jalbert, P., Voelckel, M. A., Oberle, I., and Mandel, J. L. 1991. Direct diagnosis by DNA analysis of the fragile X syndrome of mental retardation. *New England Journal of Medicine* 325:1673–1681.

Rovet, J., and Netley, C. 1982. Processing deficits in Turner's syndrome. *Developmental Psychology* 18:77–94.

———. 1983. The triple X chromosome syndrome in childhood: Recent empirical findings. *Child Development* 54:831–845.

Rubinstein, A. 1986. Pediatric AIDS. *Current Problems in Pediatrics* 16:361–409.

Rubinstein, A., Sicklick, M., Gupta, A., Bernstein, L., Klein, N., Rubinstein, E., Spigland, I., Fruchter, L., Litman, N., Lee, H., and Hollander, M. 1983. Acquired immunodeficiency with reversed T4t8 ratios in infants born to promiscuous and drug addicted mothers. *Journal of the American Medical Association* 249:2350–2356.

Rudel, R. 1982. The oblique mystique. In M. Potegal (Ed.), *Spatial Abilities: Development and Physiological Foundations,* pp. 129–146. New York: Academic Press.

Ruff, H. A. 1986. The measurement of attention in high-risk infants. In

P. Bietye and H. C. Coughan (Eds.), *Early Identification of Infants at Risk for Mental Retardation*. New York: Grune & Stratton.

Ruff, H. A., McCarton, C., Kurtzburg, D., and Vaughan, H. C. 1984. Preterm infants' manipulative exploration of objects. *Child Development* 55:1166–1173.

Sameroff, A., and Chandler, M. 1975. Reproductive risk and the continuum of caretaking casualty. In F. D. Horowitz, M. Hetherington, S. Scarr-Salapatek, and G. Siegel (Eds.), *Review of Child Development Research*, Vol. 4, pp. 187–244. Chicago: University of Chicago Press.

Samuelsson, B., and Riccardi, V. M. 1989. Neurofibromatosis in Gothenberg, Sweden: II. Intellectual compromise. *Neurofibromatosis* 2:78–83.

Sand, P. L., Taylor, N., Rawlings, M., and Chitnis, S. 1973. Performance of children with spina bifida manifesta on the Frostig Developmental Test of Visual Perception. *Perceptual and Motor Skills* 37:539–546.

Sanders, R. J. 1989. Sentence comprehension following agenesis of the corpus callosum. *Brain and Language* 37:59–72.

Sassaman, E. A., and Zartler, A. S. 1982. Mental retardation and head growth abnormalities. *Journal of Pediatric Psychology* 7:149–156.

Satz, P., and Fletcher, J. 1982. *Florida Kindergarten Screening Battery*. Odessa, Fla.: Psychological Assessment Resources.

Satz, P., Strauss, E., Wada, J., and Orsini, D. L. 1988. Some correlates of intra-and interhemispheric speech organization after left focal brain injury. *Neuropsychologia* 26:345–350.

Saul, R. E., and Sperry, R. W. 1968. Absence of commissurotomy symptoms with agenesis of the corpus callosum. *Neurology* 18:307.

Scanlon, K. B., Scanlon, J. W., and Tronick, E. 1984. The impact of perinatal and neonatal events on the early behavior of the extremely premature human. *Developmental and Behavioral Pediatrics* 3:65–73.

Schapiro, M. B., Rosman, N. P., and Kemper, T. L. 1984. Effects of chronic exposure to alcohol on the developing brain. *Neurobehavioral Toxicology and Teratology* 6:351–356.

Scheibel, A., Conrad, T., Perdue, S., Tomiyasu, U., and Wechsler, A. 1990. A quantitative study of dendrite complexity in selected areas of human cerebral cortex. *Brain and Cognition* 12:85–101.

Scheibel, A., Paul, L., Fried, I., Forsythe, A., Tomiyasu, U., Wechsler, A., Kao, A., and Slotnick, J. 1985. Dendritic organization of the anterior speech area. *Experimental Neurology* 87:109–117.

Schneider, B. F., and Norton, S. 1980. Development of neurons in the forebrains of rats following prenatal irradiation. *Neurotoxicology* 1:525–532.

Schneider, G. E. 1973. Early lesions of superior colliculus: Factors affecting the formation of abnormal retinal projections. *Brain, Behavior and Evolution* 8:3–109.

———. 1979. Is it really better to have your brain lesion early? A revision of the "Kennard principle." *Neuropsychologia* 17:557–583.

Schull, W. J., Norton, S., and Jensh, R. P. 1990. Ionizing radiation and the developing brain. *Neurotoxicology and Teratology* 12:249–260.

Schull, W. J., Otake, M., and Yoshimaru, H. 1988. Effect on intelligence test score of prenatal exposure to ionizing radiation in Hiroshima and Nagasaki: Comparison of the T65DR and DS86 dosimetry system. Radiation Effects Foundation Technical Report 3–88.

Schulte, F. J. 1988. Pathophysiological mechanisms leading to permanent brain damage in surviving children. In F. Kubli, N. Patel, W. Schmidt, and O. Lindercamp (Eds.), *Perinatal Events and Brain Damage in Surviving Children*, pp. 59–63. New York: Springer-Verlag.

Seemanova, E., Passarge, E., Beneskova, D., Housstek, J., Kasal, P., and Sevcikova, M. 1985. Familial microcephaly with normal intelligence, immunodeficiency and risk for lymphoreticular malignancies: A new autosomal recessive disorder. *American Journal of Medical Genetics* 20:639–648.

Seidel, U. P., Chadwick, O., and Rutter, M. 1975. Psychological disorders in crippled children with and without brain damage. *Developmental Medicine and Child Neurology* 17:563–573.

Sell, E. J., Luick, A., Poisson, S. S., and Hill, S. 1980. Outcome of very low birthweight (VLBW) infants. I. Neonatal behavior of 188 infants. *Developmental and Behavioral Pediatrics* 1:78–85.

Sells, C. J. 1977. Microcephaly in a normal school population. *Pediatrics* 59:262–265.

Selzer, S. C., Lindgren, S. D., and Blackman, J. A. 1992. Long-term neuropsychological outcome of high risk infants with intracranial hemorrhage. *Journal of Pediatric Psychology* 17:407–422.

Sengelaub, D. R., and Finlay, B. L. 1981. Early removal of one eye reduces normally occurring cell death in the remaining eye. *Science* 213:573–574.

Shaffer, J., Friedrich, W. N., Shurtleff, D. B., and Wolf, L. 1985. Cognitive and achievement status of children with myelomeningocele. *Journal of Pediatric Psychology* 10:325–336.

Share, D. L., Moffitt, T. E., and Silva, R. A. 1988. Factors associated with arithmetic and reading disability and specific arithmetic disability. *Journal of Learning Disabilities* 21:313–320.

Shepard, R. N., and Metzler, J. 1971. Mental rotation of three-dimensional objects. *Science* 171:701–703.

Sherman, G. F., Galaburda, A. M., and Geschwind, N. 1985. Cortical anomalies in brains of New Zealand mice: A neuropathologic model of dyslexia. *Proceedings of the National Academy of Sciences of the United States of America* 82:8072–8074.

Sherman, S. 1991. Epidemiology. In R. J. Hagerman and A. C. Cronister (Eds.), *The Fragile X Syndrome: Diagnosis, Treatment, and Research*. Baltimore: Johns Hopkins University Press.

Shprintzen, R. J., and Goldberg, R. B. 1986. Multiple anomaly syndromes and learning disabilities. In S. D. Smith (Ed.), *Genetics and Learning Disabilities*, pp. 153–174. San Diego: College-Hill Press.

Shprintzen, R. J., Goldberg, R. B., Lewin, M. L., Sidoti, E. J., Berkman, M. D., Argamaso, R. V., and Young, D. 1978. A new syndrome involving cleft palate, cardiac anomalies, typical facies, and learning disabilities: Velo-cardio–facial syndrome. *Cleft Palate Journal* 15:56–62.

Shprintzen, R. J., Goldberg, R. B., Young, D., and Wolford, L. 1981. Velo-cardio-facial syndrome: A clinical and genetic analysis. *Pediatrics* 67:167–172.

Shprintzen, R. J., Siegel-Sadewitz, V. L., Amato, J., and Goldberg, R. B. 1985. Anomalies associated with cleft lip, cleft palate, or both. *American Journal of Medical Genetics* 20:585–596.

Shuman, R. M., and Selednik, L. J. 1980. Periventricular leucomalacia. *Archives of Neurology* 37:231–235.

Shurtleff, D. B. 1986. Meningomyelocele: A new or vanishing disease? *Zeitschrift fur Kinderchirurgie* 41(Suppl.):5–9.

Shurtleff, D. B., Foltz, E. K., and Loesser, J. B. 1973. Hydrocephalus: A definition of its progression and relationship to intellectual function, diagnosis and complications. *American Journal of Diseases of Childhood* 125:688–693.

Siegel, L. S. 1983. The prediction of possible learning disabilities in preterm and full-term children. In T. Field and A. Sostek (Eds.), *Infants Born at Risk: Physiological, Perceptual and Cognitive Processes*, pp. 295–315. New York: Grune & Stratton.

Siegel, L. S., Saigal, S., Rosenbaum, P., Morten, R. A., Young, A., Berenbaum, S., and Stoskopf, B. 1982. Predictors of development in preterm and full-term infants: A model for detecting the at risk child. *Journal of Pediatric Psychology* 7:135–148.

Siesjo, B. K. 1981. Cell damage in the brain: A speculative synthesis. *Journal of Cerebral Blood Flow Metabolism* 1:155.

Sigman, M., and Parmelee, A. H. 1974. Visual preferences of four month old premature and full-term infants. *Child Development* 45:959–965.

Silbert, A., Wolff, P. H., and Lilienthal, J. 1977. Spatial and temporal processing in patients with Turner's syndrome. *Behavior Genetics* 7:11–21.

Simms, B. 1986. Learner drivers with spina bifida and hydrocephalus: The relationship between perceptual-cognitive deficit and driving performance. *Zeitschrift fur Kinderchirurgie* 41(Suppl.):51–55.

———. 1987. Route learning ability of young people with spina bifida and hydrocephalus and their able-bodied peers. *Zeitschrift fur Kinderchirurgie* 42(Suppl.):53–56.

Simonds, R., and Scheibel, A. 1988. The postnatal development of the motor speech area: A preliminary report. *Brain and Language* 37:42–58.

Sinha, S. K., Davies, J. M., Sims, D. G., and Chiswick, M. L. 1985. Relation between periventricular haemorrhage and ischaemic brain lesions diagnosed by ultrasound in very preterm infants. *Lancet* 2:1154–1156.

Skoutelli, H. N., Dubowitz, L. M. S., Levene, M. I., and Miller, G. 1985. Predictors of survival and normal neurodevelopmental outcome of infants weighing less than 1001 grams at birth. *Developmental Medicine and Child Neurology* 27:588–595.

Smith, J. F., Reynolds, E. O. R., and Taghizadeh, A. 1974. Brain maturation and damage in infants dying from chronic pulmonary insufficiency in the postnatal period. *Archives of Diseases in Childhood* 49:359–366.

Smith, R. A., Sibert, J. R., and Harper, P. S. 1990. Early development of boys with Duchenne muscular dystrophy. *Developmental Medicine and Child Neurology* 32:519–527.

Smith, W. W. 1976. How Soon Is Early? United Kingdom: East Grinstead and District Society for Mentally Handicapped Children.

Smithells, R. W., Seller, M. J., Harris, R., Fielding, D. W., Schorah, C. J., Nevin, N. C., Sheppard, S., Read, A. P., Walker, S., and Wild, G. 1983. Further experience of vitamin supplementation for prevention of neural tube defect recurrences. *Lancet* 1:1027–1031.

Soare, P., and Raimondi, A. 1977. Intellectual and perceptual-motor characteristics of treated myelomeningocele children. *American Journal of Diseases in Childhood* 131:199–204.

Sobesky, W. E. 1991. The emotional phenotype of fragile X heterozygotes. Paper presented at the International X-linked Mental Retardation Workshop, Bischenberg, France.

Sokol, R. J., Miller, S. I., and Reed, G. 1980. Alcohol abuse during pregnancy: An epidemiological study. *Alcoholism: Clinical and Experimental Research* 4:135–145.

Sollee, N. D., Latham, E. E., Kindlon, D. J., and Bresnan, M. J. 1985. Neuropsychological impairment in Duchenne muscular dystrophy. *Journal of Clinical and Experimental Neuropsychology* 7:486–496.

Soper, H. V., Satz, P. S., Orsini, D. L., Van Garp, W., and Green, M. F. 1987. Handedness distribution in a residential population with severe or profound mental retardation. *American Journal of Mental Deficiency* 92:94–102.

Sostek, A., Smith, Y., Katz, K., and Grant, E. 1987. Developmental outcome of preterm infants with intraventricular hemorrhage at one and two years of age. *Child Development* 58:779–786.

Sovik, O., Van der Hagen, C. B., and Loken, A. C. 1977. X-linked aqueductal stenosis. *Clinical Genetics* 11:416–420.

Spain, B. 1974. Verbal and performance ability in preschool children with spina bifida. *Developmental Medicine and Child Neurology* 16:773.

Sperry, R. W. 1986. Consciousness, personal identity and the divided brain. In F. Lepore, M. Ptito, and H. H. Jaspers (Eds.), *Two Hemispheres—One Brain: Functions of the Corpus Callosum*, pp. 3–20. New York: Alan R. Liss.

Spohr, H. L., and Steinhausen, H. C. 1984. A retrospective four-year follow-up study of children with fetal alcohol syndrome: Clinical, psychopathological and developmental aspects. *CIBA Foundation Symposium* 105:197–217.

Sprecher, S., Soumenkoff, G., Puissant, F., and Degueldre, M. 1986. Vertical transmission of HIV in 15-week fetus. *Lancet* 2:288–289.

Spungen, L. B., Kurtzburg, D., and Vaughn, H. G. 1985. Patterns of looking behavior in full-term and low birth weight infants at 40 weeks postconceptional age. *Journal of Developmental and Behavioral Pediatrics* 6:287–294.

Stehbens, J. A., and Kisker, C. T. 1984. Intelligence and achievement testing in childhood cancer: Three years postdiagnosis. *Developmental and Behavioral Pediatrics* 5:184–188.

Steinhausen, H. S., Gobel, D., and Nestler, V. 1984. Psychopathology in the offspring of alcoholic parents. *Journal of the American Academy of Child Psychiatry* 23:465–471.

Stellman, G. R., and Bannister, C. M. 1985. Factors predicting developmental outcome in premature infants with hydrocephalus due to intraventricular haemorrhage. *Zeitschrift fur Kinderchirurgie* 40(Suppl.):24–26.

Stellman, G. R., Bannister, C. M., and Hillier, V. 1986. The incidence of seizure disorder in children with acquired and congenital hydrocephalus. *Zeitschrift fur Kinderchirurgie* 41 (Suppl.):38–41.

Stewart, A., and Hope, P. 1988. Prediction of outcome: Periventricular hemorrhage versus ischemia. In F. Kubli, N. Patel, W. Schmidt, and O. Lindercamp (Eds.), *Perinatal Events and Brain Damage in Surviving Children*, pp. 257–264. New York: Springer-Verlag.

Stewart, A., and Reynolds, E. O. R. 1974. Improved prognosis for infants of very low birthweight. *Pediatrics* 54:724–735.

Stewart, A. L., Reynolds, E. O. R., and Lipscomb, A. R. 1981. Outcome for infants of very low birthweight: Survey of world literature. *Lancet* 1:1038–1041.

Stewart, A. L., Thorburn, R. J., and Hope, P. L. 1983. Ultrasound appearance of the brain in very preterm infants and neurodevelopmental outcome at 18 months of age. *Archives of Diseases in Childhood* 58:598–604.

Steyaert, J., Borghgraef, M., Gaulthier, C., Fryns, J. P., and Van den Berghe, H. 1992. Cognitive profile in adult, normal intelligent female fragile X carriers. *American Journal of Medical Genetics* 43:116–119.

Stiles-Davis, J., Janowsky, J., Engel, M., and Nass, R. 1988. Drawing ability in four young children with congenital unilateral brain lesions. *Neuropsychologia* 26:359–371.

Stiles-Davis, J., Sugarman, S., and Nass, R. 1985. The development of spatial class relations in four young children with right-cerebral-hemisphere damage: Evidence for an early spatial constructive deficit. *Brain and Cognition* 4:388–412.

Stine, S. R., and Adams, W. V. 1989. Learning problems in neurofibromatosis patients. *Clinical Orthopaedics and Related Research* 245:43–48.

Stoltenburg-Didinger, G., and Spohr, H. L. 1983. Fetal alcohol syndrome and mental retardation: Spine distribution of pyramidal cells in prenatal alcohol-exposed rat cerebral cortex. *Developmental Brain Research* 11:119–123.

Strang, J. D., and Rourke, B. P. 1985. Arithmetic disability subtypes: The

neuropsychological significance of specific arithmetic impairment in childhood. In B. P Rourke (Ed.), *Neuropsychology of Learning Disabilities: Essentials
of Subtype Analysis*, pp. 167–183. New York: Guilford Press.

Streeter, G. L. 1951. Developmental horizons in human embryos: Description
of age groups XIX, XX, XXII, XXIII. Carnegie Institute of Washington
Publication 592. *Contributions to Embryology* 34:165–197.

Streissguth, A. P. 1986. The behavioral teratology of alcohol: Performance,
behavioral, and intellectual deficits in prenatally exposed children. In J. R.
West (Ed.,), *Alcohol and Brain Development*, pp. 3–44. New York: Oxford
University Press.

Streissguth, A. P., Barr, H. M., and Martin, D. C. 1983. Maternal alcohol use
and neonatal habituation assessed with the Brazelton scale. *Child Development* 54:1109–1118.

———. 1984. Alcohol exposure in utero and functional deficits in children
during the first four years of life. *CIBA Foundation Symposium* 105:254-274.

Streissguth, A. P., Barr, H. M., Martin, D. C., and Herman, C. S. 1980. Effects
of maternal alcohol, nicotine and caffeine use during pregnancy on infant
mental and motor development at 8 months. *Alcoholism: Clinical and Experimental Research* 4:152–164.

Streissguth, A. P., Barr, H. M., Sampson, P. D., Darby, B. L., and Martin, D.
C. 1989. IQ at age 4 in relation to maternal alcohol use and smoking during
pregnancy. *Developmental Psychology* 25:1–11.

Streissguth, A. P., Barr, H. M., Sampson, P. D., Parrish-Johnson, J. C., Kirch-
ner, G. L., and Martin, D. C. 1986. Attention, distraction and reaction time
at age 7 years and prenatal alcohol exposure. *Neurobehavioral Toxicology and
Teratology* 8:717–725.

Streissguth, A. P., Bookstein, F. L., Sampson, P. D., and Barr, H. M. 1989.
Neurobehavioral effects of prenatal alcohol: Part III. PLS analyses of neuropsychologic tests. *Neurotoxicology and Teratology* 11:493–507.

Streissguth, A. P., Herman, C. S., and Smith, D. W. 1978. Intelligence, behavior and dysmorphogenesis in the fetal alcohol syndrome: A report on 20
patients. *Journal of Pediatrics* 92:363–367.

Streissguth, A. P., Van Derveer, B. B., and Shepard, T. H. 1970. Mental
development of children with congenital rubella syndrome. *American Journal of Obstetrics and Gynecology* 108:391–399.

Sudhalter, V., Cohen, I. L., Silverman, W., and Wolf-Schein, E. G. 1990.
Conversational analyses of males with fragile X, Down syndrome, autism:
Comparison of the emergence of deviant language. *American Journal of
Mental Retardation* 94:431–441.

Sudhalter, V., Marianon, M., and Brooks, P. 1992. Expressive semantic deficit
in the productive language of males with fragile X syndrome. *American
Journal of Medical Genetics* 43:65–71.

Sudhalter, V., Scarborough, H. S., and Cohen, I. 1991. Syntactic delay and
pragmatic deviance in the language of fragile X males. *American Journal of
Medical Genetics* 38:493–497.

Sullivan, W. C. 1899. A note on the influence of maternal inebriety on the offspring. *Journal of Mental Science* 45:489–503.

Sutherland, R. J., Kolb, B., Schoel, W. M., Whishaw, I. Q., and Davies, D. 1982. Neuropsychological assessment of children and adults with Tourette syndrome: A comparison with learning disabilities and schizophrenia. In A. J. Friedhoff and T. N. Chase (Eds.), *Gilles de la Tourette Syndrome*, pp. 311–322. New York: Raven Press.

Takashima, S., and Tanaka, K. 1978. Development of cerebrovascular architecture and its relationship to periventricular leucomalacia. *Archives of Neurology* 35:11–16.

Tallal, P. 1980a. Auditory temporal perception, phonics, and reading disabilities in children. *Brain and Language* 9:182–198.

———. 1980b. Language and reading: Some perceptual prerequisites. *Bulletin of the Orton Society* 30:170–178.

Tallal, P., and Piercy, M. 1973. Defects of non-verbal auditory perception in children with developmental aphasia. *Nature* 241:468–469.

Taylor, E. M. 1961. *Psychological Appraisal of Children with Cerebral Defects*. Cambridge: Harvard University Press.

Taylor, N., Sand, P. L., and Jebson, R. 1973. Evaluation of hand function in children. *Archives of Physical Medicine* 54:129–135.

Teebi, A. S., Al-Awadi, S. A., and White, A. G. 1987. Autosomal recessive nonsyndromal microcephaly with normal intelligence. *American Journal of Medical Genetics* 26:355–359.

Tekolste, K. A., Bennett, F. C., and Mack, L. A. 1985. Follow-up of infants receiving cranial ultrasound for intracranial hemorrhage. *American Journal of Diseases of Children* 139:299–303.

Temple, C. M., Jeeves, M. A., and Villaroya, O. 1989. Ten pen men: Rhyming skills in two children with callosal agenesis. *Brain and Language* 37:59–72.

Tew, B. 1979. The cocktail party syndrome in children with hydrocephalus and spina bifida. *British Journal of Disorders of Communication* 14:89–101.

Tew, B. J., and Laurence, K. M. 1972. The ability and attainments of spina bifida patients born in South Wales between 1956–1972. *Developmental Medicine and Child Neurology* 14(Suppl.):124–131.

———. 1975. The effect of hydrocephalus on intelligence, visual perception and school attainment. *Developmental Medicine and Child Neurology* 35(Suppl.):129–134.

———. 1979. The clinical and psychological characteristics of children with the "cocktail party" syndrome. *Zeitschrift fur Kinderchirurgie* 28:360–367.

———. 1983. Spina bifida children's intelligence test scores on school entry and at school leaving. *Child Care Health and Development* 9:13–17.

———. 1984. The relationship between intelligence and academic achievements in spina bifida adolescents. *Zeitschrift fur Kinderchirurgie* 39(Suppl.): 122–124.

Thorley, B. S., and Wood, V. M. 1979. Early number experiences for preschool Down's syndrome children. *Australian Journal of Early Childhood* 4:15–20.

Tilson, H. A., Jacobson, J. L., and Rogan, W. J. 1990. Polychlorinated biphenyls and the developing nervous system: Cross-species comparisons. *Neurotoxicology and Teratology* 12:239–248.

Towbin, A. 1978. Cerebral function related to perinatal organic damage: Clinical-neuropathologic correlations. *Journal of Abnormal Psychology* 87:617–635.

Tucker, T. J., and Kling, A. 1967. Differential effects of early and late lesions of frontal granular cortex in the monkey. *Brain Research* 5:377–389.

Tudehope, D. I., Burns, Y., O'Callaghan, M., Mohay, H., and Silcock, A. 1983. The relationship between intrauterine and postnatal growth on the subsequent psychomotor development of very low birthweight (VLBW) infants. *Australian Paediatric Journal* 19:3–8.

Ultmann, M. H., Belman, A. L., Ruff, H. A., Novick, B. E., Cone-Wesson, B., Cohen, H. J., and Rubinstein, A. 1985. Developmental abnormalities in infants and children with acquired immune deficiency syndrome (AIDS) and AIDS-related complex. *Neurology* 27:563–571.

Ultmann, M. H., Diamond, G. W., Ruff, H. A., Belman, A. L., Novick, B. E., Rubinstein, A., and Cohen, H. J. 1987. Developmental abnormalities in children with acquired immunodeficiency syndrome (AIDS): A follow-up study. *International Journal of Neuroscience* 32:661–667.

U.S. Department of Health and Human Services, Centers for Disease Control. March 1992. *HIV/AIDS Surveillance Report.*

U.S. Environmental Protection Agency. 1986. *Air Quality Criteria for Lead.* EPA Report EPA-600/8-83/028af-df.4v. Research Triangle Park, N.C.: Office of Health and Environmental Assessment, Environmental Criteria and Assessment Office.

———. 1989. Supplement to the 1986 EPA air quality for lead: Volume I addendum (pages A1–67). EPA Report EPA-600/8-89/049A. Washington, D.C.: Office of Research and Development, Office of Health and Environmental Assessment.

van Bel, F., den Ouden, L., van de Bor, M., Stijnen, T., Baan, J., and Ruys, J. H. 1989. Cerebral blood flow in the first week of life of preterm infants and neurodevelopment at two years. *Developmental Medicine and Child Neurology* 31:320–328.

Van de Bor, M., Ens-Dokkum, M., Schreuder, A. M., Jeen, S., Brand, R., and Verloove-Vanhorick, S. P. 1993. Outcome of periventricular-intraventricular haemorrhage at five years of age. *Developmental Medicine and Child Neurology* 35:33–41.

Van der Vlugt, J., and Satz, P. 1985. Subgroups and subtypes of learning disabled and normal children: A cross-cultural replication. In B. P. Rourke (Ed.), *Neuropsychology of Learning Disabilities: Essentials of Subtype Analysis,* pp. 212–227. New York: Guilford Press.

Vanucci, R. C., and Duffy, T. E. 1977. Cerebral metabolism in newborn dogs during reversible asphyxia. *Annals of Neurology* 1:528.
Vargha-Khadem, F., O'Gorman, A. M., and Watters, G. V. 1985. Aphasia and handedness in relation to hemispheric side, age at injury and severity of cerebral lesion during childhood. *Brain* 108:677–696.
Vargha-Khadem, F., Watters, G. V., and O'Gorman, A. M. 1985. Development of speech and language following bilateral frontal lesions. *Brain and Language* 25:167–183.
Vauclair, J., Fagot, J., and Hopkins, W. D. 1993. Rotation of mental images in baboons when the visual input is directed to the left cerebral hemisphere. *Psychological Science* 4:99–103.
Venter, P. A., Op't Hof, J., Coetzee, D. J., Van der Walt, C., and Retief, A. E. 1984. No marker (X) syndrome in autistic children. *Human Genetics* 67:107.
Verkerk, A. J., Pierette, M., Sutcliffe, J. S., Fu, Y. H., Kuhl, D. P., Pizzuti, A., Reiner, O., Richards, S., Victoria, M. F., Zhang, F., Eussen, B. E., Van Ommen, G. J., Blonden, L. A. J., Riggins, G. J., Chastain, J. L., Kunst, C. B., Galjaand, H., and Caskey, C. T. 1991. Identification of a gene (FMR-1) containing a CGG repeat coincident with a breakpoint cluster region exhibiting length variation in fragile X syndrome. *Cell* 65:905–914.
Villablanca, J. R., Burgess, J. W., and Sonnier, B. J. 1984. Neonatal cerebral hemispherectomy: A model for postlesion reorganization of the brain. In S. Finger and D. G. Stein (Eds.), *Early Brain Damage*, Vol. 2: *Neurobiology and Behavior*, pp. 179–210. New York: Academic Press.
Vogt, M. W., Witt, D. J., Craven, D. E., Byington, R., Crawford, D. F., Hutchinson, M. F., Schooley, R. T., and Hirsch, M. S. 1987. Isolation patterns of the human immunodeficiency virus from cervical secretions during the menstrual cycle of women at risk for the acquired immunodeficiency syndrome. *Annals of Internal Medicine* 106:380–382.
Vohr, B. R., and Garcia Coll, C. T. 1985. Neurodevelopmental and school performance of very low birthweight infants: A seven year longitudinal study. *Pediatrics* 76:345–350.
Volcke, P., Dereymaeker, A. M., Fryns, J. P., and Van den Berghe, H. 1990. On the nosology of moderate mental retardation with special attention to X-linked mental retardation. *Genetic Counseling* 1:47–56.
Volpe, J. J. 1987. *Neurology of the Newborn*, 2nd Edition. Philadelphia: W. B. Saunders.
Waber, D. 1979. Neuropsychological aspects of Turner's syndrome. *Developmental Medicine and Child Neurology* 21:58–70.
Waber, D. P. 1977. Sex differences in mental abilities: Hemispheric lateralization and rate of physical growth in adolescence. *Developmental Psychology* 13:29–38.
Wadshy, M., Lindehammer, H., and Feg-Olofsson, O. 1989. Neurofibromatosis in childhood: Neuropsychological aspects. *Neurofibromatosis* 2:251–260.
Walzer, S. 1985. X chromosome abnormalities and cognitive development:

Implications for understanding normal human development. *Journal of Child Psychology and Psychiatry* 26:177–184.

Walzer, S., Wolff, P. H., Bowen, D., Silbert, A. R., Bashir, A. S., Gerald, P. S., and Richmond, J. B. 1978. A method for the longitudinal study of behavioral development in infants and children: The early development of XXY children. *Journal of Child Psychology and Psychiatry* 19:213–229.

Warkany, J., and Dignan, P. St.J. 1973. Congenital microcephaly. In J. Wortis (Ed.), *Mental Retardation: Annual Review*, Vol. 5, pp. 113-135. New York: Brunner/Mazel.

Warkany, J. L., Lemire, R. J., and Cohen, M. M. 1981. *Mental Retardation and Congenital Malformations of the Central Nervous System*. Chicago: Year Book Medical Publishers.

Watson, J. D., and Crick, F. H. C. 1953. Molecular structure of nucleic acids: A structure for deoxyribose nucleic acid. *Nature* 171:737–738.

Weller, T. H., and Hanshaw, J. B. 1962. Virologic and clinical observations on cytomegalic inclusion disease. *New England Journal of Medicine* 266:1233–1244.

Welsh, M. C., Pennington, B. F., Ozonoff, S., Rouse, B., and McCabe, F. R. 1990. Neuropsychology of early-treated phenylketonuria: Specific executive function deficits. *Child Development* 61:1697–1713.

Whelan, T. B. 1987. Neuropsychological performance of children with Duchenne muscular dystrophy and spinal muscular atrophy. *Developmental Medicine and Child Neurology* 29:212–220.

White, J. L., Moffitt, T. E., and Silva, P. A. 1992. Neuropsychological and socioemotional correlates of specific arithmetic disability. *Archives of Clinical Neuropsychology* 7:1–16.

Wigglesworth, J. S. 1984. *Perinatal Pathology*. Philadelphia: W. B. Saunders.

———. 1988. Trauma and the developing brain. In F. Kubli, N. Patel, W. Schmidt, and O. Lindercamp (Eds.), *Perinatal Events and Brain Damage in Surviving Children*, pp. 64–69. New York: Springer-Verlag.

Wigglesworth, J. S., Davies, P. A., Keith, I. H., and Slade, S. A. 1977. Intraventricular haemorrhage in the preterm infant without hyaline membrane disease. *Archives of Diseases in Childhood* 52:447–451.

Wigglesworth, J. S., and Pape, K. E. 1978. An integrated model for hemorrhagic and ischemic lesions in the newborn brain. *Early Human Development* 2:179–199.

Willerman, L., Schultz, R., Rutledge, J. N., and Bigler, E. D. 1991. In vivo brain size and intelligence. *Intelligence* 15:223–228.

———. 1992. Hemisphere size asymmetry predicts relative verbal and nonverbal intelligence differently in the sexes: An MRI study of structure-functional relations. *Intelligence* 16:315–328.

Williams, J., Richman, L., and Yarbrough, D. 1991. A comparison of memory and attention in Turner syndrome and learning disability. *Journal of Pediatric Psychology* 16:585–593.

Williams, J. C. P., Barrett-Boyes, B. G., and Lowe, J. B. 1961. Supravalvular aortic stenosis. *Circulation* 24:1311–1318.

Williamson, M. L., Koch, R., Azen, C., and Chang, C. 1981. Correlates of intelligence test results in treated phenylketonuric children. *Pediatrics* 68:161–167.

Williamson, W. D., Desmond, M. M., Wilson, G. S., Andrew, L. P., and Garcia-Prats, J. A. 1982. Early neurodevelopmental outcome of low birthweight infants surviving neonatal intraventricular hemorrhage. *Journal of Perinatal Medicine* 10:34–41.

Wishart, J. G. 1991. Learning difficulties in infants with Down's syndrome. *International Journal of Rehabilitation Research* 14:251–255.

Wisniewski, K. E., Laure-Kamionowska, M., Connell, F., and Wen, G. Y. 1986. Neuronal density and synaptogenesis in the postnatal stage of brain maturation in Down syndrome. In J. Epstein (Ed.), *The Neurobiology of Down Syndrome*, pp. 29–44. New York: Raven Press.

Witelson, S. F. 1986. Wires of the mind: Anatomical variation in the corpus callosum in relation to hemispheric specialization and integration. In F. Lepore, M. Ptito, and H. H. Jaspers (Eds.), *Two Hemispheres—One Brain: Functions of the Corpus Callosum*, pp. 117–137. New York: Alan R. Liss.

———. 1987. Neurobehavioral aspects of language in children. *Child Development* 58:653–688.

Wolf, M. 1984. Naming, reading and the dyslexias: A longitudinal overview. *Annals of Dyslexia* 34:87–115.

Wood, J. W., Johnson, K. G., and Omori, Y. 1965. In utero exposure to the Hiroshima atomic bomb: A follow-up at twenty years. Atomic Bomb Casualty Commission Technical Report 9-65.

Wood, J. W., Johnson, K. G., Omori, Y., Kawamoto, S., and Keehn, R. 1966. Mental retardation in children exposed in utero. Hiroshima-Nagasaki Atomic Bomb Casualty Commission Technical Report 10-19.

Woods, B. T., and Carey, S. 1979. Language deficits after apparent clinical recovery from childhood aphasia. *Annals of Neurology* 6:405–409.

Woods, B. T., and Teuber, H.-L. 1978. Changing patterns of childhood aphasia. *Annals of Neurology* 3:273–280.

World Health Organization. 1948–49. *Manual of the International Statistical Classification of Diseases, Injuries and Causes of Death.* Geneva: World Health Organization.

———. 1961. *Public Health Aspects of Low Birthweight.* 3rd Report, Expert Committee on Maternal and Child health, Technical Report Series, No. 217. Geneva: World Health Organization.

Wynn, M., and Wynn, A. 1979. *Prevention of Handicap and the Health of Women.* London: Routledge & Kegan Paul.

Yakovlev, P. I., and Lecours, A-R. 1967. The myelogenetic cycles of regional maturation of the brain. In A. Minkowski (Ed.), *Regional Development of the Brain in Early Life*, pp. 3–65. Oxford: Blackwell Scientific Publications.

Yakovlev, P. I., and Rakic, P. 1966. Patterns of decussation of bulbar pyramids and distribution of pyramidal tracts on two sides of the spinal cord. *Transactions of the American Neurological Association* 91:366–367.

Yu, S., Pritchard, M., Kremer, E., Lynch, M., Nancarrow, J., Baker, E., Holman, K., Mulley, J. G., Warren, S. T., Schlessinger, D., Sutherland, G. R., and Richards, R. I. 1991. Fragile X genotype characterized by an unstable region of DNA. *Science* 252:1179–1181.

Zaidel, E. 1986. Callosal dynamics and right hemisphere language. In F. Lepore, M. Ptito, and H. H. Jaspers (Eds.), *Two Hemispheres—One Brain: Functions of the Corpus Callosum*, pp. 435–459. New York: Alan R. Liss.

Zang, K. D. 1984. Genetics and cytogenetics of Klinefelter's syndrome. In H. J. Bandmann and R. Breit (Eds.), *Klinefelter's Syndrome*, pp. 12–23. New York: Springer-Verlag.

Zeiner, H. K., and Prigatano, G. P. 1982. Information processing deficits and letter reversal in hydrocephalic children. *Neuropsychologia* 20:483–492.

Ziegler, J. B., Cooper, D. A., Johnson, R. O., and Gold, J. 1985. Postnatal transmission of AIDS-associated retrovirus from mother to infant. *Lancet* 1:896–898.

Zuckerman, B. S., and Hingson, R. 1986. Alcohol consumption during pregnancy: A critical review. *Developmental Medicine and Child Neurology* 28:649–654.

Indexes

Synaptogenesis, 23, 24; in Down syndrome, 55, 57

Tourette syndrome: and attention deficit hyperactivity disorder, 44, 45; and dopamine, 32, 45; incidence of, 44; intelligence in, 45, 46; learning disabilities in, 45; and prefrontal cortex, 32; prevalence of, 44; visual perceptual skills in, 46; and Wisconsin Card Sorting Test, 46

Turner syndrome, 47; attention in, 53; chromosome defect in, 29; hyperactivity in, 53; intelligence in, 47, 53, 220; language in, 47, 52, 53; learning disabilities in, 53; mathematical ability in, 52

Vascularization, cerebral: of basal ganglia, 18; and brain injury, 15, 17–20, 22; of cerebral cortex, 16–18; in embryonic period, 15, 16; in fetal period, 15–18; in germinal matrix tissue, 17, 18, 20; of midbrain and cerebellum, 18

Velocardiofacial syndrome, 66, 67; abstract reasoning in, 111, 112; hearing loss in, 111, 112; intelligence in, 111, 112; learning disabilities in, 111, 112; and microcephaly, 111, 112; visual perceptual skills in, 111

Williams syndrome, 66, 67, 79, 102; and cocktail party syndrome, 104, 105; intelligence in, 103, 220; language in, 103, 104; learning disabilities in, 103; motor skills in, 103, 104; visual perceptual skills in, 103, 104, 220, 222

X-Linked inheritance, 29, 216; in fragile X syndrome, 36, 37; in microcephaly, 106; and reading, 256

47XXX: intelligence in, 47; language in, 47, 49, 54; learning disabilities in, 54; memory in, 54; motor skills in, 47; spatial skills in, 47, 49, 54

47XYY: handedness in, 49; intelligence in, 47, 50, 52; language in, 47, 49, 220; reading in, 52; spatial skills in, 47, 49, 52, 220; testosterone in, 49, 50

Author Index

Library of Congress Cataloging-in-Publication Data

Dorman, Casey.
  Cognitive effects of early brain injury / Casey Dorman and Bilha Katzir.
    p.   cm. — (The Johns Hopkins series in psychiatry and neuroscience)
  Includes bibliographical references and index.
  ISBN 0-8018-4856-3 (hc : alk. paper)
    1. Brain-damaged children.   2. Cognition disorders in children.   3. Brain—
  Wounds and injuries—Complications.   I. Katzir, Bilha.   II. Title.   III. Series.
    [DNLM: 1. Brain Injuries—congenital.   2. Brain Injuries—complications.
  3. Cognition Disorders—etiology.   WS 340 D712c 1994]
  RJ496.B7D67   1994
  617.4'81044'083—dc20
  DNLM/DLC
  for Library of Congress   94-6782

DATE DUE

JUN 1 4 1998	
NOV 1 2 2003	

BRODART   Cat. No. 23-221

SPEAKING OF LIFE

COMMUNICATION AND SOCIAL ORDER

An Aldine de Gruyter Series of Texts and Monographs

Series Editor

David R. Maines, Wayne State University

Advisory Editors

Bruce Gronbeck • Peter K. Manning • William K. Rawlins

David L. Altheide and Robert Snow, **Media Worlds in the Postjournalism Era**

Joseph Bensman and Robert Lilienfeld, **Craft and Consciousness: Occupational Technique and the Development of World Images** (*Second Edition*)

Valerie Malhotra Bentz, **Becoming Mature: Childhood Ghosts and Spirits in Adult Life**

Jörg R. Bergmann, **Discreet Indiscretions**

Herbert Blumer, **Industrialization as an Agent of Social Change: A Critical Analysis** (*Edited with an Introduction by David R. Maines and Thomas J. Morrione*)

Dennis Brissett and Charles Edgley (*editors*), **Life as Theater: A Dramaturgical Sourcebook** (*Second Edition*)

Richard Harvey Brown (*editor*), **Writing the Social Text: Poetics and Politics in Social Science Discourse**

Norman K. Denzin, **Hollywood Shot by Shot: Alcoholism in American Cinema**

Irwin Deutscher, Fred P. Pestello, and H. Frances G. Pestello, **Sentiments and Acts**

Pasquale Gagliardi (ed), **Symbols and Artifacts: Views of the Corporate Landscape** (paperback)

Bryan S. Green, **Gerontology and the Construction of Old Age: A Study in Discourse Analysis**

Jaber F. Gubrium, **Speaking of Life: Horizons of Meaning for Nursing Home Residents**

J. T. Hansen, A. Susan Owen, and Michael Patrick Madden, **Parallels: The Soldiers' Knowledge and the Oral History of Contemporary Warfare**

Emmanuel Lazega, **The Micropolitics of Knowledge: Communication and Indirect Control in Workgroups**

Niklas Luhmann, **Risk: A Sociological Theory**

David R. Maines (*editor*), **Social Organization and Social Process: Essays in Honor of Anselm Strauss**

Peter K. Manning, **Organizational Communication**

Stjepan G. Meštrović, **Durkheim and Postmodernist Culture**

R. S. Perinbanayagam, **Discursive Acts**

William K. Rawlins, **Friendship Matters: Communication, Dialectics, and the Life Course**

Dmitry Shlapentokh and Vladimir Shlapentokh, **Soviet Cinematography, 1918–1991: Ideological Conflict and Social Reality**

Anselm Strauss, **Continual Permutations of Action**

Jacqueline P. Wiseman, **The Other Half: Wives of Alcoholics and Their Social-Psychological Situation**

SPEAKING OF LIFE

Horizons of Meaning for
Nursing Home
Residents

Jaber F. Gubrium

ALDINE DE GRUYTER
New York

About the Author

Jaber F. Gubrium is Professor in the Department of Sociology at the University of Florida. He has conducted research on the social organization of care in diverse treatment settings, including nursing homes, physical rehabilitation, caregiver support groups, and family counseling. His continuing fieldwork on the organizational embeddedness of social forms serves as a basis for comparative interpretive ethnography and a sociology of description.

Professor Gubrium is the editor of *Journal of Aging Studies* and the author of *Living and Dying at Murray Manor, Oldtimers and Alzheimer's, Analyzing Field Reality,* and *The Mosaic of Care*. His recently coauthored books (with J. Holstein) *What is Family?* and *Constructing the Life Course* present constructionist approaches to domestic order and the life course.

ALDINE DE GRUYTER
A division of Walter de Gruyter, Inc.
200 Saw Mill River Road
Hawthorne, New York 10532

This publication is printed in acid-free paper ⊚

Library of Congress Cataloging-in-Publication Data

Gubrium, Jaber F.
    Speaking of life : horizons of meaning for nursing home residents
/ Jaber F. Gubrium.
        p.   cm. — (Communication and social order)
    Includes bibliographical references and index.
    ISBN 0-202-30481-7 (alk. paper). — ISBN 0-202-30482-5 (pbk. :
alk. paper)
        1. Nursing home care.   2. Nursing home patients.   I. Title.
II. Series.
RC954.3.G83   1993
362.1'6—dc20   93-28591
                                                                      CIP

Manufactured in the United States of America

10 9 8 7 6 5 4 3 2 1

FOR THE STORYTELLERS

Jake Bellows
Rebecca Bourdeau
Lula Burton
Mary Carter
Ruby Coplin
Martha Gilbert
Karen Gray
Sue and Don Hughes
Myrtle Johnson
Bea Lindstrom
Jane and Tom Malinger
Julia McCall
Jane Nesbit
Opal Peters
Betty Randolph
Peter Rinehart
Lily Robinson
Roland Snyder
Alice Stern
Celia Turner
Rita Vandenberg
Grace Wheeler

Contents

Foreword

There has been only one paradigm shift during the past century in sociological thought that has meant much. That was when, under the influence of Thomas and Znaniecki's *Polish Peasant* research, instinct theories were forever replaced by social ontologies. Genetics was out, social forces and social processes were in, and sociology flourished as a result.

But a weariness now permeates the field. Formula sociology (do a survey, run some statistics, test a model), which also flourished, worked well for awhile, but we now understand that it worked best as an ideological and administrative practice. It went a long way toward legitimating sociology, but in the process it ironically became an orthodoxy that retarded scholarship. And so now, with the limits of the orthodoxy reached, the discipline is tired.

That disciplinary weariness has created an intellectual space that is now being filled by the renewed vigor of interpretive approaches. On its surface, this renewal looks like a second major paradigm shift: witness the rise of cultural studies, both American and European; the collage of postmodernist and poststructuralist debates, the increased attention to narrative the rhetoric; the wide-spread advocacy of multi-method research designs, the broader base of interactionist scholarship throughout the social sciences, let alone the increased blurring of genres that Geertz wrote about. I suspect, though, that there is more continuity and less of a shift in these approaches than one might think. What we have is merely a sharper and more articulate framing of ideas, perspectives, and concepts that have been around for decades and that these new framings have mobilized a new energy, excitement, and set of promises.

Jay Gubrium has represented a central and sustaining voice in and of that continuity. He has brought imagination, intellect, and an admirable tenacity to his scholarly endeavor, and he has justly become internationally known for his qualitative research is gerontology. When others were torturing the details of topics such as the demographic conditions for the emergence of nursing homes, Gubrium was publishing *Living and Dying at Murray Manor* and providing a masterly account of the living among the dying. When others sought to chart sequences along the life course, he told us of the biographies and lived experiences that cut across those sequences. For over twenty years, he has reminded us that sociology ought to study what people actually do; that people are creatures who communicate through symbols and are part of the very environments they create, and that their essence (in Dewey's sense of the term) rests in a selved, ongoing, and always partially formed inter-subjectivity. Science, with its methods and theories, and policy, with its attempts to structure human contact, must both eventually make their peace with these human conditions.

With the publication of *Speaking of Life*, Gubrium enters the apparent paradigm shift, sometimes called the interpretive turn, sometimes the narrative turn. In so doing, he exemplifies the continuity of scholarship in which these "turns" are grounded. He emphasizes meaning, context, time, reasonable accounts, the normalcy of inconsistency, and emotionality, which have been the bread and butter of interpretive, qualitative research all along. But he sharpens these traditional issues by emphasizing narrativity and what he calls horizons of meaning. He focuses attention on lifelong biographical linkages among nursing home residents that can be rendered only in the form of life narratives. Within these narrative renditions, horizons of meaning are discovered: worry, disappointment, regret, death, hope, joy. The nursing home is not a mere set of role arrangements, nor merely a setting containing people who can tell life narratives. Rather, it is like any other site of human collectivities—storied, transacted, layered with ambiguity, permeated by contingency, and ultimately, given life through perspectives of interpretation.

Gubrium takes these sorts of things seriously in giving us a realist narrative of nursing home residents' lives. He brilliantly accomplishes the task he sets out upon by providing stories to residents' faces, but I think he really goes further by telling us that there must be faces to the sociological storyteller. For, indeed, our professional accounts are the only *one* narrative version subject, like all stories, to group conventions of storytelling. Here, he warns us of the undesirable consequences of conceptual dogma, of the inhumane and impractical implications of univocal policy, of the inevitable reactivity in social research, of the observed and rendered fact that nursing home residents are not always "residents' " when they talk to us. In *Speaking of Life*, Jay Gubrium speaks again of life among the dying. But, he also speaks of the continuity of interpretive research and thereby contributes a considerable dose of energy to our tired discipline.

David R. Maines

Acknowledgments

It is the narratives of those whose experience we study that make it possible to do social science. This book is dedicated to the men and women, resident in nursing homes, whose stories form the basis of what I have written. I am deeply grateful to them for affording me and my assistant both the time and the pain to convey the meanings of their lives and care in residence.

Carol Ronai, my doctoral student, assisted in the interviewing. She was an invaluable source of insights and efficiently moved the project along. I thank the University of Florida's Institute for Community Studies for administering the project, whose staff competently completed the transcriptions and managed the narrative material.

A number of colleagues and friends read the manuscript and made helpful comments. My good friend and collaborator Jim Holstein, with whom it is always a pleasure to work, identified strengths and weaknesses and in his invariably supportive manner advised me how to improve and sharpen the presentation. Florida colleague Anne Wyatt-Brown brought a critical humanist's eye to the text and informed me of the many ways in which what I had to say paralleled literary themes. David Maines, this book's series editor, offered useful advice.

Sharon Kaufman's research on the aging self and Robert Rubinstein's work on personal meaning have been sources of inspiration. I have extended some of their insights into the nursing home setting. Suzanne Gubrium, Steve Golant, R. Satyanarayana, and Camille Van Kirk were most encouraging throughout the project. As usual, my loving daughters, Aline and Erika, pummeled me with approving sarcasm. And, last but not least, the people I worked with at Aldine—Richard Koffler, Arlene Perazzini, and Mike Sola—were a first-rate editorial and production team.

The larger study of which this project was a part was supported by a two-year grant from the National Institute on Aging (R01 AG07985).

Introduction

Quality assurance has become a leading goal of health care delivery, the effect of public alarm over the high cost of care and the aim of offering the best care for the fewest dollars. One outcome has been the development of systems of quality management to assess quality on several fronts, from the quality of care provided to the resulting quality of life for care receivers.

This is increasingly evident in long-term care. In the past, nursing homes were besieged by journalistic exposes of poor-quality care; the leading assault now is being rationalized into the formal documentation of the quality of care provision and the quality of life for residents. A quality assurance industry is emerging to design assessment instruments, offer data management services, and monitor results and compliance activity.

Yet, for all the alarm and rationalization, few are asking what the subjective meaning of quality of care and quality of life is for those whose lives are affected. In contrast to the relatively short stays of hospital patients, nursing home residents are typically "long stayers" and, for better or worse, are likely to encounter the nursing facility as a final household. Matters of home, family, interpersonal ties, life history, self-worth, dependence, disappointment, and destiny confront residents in ways irrelevant to hospital patients or other short-stay care receivers. The matters significantly mediate the meaning of quality of care and quality of life.

This book examines the subjective meaning of the nursing home's quality of care and quality of life. A sample of residents has been given the opportunity to tell their stories, to speak of life and to convey in their own terms the meaning of the qualities in their facilities in relation to the significant matters of long stays. Meanings are presented from residents' points of view, revealing where and, if so, how in their lives the qualities figure in. It is a bottom-up rather than a top-down look and shows how what may be administratively deemed the qualities of care and life do not reflect what the qualities appear to be to care receivers.

The thesis is that the qualities are narratively organized by horizons of meaning: Residents convey the meaning of the quality of care and quality of life in terms of the differential linkages they make with lifelong experiences. For example, for residents whose horizons show them to be "worried to death" or who demonstrate otherworldly linkages, such as being engrossed with "lovin' the Lord," the quality of the facility's care is not as significant as it is for residents whose horizons articulate a vigilance for equity and justice in interpersonal relations. Among the former residents, the quality of care is at worst a source of daily irritations and at best a gamut of mere comforts. Against the horizon of vigilance, however, the quality of care becomes an all-consuming matter.

This thesis relates to a long-standing theoretical concern with how experience is given voice in everyday life, part of a broader interest in the sociology of description. For many years, the interest focused empirically on how organizations condition the way participants convey experience. For instance, ethnographic material gathered in fieldwork in a nursing home called Murray Manor was interpreted to reveal that a single nursing home, in practice, was three different "worlds" of living and dying. I argued then that differences in attitudes, sentiments, and behavior among administrators, frontline workers, and residents could not be understood unless their respective worlds were taken into account (Gubrium 1975). Recently, I have turned this around a bit theoretically to highlight participants (in this case, nursing home residents) as more active conveyers of meaning, less conditioned by circumstances than taking circumstances into account in telling their stories. It has not been a complete turnabout, inasmuch as residents' narratives are not viewed as conveyed with total disregard for leading orientations to the qualities of care and life, the special circumstances that distinguish residents from each other, and the broader experiential significances of long-term care and stays in a nursing home. But it is a definite turn to narrative as grounds for interpretation.

As far as possible in the following chapters, I present residents' stories in their own voices. Overall, the reader will not find the stories particularly gripping. They are only occasionally vividly packaged or poignantly ironic. Some are dishearteningly sad; others are glib or comical. Reading them, from chapter to chapter, is an emotional roller coaster. A few of the stories are repetitive, digressive, even confused. Yet they are categorizable into narrative types, revealing the storytellers to be meaningfully oriented in different ways to matters of life and care. Their tellers link the present qualities of care and nursing home life with experiences long past and with what is foreseen well beyond the days ahead. Mundane as the stories are, they inform the reader that quality of life and quality of care, in residents' voices, are not so much rationally assessable conditions, as they are horizoned, ordinary, and biographically active renderings of lifelong experience.

1

Faces without Stories?

Twenty years ago, I completed fieldwork that led to the publication of *Living and Dying at Murray Manor* (Gubrium 1975), an ethnography of a nursing home. I can't say that horizons of meaning for nursing home residents or more particular concerns such as the quality of care and the quality of life were uppermost in my mind at the time. If anything, these matters were simmering at the sidelines of research focused on life worlds within institutional settings. It would be in the course of studies that followed much later that the matters' subjective meaning for residents would become the full-blown project reported here. Even so, the project has critical roots in the earlier work, which is where I will begin.

The fieldwork for the ethnography had an unexpected yet propitious start. Trained as a survey researcher and having just finished a study of life satisfaction among noninstitutionalized elderly, I planned to investigate the ingredients of life satisfaction for elderly in nursing homes. Methodologically, the plan seemed straightforward enough: Take the concepts and the skills learned in the community study and apply them in the nursing home setting.

But I had never set foot in a nursing home, and I knew no one who was resident in one nor anyone who worked there. The research literature on the social organization of nursing homes was meager. Anthropologist Jules Henry (1963) provided a comparative view of a hospital and two nursing homes. He called one of the nursing homes "hell's vestibule" because it offered residents filth and neglect. A few articles by sociologists were forthcoming, such as Elizabeth Gustafson's (1972) paper on the moral career of the nursing home patient and Charles Stannard's (1973) on the social conditions for patient abuse in a nursing home. Fiction writer May Sarton's (1973) eloquently written and touching account, *As We Are Now,* of seventy-six-year-old protagonist Caro Spencer's experience as a resident in a rural nursing home called Twin Elms was a year from publication.

From the media, I had gotten a quite negative sense of what nursing home life was like. There were the frequent exposés of poor nursing

home care I read in newspapers and magazines and watched on television public affairs programs. I could hardly mention my new research
interest without being told things such as "Those awful places you read
about," "I would never put my mother in one of them," and "That's the
end of the road."

It all suggested that I take a look for myself, to get a firsthand view of
the situation within which my survey questions were to be asked. I
contacted seven nursing homes and arranged to speak with the administrators about my research plans, especially the need to spend time in a
few homes to get a handle on the rhythms of everyday life and caregiving. The administrators expressed interest in the study, but some were
understandably wary of my intentions because of what one called the
"bad press" nursing homes were getting.

One administrator, whose name I fictionalized as Mr. Filstead in *Living
and Dying at Murray Manor*, showed the kind of concern that I later
realized was an ethnographer's dream. Filstead prided himself on being
research-oriented and hoped to effect improved living conditions not
only for the residents of his facility, which became Murray Manor, but
for nursing home residents everywhere. He admired the aim of getting a
firsthand view before launching the survey. I recall him explaining that
things can't be "just labeled as all bad or all good and leave it at that, like
you read in the papers." I had mentioned how I felt about the need to
understand the complexities of life satisfaction and wanted to avoid
rushing to judgment about what would be asked in a survey. I admired
Filstead's commitment to the welfare of residents and his decided preference for seeing "all sides" of circumstances.

Inviting me to "take a look" at Murray Manor, Filstead eased my way
into various units, introducing me to the floor staff and some of the
residents. I soon found myself comfortably ensconced at nurses' sta-
tions, walking unit floors, visiting residents' rooms, sitting and chatting
in lounges, participating in the activities area and in occupational therapy, and sharing meals with residents and the staff. On the floors, I
became acquainted with the enduring tension between caring and completing a job. Off the floors, I was invited to participate in the activities
of those whom I eventually called "top staff," which included the administrator, director and assistant director of nursing, the medical director, the in-service coordinator, the social worker, the activity supervisor,
an occupational therapist, a chaplain, and the dietitian. I made a special
point of attending patient care planning conferences, the purpose of
which was to review residents' conditions with the aim of setting short-
and long-term goals for their care.

Interacting with top staff, floor staff, and the residents, I began to
think that their daily lives and worlds offered quite different perspec-

tives on the meaning of care and caregiving. It occurred to me that a single nursing home might be three different organizations in practice, depending on the point of view. I actually used the term *worlds* to convey the difference because the term suggested something separate and distinct, yet equally compelling. What top staff saw as good and efficient caregiving, floor staff could consider "just getting the job done." What a resident felt was time well spent chatting with a friendly aide, from the aide's point of view could be less time to complete other duties.

The idea that whatever went on in the nursing home had to be understood within the context of particular worlds informed my growing inclination to turn the planned nursing home survey into a different project. I presented the idea to Filstead of conducting what I described as an "in-depth" sociological study of a single nursing facility. It needed doing, I explained, because the social organization of work and life in such settings had not been documented. It wasn't long before Filstead formally welcomed me to "join the team." So began the research for *Living and Dying at Murray Manor* and the background work for a study of the subjective meaning of the qualities of care and life.

RETRIEVED KNOWLEDGE

Twenty years later, there is a literature presenting the complexities. The accounts have documented knowledge that could not have been retrieved by the conventional survey or quality assessment. A cross-cultural view is offered by Jeanie Kayser-Jones (1981), who compares two facilities, one in California and the other in Scotland, to show the cultural mediations of life satisfaction and quality of care. Anthropologist Renee Shield (1988) describes how everyday life and care at the Franklin Nursing Home, a Jewish facility, are affected by ethnicity and the cultural contradictions of orienting to the environs as both a home and a hospital. Joel Savishinsky (1991) illustrates meanings and losses, memories and symbols, through the voices of individual residents, comparing his material with other nursing home ethnographies. Sociologist Tim Diamond's (1993) book, *Making Gray Gold*, based on his observations as an employed nurse's aide, tells of the broad-based complications of care work, beset as it is by the competing pressures of corporate profit-making, residents' needs, and the separate domestic experiences of the aides themselves. Other studies, equally insightful, add to our understanding (see Johnson and Grant 1985; Savishinsky 1991, chap. 1).

It is important to consider the kind of knowledge retrieved by nursing home ethnography. First, ethnography gives us anything but a static view of care, life, and death in the nursing home. Actually participating in the setting under study, the observer is witness to the practical fate of residents' and staff members' responses to events. Time spent with residents, for example, has a way of showing how what is said about the quality of care on one occasion can contradict what is said on another, even while the responses may be equally reasonable expressions in their separate contexts. In this regard, varied as they are, the narrative linkages made by residents in the following chapters are in-depth interview meanings, just as, say, standardized quality of care assessments are measurement-situated accounts.

When a frail elderly resident comments in the morning to an inquiring charge nurse that she, the resident, is well taken care of, compliments her assigned aide for the quality of her care on the afternoon of the same day, and later in the evening tearfully complains to a visiting daughter that the quality of care in the facility leaves much to be desired, time and context have a way of sorting the difference. We have an empirical basis for entertaining the possibility that the concern as addressed to a charge nurse or an aide is different in kind, not just degree, from the concern expressed to a daughter. In the former context, we may learn that what is at stake is continued good relations with staff members, while in the latter, it may be an interpersonal history of emotional blackmail.

Second, ethnography retrieves point of view in the documentation of experience. I have tried to underscore this by using the terms *story* and *version* to illustrate how an event takes on different meanings when examined from the viewpoints of separate parties or witnesses (Gubrium 1991). Listening to stories about an event such as a resident's alleged hostility suggests that the event necessarily comes in different versions because those who tell their stories do so in connection with their particular ties to, and interests in, the event. The hostility toward others that is warranted as perfectly reasonable from the standpoint of the resident who wishes "peace and quiet" during the night and believes peace and quiet to be a matter of residents' rights, may be seen as a sign of confusion and agitation, possibly dementia, by staff or family members worried about the resident's lucidity. Ethnographically, there is nothing contradictory about the difference, natural as it is to its points of view.

Consideration of viewpoint sheds critical light on the growing interest in quality assurance in health care. The nursing home industry is responding to nursing home reform legislation that makes quality of care and quality of life targets of national policy (Institute of Medicine 1986). An important feature of quality assurance is that care deal with the psychosocial needs of residents, which purports to take account of the whole person, not just physical health and functional capacity.

Resident assessment systems for nursing homes are in use or under development nationwide (see, for example, Morris et al. 1990; *NHCMQ*

Training Manual 1991). The knowledge retrieved by ethnographic research makes it evident, however, that such systems, which produce information in the form of so-called minimum data sets and other standardized measures, are applied without regard to viewpoint. They can hardly uncover differences in the interpretation of quality that emerge when viewpoint is taken into account. The systems are constructed from one-dimensional, typically administrative, definitions of quality. Their assessment instruments are designed accordingly and portend subjectively biased outcomes from the start.

Researchers Rosalie and Robert Kane (1988) caution those who would enter especially into the assessment of social functioning without taking its complexity into account. Well aware of the subjective, cultural, interactive, perspectival, and otherwise exceedingly general nature of the concepts of social health and social functioning, the Kanes write:

> Rhetoric about "treating the whole person" pervades today's medical world, especially primary-care fields. Nevertheless, holistic person-centered health care remains a vague ideal. The term holistic, which is rarely well specified, connotes caregivers who are mindful of the patient's physical, emotional, and social circumstances when making a diagnosis or recommending a course of action. Providers with this philosophy are expected to remember that patients are not diseased objects but people with families who live in communities and who view their health needs in the larger context of their social structure and personal life. . . . The hallmark of long-term care is a fusion (and sometimes a confusion) of health and social care. . . . Finding an efficient and accurate way of assessing the social well-being of elderly patients is a formidable challenge. (p. 133)

The Kanes' (1988) own pioneering research in the area has shown how varied the meanings of quality of care and quality of life can be when point of view is considered. Comparing the views of social workers and nursing home administrators in a different study, Betsy Vourlekis and her associates (1992) found that while there is consensus on priority psychosocial needs, there are different understandings of how psychosocial needs are to be met. Such findings lead us to ask, Whose view of quality is the basis of assessment?

Third, ethnography displays subjective complexity, avoiding the reduction of experience into undifferentiated scores such as a summary index of personal initiative. Anyone who has taken the time to observe people and listen to what they say knows that consistent behaviors, thoughts, and feelings are hardly more in evidence than behavior at odds with itself, sea changes of mind, and mixed emotions. Personal initiative, for example, has stories associated with it, which if we listened to carefully would show initiative to be a matter of judgment, sensitive to discretionary comparisons with others, the subject's earlier life, and expectations for his or her future. Ordinary caveats conveyed in formal interviews and in casual conversation highlight the complications. Cautionary utterances made by respondents, such as "it depends," "I've never thought about that before," "thinking ahead," "talking about it makes me . . . ," and "compared with earlier in life," indicate experience (and data) in the making and reflect matters that are far from the simple traits of individuals. Meaning is not necessarily made on the spot, but is mediated by comparative, retrospective, and prospective considerations.

The interpretive contingencies and narrative complications of social functioning have a way of making rather shallow the sorting of conduct, attitudes, and sentiments into either/or, yes/no, agree/disagree, or more or less. Such response options register the mere surface of the qualities of care and life. To represent this in the rationalized form of indexes, scales, or Likert-type responses (strongly agree, agree, neutral, disagree, strongly disagree) is to render subjective complexity invisible. As researchers, we diversely construct, deliberate over, debate, and periodically reformulate our own ideas about the lives we study. Why should we suppose that those studied don't do likewise?

A NARRATIVE TURN

A mark of the newest ethnography is that the many faces seen in a field setting have their own stories. Whether the setting is a small, nonliterate society, a retirement community, a household, or a nursing home, fieldwork is increasingly a matter of documenting narrative and its organization.

The history of ethnography shows considerable variation in the extent that story and narrative are taken as metaphors for orienting to the field. Whether anthropological or sociological, early ethnography tended to ignore native authorship. In realist styles of writing, ethnographers wrote more or less colorfully of the social organization of this or that people, community, or other recognizable grouping with little regard for point of view (Geertz 1988; Van Maanen 1988). There has been a decided turn to authorship and narrativity in recent ethnography, indeed to the writing of ethnography itself (Clifford and Marcus 1986; Atkinson 1990; Clough 1992; Maines 1993; Maines and Ulmer 1993). Especially pertinent in the new ethnography is the way the style of ethnographic writing shapes the reader's response to the experiences and worlds written about. We are apt now to be told as much about the story behind ethnographers' own faces as about the stories of those studied.

This book does not represent as radical a turn, but it does take the nursing home resident's life narrative or story of life as a point of departure for uncovering the subjective meaning of the nursing home experience in relation to the life as a whole (see Kaufman 1986; Rubinstein 1988, 1989, 1990, 1992). Thinking back on the Murray Manor fieldwork in this way, I would say that my observations did orient to stories of work and life there as authored out of different perspectives. The concept "worlds" helped me to interpret a nurse's aide's story, for example, as grounded in the local experiences of a rather different author (and world) than the story, say, of an administrator or a resident. I did not evaluate the different stories for their comparative accuracy in depicting events in the life of the nursing home, but rather accepted them as perspectives and documented them from their separate angles.

Yet, if the role of field-worker as participant observer does lend itself to the storied representation of everyday life, in the versions and from the points of view life can be conveyed, participant observation's decided attention to setting and interaction makes it partial to stories about the present, even while it does not ignore stories about the past. At Murray Manor, my observations were centered on what was inferred from, done, or said about the daily events, thoughts, and feelings of staff members and residents, not on the subjective meaning of such matters in the context of a concerted interest in lifelong experiences. I was not as much concerned, for example, with how the nurse's aide's personal history, especially her family, class, or ethnic background, related to her feelings about what I called the "bed-and-body" work she was responsible for completing. Rather, as participant observer, I approached the aide's story as a narrative of current social relations with co-workers, employers, residents, and family members. Residents' stories were heard likewise, as narratives about living and dying at Murray Manor.

Taking the role of in-depth interviewer in this latest project and focusing on subjective meaning helps to uncover lifelong biographical linkages and locate them in relation to interpretations of current experience. What can be learned about the meaning of the resident's nursing home situation when it is examined in the context of his or her life narrative? How does a life story inform the relevance of care quality? The questions turn us to an alternative sense of story, one less centered on the present—nursing home living—than broadened to take account of meaning in relation to life as a whole.

Whether in the short or the long run, residents do bring life experiences with them to the facilities in which they live. They do not cease being Roland Snyder, Martha Gilbert, Ruby Coplin, Jake Bellows, Lula Burton, Alice Stern, Grace Wheeler, Julia McCall, or Karen Gray after checking in. They are not just more or less sick, alert, oriented, and ambulatory, but in their words "as well as can be expected for a man who's been ill much of my life," "not as confused as most of them are here," "feeling more at home than ever before," and "crying my eyes out because it's come to this," among other expressions that communicate what life has become in relation to what it was. It is these linkages that are now my concern.

BIOGRAPHICALLY ACTIVE RESPONDENTS

The narrative turn relates to a new perspective on an important concept. Sociologists commonly categorize those researched in terms of *roles*. Theirs are not individual studies of Jake Bellows, Julia McCall, Alice Stern, and others, but of their place and experience in the world as, say, frail elderly or nursing home residents. Sociologists trace patterns in role relationships, for example, the relationship between marital status and nursing home residence or between gender and caregiving. More complicated relationships may be investigated, such as the connection between gender and caregiving in historical context or in rural and urban comparison. Regardless of the relationship studied, experience is analytically appropriated to role, not to the individual. The concept role is used to explain the experience of those who occupy roles, as in the finding that the nature of caregiving is explained by the fact that it is centered in women's experience.

Concepts can be a disciplinary hazard. Anthropologists instinctively think in terms of culture to organize their observations, even while they differ among themselves on its connotation. Psychologists readily use the concept of the person, even if some colleagues prefer a less global notion. Sociologists are inclined to view experience in terms of roles, although they recognize alternative senses of the concept. The hazard comes in mechanical application, usage that does not stop to consider how experience will be conveyed in the process. This prompted Herbert Blumer (1969) somewhat reluctantly to reflect on the possibility of a science without concepts. Assuring his reader that such a science was inconceivable, Blumer still complained of concepts that unnaturally colored the empirical world or concepts so set in stone as to endure long after they proved empirically useful.

The concept role as applied by gerontological specialists can be particularly mechanical. Does the specialized purview serve to present the experiences of the later years chiefly in terms of the elderly role, as anthropologist Sharon Kaufman (1986) asks in her study of the self in aging? Kaufman shows how elders, allowed to tell their stories in their own terms, categorically transcend age as a framework for conveying experience. More to the point, are the lifelong experiences of the nursing home resident primarily understood according to the parameters of institutionalization? Does twelve-year nursing home resident Julia McCall, for instance, convey details of her life solely from the perspective of the official resident? Given the opportunity to tell her story in the open format of an in-depth interview, to what roles does *she* appropriate her experience? How does her life in a nursing facility and her status as a resident color her story, if at all?

The questions direct us to residents who are biographically active, providing space from the outset for them to narrate the informing roles they deem pertinent for understanding the meaning of the past and future in relation to the present (Gubrium and Lynott 1985; Gubrium, Holstein, and Buckholdt 1994). These are respondents who are not, a priori, experientially framed as residents, whose lives are not predefined primarily in terms of institutional contingencies.

Viewing residents as biographically active is not to see them, even under the most favorable of research conditions, as purely telling the individual truths of their lives. Narrative, after all, is eminently social, conveyed by someone to another, who together collaborate in its production (Bauman 1986; Frank 1980). Knowledge of nursing home resident Lula Burton's life story requires the researcher to ask about it, and the asking itself helps to shape the story. What Burton shares responds to the request to tell her story (Wallace 1992). She may never have been asked this before, nor have considered how to organize lifelong experiences in this way. The researcher (any researcher), too, is biographically active from the start, implicated as he or she questions, frames experience, prompts, and moves on to other questions.

HORIZONS AND THEIR NARRATIVE LINKAGES

Listening to Lula Burton and others speak of the qualities of care and life is hearing more than words and deeds. Also conveyed are horizons of meaning drawn by the patterns of narrative linkages each makes with experiences in and out of nursing homes. In referring to meaning as having horizons, I take it that what residents say about matters such as the quality of care needs to be understood in relation to the linkages. It is the linkages that give the qualities subjective meaning (see Gadamer 1993; Goffman 1974; Schutz 1967).

As Chapter 8 will show, for example, the subjective meaning of the quality of care and nursing home life for Lula Burton is conveyed in her interview through repeated linkages with the special circumstance of having grown up and grown old alongside her twin sister Lily, who now shares a room with Lula in a nursing home. Against this horizon of meaning, Burton's orientation to the quality of care and nursing home life contrasts with others who lack close and continuing relationships or whose relationships have been troublesome.

Horizons of meaning divide the book into parts and chapters. Part I shows the ways in which various horizons orient residents to the qualities of care and life in the nursing home. Residents Martha Gilbert and Jane Nesbit of Chapter 3, for instance, do not just convey the chronological facts of their lives past and present, but speak of the quality of nursing home life in terms of new meanings of home. Residents Myrtle Johnson and Alice Stern of Chapter 4 not only tell us how the present situation relates to their pasts, but are repeatedly amazed that their lives have "come to this," referring to the fated emptiness of a nursing home existence.

Special circumstances, such as having a lifelong disability or living in the nursing home with a spouse or sister, further specify horizons of meaning and are the subject matter of Part II. In such cases, a significant past event, an extraordinary experience, or special relationship becomes a primary narrative linkage for the present. For example, the long-standing conversation that marriage has been for spouses who now live together intimately in a nursing facility offers a special experiential continuity that other residents, many widowed or sole survivors, do not have and contrastingly horizons their respective senses of the quality of nursing home life (see Berger and Kellner 1970).

The orientations and special circumstances presented are not exhaustive of horizons of meaning for nursing home residents. Rather, they exemplify the varied narrative linkages of experience to reveal subjective meanings of the qualities of care and life.

THE STUDY AND THE RESIDENTS

Nursing home life typically is studied for its negative impact on the person. In Colleen Johnson and Leslie Grant's (1985) overview of the effects of institutionalization, the negative impact is said to vary according to institutional "totality" (Goffman 1961), that is, with the degree of confinement and life engrossment of a setting. In that respect, a prison would seem to be more confining and engrossing of self and daily life than, say, a public school or a support group. To the extent a nursing home is a total institution, it is said to depersonalize the self. Identity and self-worth become matters of institutional definition and management (Coe 1965). A social blandness overshadows individual differences

(Gottesman and Bourstrom 1974; Watson and Maxwell 1977). Leon Pastalan (1970) has portrayed this as a loss of privacy stemming from the environmental encapsulation of personal autonomy. This combines with the estrangement and isolation resulting from a lost home and the death of kindred or withdrawal of support from significant others. According to Richard Zusman (1966), it forms a "social breakdown syndrome," which Russell Ward describes as "the individual becoming increasingly oriented to the world of the institution and isolated from the outside world, thereby losing the capacity to exist independent of the institution" (1979, p. 402).

The negative view does not reveal how residents themselves assign meaning to institutional living. To find out and to learn how lives as a whole figure in, I contacted six nursing homes recognized as comparable in the quality of the care they offered. After a series of meetings to explain the research rationale and its goals, the homes' administrators agreed to participate in the study. The administrator of one of the nursing homes contacted was on target when he offered this understanding of what I aimed to accomplish:

> I think it's a very good idea, getting these folks' life stories. Ya walk in here day after day and it's easy to think that all there is to their lives is sitting in wheelchairs, eating, sleeping, and being sick. That's pretty negative. They're just faces in the hall, without any stories. I would guess that if you took the time to listen, they'd have a lot of interesting things to say about their lives . . . not that I would want you to paint a glowing picture. I know that a lot of them are very sick, more than ever, given the current trend of things, and nursing homes have their share of problems, as you know. But residents are people too and I like the way you're going to try and bring that out—give them a chance to tell their stories.

The phrase "faces without stories" was his, but I used it effectively from then on to describe the study.

The nursing homes were located in Florida. The state's population is a mix of natives and immigrants, typically from midwestern and eastern states, which was reflected in the backgrounds of the residents who became the subjects of the study. Whether from the North or the South, many had spent childhoods in small towns or rural settings. This was a generation of people, now mostly in their seventies, eighties, and nineties, who grew up in large families. Residents commonly spoke of having had five, six, up to ten or twelve siblings. They were quick to add that many of the siblings had died and, as a result, they had experienced a great deal of sickness and death among loved ones in their lifetimes.

It is perhaps the last generation to take for granted the place of religion in daily living. Not that all the residents were religious or had

become so in later life. Rather, surrounding their attitudes and preferences were everyday vocabularies that routinely referred to religious
practices, the deity, and moral life, something that now seems to typify
public life only on special occasions. It also is a generation for which an
ethic of hard work is a matter of open pride. In the interviews, it was
rare for work and its difficulties not to be mentioned, even by those who
had had stable and fairly well-paid jobs.

Typical of the nursing home population as a whole, most of the residents interviewed were widowed, female, and white, with some African
Americans. While a few residents had had extensive formal education,
such as the rare professional and graduate degree, many had only six,
seven, or eight years of schooling. This, too, was not unusual for this
generation. As one resident reminded me, "We didn't much go beyond
the eighth grade back then because you didn't need it and, if you
wanted it and the family could afford it, you had to ride all the way
across the county or into town."

Respondent selection was affected by health and communicative ability. The comatose, intermittently conscious, and demented were not interviewable. We were not prepared to interview the deaf or the alert but
orally noncommunicative. Staff and family members sometimes informed us that they preferred particular residents not be interviewed
because the residents were too ill for prolonged interaction. If the study
sample is biased, it is toward the relatively less sick and the more communicative.

A total of fifty-eight residents completed interviews, twenty-four of
whom are represented in the following chapters. Thirty-three of the
fifty-eight completed interviews were with so-called long-stayers, who
had resided in a facility for over a year. Twenty-two of the long-stayers
had lived in their nursing home for over two years and seven for more
than five years. Among the latter was Julia McCall, a twelve-year resident. All thirty-three long-stayers were interviewed once in the course
of the study.

The other twenty-five completed interviews were with residents
whom we followed for a year from their time of admission. I wanted to
explore how horizons of meaning changed following placement, whether in a stepwise or more complex fashion. Each of these residents was
interviewed within two months of admission. They were not all new to
nursing home living, however. Several had been residents of other nursing homes before coming to reside in their current ones. Some of the
twenty-five residents died before their second or third interviews, which
were scheduled, respectively, six months and one year after the first
interview. Some became too ill to be reinterviewed. Some were discharged and moved too far away to make an interview feasible. A few

refused to be reinterviewed. Of the twenty-five residents followed, ten were reinterviewed six months later and, for the reasons stated, did not complete their scheduled third interview. Seven of the twenty-five completed a third interview one year after admission. Eight of the twenty-five were discharged before being reinterviewed in the nursing home, but were interviewed again following their return to the community.

THE INTERVIEWS

The in-depth interviews, conducted by myself and my assistant Carol Ronai, ranged in duration from a half hour to two hours. Each interview was flexibly focused on commonplace considerations of life in nursing homes—questions about the fate of life, daily living in the facility, the meaning of home and family, self-perception, health, aging, and death. To accent the biographical and following psychologist Jerome Bruner's (1986) practice, respondents were asked at the outset to tell their life stories, even if might seem difficult to do in a relatively short time. They were encouraged to begin wherever and however they wished. Respondents were invited to address the matters under consideration in relation to lifelong and current personal experiences. They also were asked if they had the opportunity to write their life story, what the various chapters would be about. We were especially interested in how the last chapter related to their present situation and its horizons.

However brief, beginning with the telling of a life story set two narrative precedents. It served to inform the respondents that we were interested in whether and, if so, how their lives as a whole related to their current situations. We wanted to see if the distant personal past and both the foreseeable and imagined future were narratively linked with the present qualities of care and life in the nursing home to make meaning in relation to lifelong experience. While some residents warned us that their lives weren't very interesting or claimed that there was little to tell, we nonetheless assured them that we would listen to whatever linkages they cared to make between the present and the past in speaking of their lives. Beginning with the life story also offered us an empirical basis for suggesting to the residents possible linkages between the past, the future, and the present, which we reminded them they were free to ignore or recast in their own terms.

An interview guide was constructed early on (see Appendix). The plan was to use it more as a conversational agenda than as a procedural directive. We hoped this would enhance the interview's interactive format. In some interviews, certain guide items became the crux of conversations. For instance, resident Karen Gray's background in health care administration and regulation turned many topics of conversation in her interview into quality assessment discussions. When Gray was not wearing her "personal hat," the narrative linkages conveyed in her interviews were articulated out of her professional experience (see Chapter 11). In other interviews, guide items receded into the background as residents set their own narrative agendas. The sequence in which interview guide items were asked was determined more by the flow of particular conversations than the order of their appearance in the guide.

Because residents were conceived as biographically active, their emphases were taken to be as important as guide items in shaping the interviews. The rule was to let the relevance of particular guide items be determined by the experiential linkages respondents made in the course of the interview, keeping in mind that many guide items nonetheless reflected public concerns thought to potentially bear on the lives of all residents.

The adage, No man or woman is an island, set another rule for the interview process. Previous research experience and a theoretical orientation to the social character of self and communication were a basis for encouraging respondents to compare their lives with others, especially other residents in the nursing home. We also interjected ourselves into the interviews by gently suggesting how one might feel or would think if one were in the resident's shoes or the resident in another's place. Residents were invited to agree or disagree and encouraged to describe differences, if any. The idea was to suggest and offer up contrasting narrative linkages as a basis for prompting the respondent to newly discover, elaborate upon, or demur from possible connotations of his or her experience.

These rules—from encouraging subjective relevancies to prompting subjective possibilities—provided a procedural basis for documenting the biographical activity of respondents. The rules helped to avoid conjuring up nursing home residents and the interviewers as narrative dopes (Garfinkel 1967).

Interviews were tape-recorded with the informed consent of the residents. The tapes were later transcribed and the transcripts checked for accuracy against the recordings. In the extracts presented in the following chapters, all personal names have been fictionalized except for my own informal first name (Jay) and my assistant's first name (Carol). While the residents and the interviewers referred to each other in various ways—sometimes by first names and other times more formally as Mr. or Ms. So-and-so—first names are used to identify speakers in all interview extracts. Where location or affiliation might reveal identities, pseudonyms also are used.

Before moving on to the interview material, it is important to keep in mind that the responses form life narratives, not life histories (see Bertaux 1981; Bertaux and Kohli 1984). Life histories are meant to be evaluated according to how accurately they reflect what actually happened in their subjects' lives. The truth of a life history lies less in its formulation than in its subject matter. Ideally, life histories should factually describe the lives they are about. Life narratives, in contrast, are communicated lives. The past, present, and future are linked together to assemble meaning. In our case, lives are communicated by nursing home residents in collaboration with the researcher. The life narratives in this book should be read accordingly, not in terms of whether, say, Jake Bellows actually was a stand-up comic on the road fifty weeks of the year, but in terms of how he links that experience to his feeling of being "at home" in the nursing facility, his way of conveying subjective meaning.

It also should be kept in mind that the life narratives are not personality profiles, even while long-standing personal traits and experiences are invoked by residents in speaking of life. The narratives do not convey the overall psychological designs of the lives they are about. As Jake Bellows and the other residents speak of life in the following chapters, they do so as agents considering their experiences in relation to their current living situation and in the context of an in-depth interview. What comes across is a retrospectively and circumstantially constructed rendition of the qualities of care and life, sparked by the opportunity to link together parts of experience and guided by a slate of public concerns.

PART

I

ORIENTATIONS

CHAPTER

2

Worried to Death

The life narratives of some nursing home residents highlight worry, disappointment, and thoughts of death. Worry can be so profoundly central to the narrative as to overwhelm the life story. The mere mention of such common life themes as family and home unleashes sobs and expressions of how it may soon come to an end. In such moments, whatever is conveyed about the past, be it family, home, or some other realm, is told in relation to thoughts of death. It is difficult to imagine no longer being with one's "wonderful and warm" family, with the children one raised, with one's "dear and caring" son or daughter. It is hard to acknowledge the possibility of becoming like one of the nursing home residents who have "lost their minds" or are totally incapacitated, who are no longer themselves. The worry is as much about the loss of identity as it is about growing frailty, as much about leaving oneself and others forever as it is about dying.

Yet those who worry to death can be ready to die. For many, the unimaginable makes it too difficult to go on. It is as if they admit, in a strange twist of an ancient maxim, The examined life is not worth living. Worry is linked by some to a sense that one either has outlived or might outlive those one should not. It is a prevalent belief that, by all rights of fate, the oldest die first, the younger die next, and the youngest last. In this connection, the worried despair that they might outlive a cherished son, daughter, or younger brother or sister. They are ready to die because of this, too, as much as from what the unimaginable confronts them with.

Among the worried, the quality of care of the nursing home is a matter reckoned in a restricted framework. For some, the quality of care is hardly the problem, as adequate or fine as care is judged to be in support of activities of daily living such as eating, dressing, and cleanliness. One can be a "good eater" but nonetheless be ready to die. One can be the active participant of the Sunshine Club, a group for spreading good cheer, yet narratively convey that as marginal to the real possibility of "never getting better." For others, quality of care may be a point of constant complaint, yet hardly matter at all in relation to what they once knew. As annoying as the quality of care might be at times, it is just a matter of daily living, the "nursing home resident" role not conveying what life is believed to really be about.

Disappointment can be conveyed in relation to oneself or others. There is the disappointment of not progressing as expected in recovering from a disabling illness or accident, turning what was foreseen as a short, rehabilitative stay in a nursing home into long-term residency. In this context, the nursing home portends the end of life as once known. There also is the disappointment associated with the need for others, often adult children, to place a frail elderly parent in a nursing home because the burdens of continued home care have become unmanageable. While the need may be acknowledged by residents, lingering doubts over failed filial responsibility cause them to be disappointed in those—their children—from whom they had come to expect much more.

RITA VANDENBERG

Our first resident, Rita Vandenberg, is ready to die. She is an eighty-two-year-old divorced white female, who has diabetes, injects insulin, suffers from congestive heart failure, and is arthritic. Now living at Bayside Nursing Home, Vandenberg has resided in institutional settings for many years, the last a three-year stint in a nursing home in another state. She keeps busy in many ways, not the least of which is trying to make Bayside a home. But it is an effort overwhelmed by a story of worry for herself and especially her surviving, middle-aged son.

Vandenberg was interviewed two weeks after she moved into Bayside and again six months later. She refused to be interviewed a third time one year after we met because she was worried about getting depressed and having heart failure.

The First Interview

We began the first interview by talking about her work life, which quickly converged on her present worries.

> Jay: Everyone has a life story. Why don't you tell me a little about your life?
> Rita: Well, there's not much. I worked in the telephone company as a telephone operator before I was married. After I got married, I moved to New Jersey and had two boys. I didn't work until he [husband] passed away, after we moved to Reading, Pennsylvania. Then I got work, mostly in the steel mill.
> It wasn't very exciting. I did a lot of work and places just seemed to have jobs lots like. That lasted a little while and then I'd go and hunt

something else to do. But my last work was . . . as I got older, I worked in a children's home, a house mother . . . oh, about ten and a half years I think. And then after that, I couldn't take that anymore. It got on my nerves a little bit as I got older. So then I worked in a nursing school as a housemother where they were teaching the nurses. I worked there eight and a half years and I retired from there. And since that, I did nothing but go out and eat with my brother, who passed away about two weeks ago. And I lost my mother. My mother first, then my sister, and then my son. And then my brother. So I'm living too long.

But I had a nice life. I had to work. I wanted to be home all the time, but I couldn't be. Had to work for the money. And I had my son, the one in the picture over there. He was in the marines for thirty years, then he went to college, and now he's teaching. But he's not too well. Has rheumatoid and the knees must be operated on. And he has some kind of disease of the nerves. They have to cut the nerves somehow for him to walk. My other son [Tom], he died. I think Tom's dead about two years now, maybe not quite two years. He had cancer of the pancreas. He was only fifty-two, just a young fellow. [Whimpers]

Jay: I'm sorry. [Pause] So you had two sons.

Rita: They're very good to me. The one here . . . I wanted to stay up in Reading because my family's up there, my brothers and sisters. But he wanted me with him. So he brought me down to Mississippi when he lived there. I was there a little while and I got a heart attack. So then they put me in a nursing home because my daughter-in-law couldn't take care of me. Then he moved to Tennessee and I been in a nursing home up there. It was nice up there. But it was Seventh Day Adventist and there was no meat, and I like meat. But they were nice. They were good people. Three years I was up there.

I presented her with the idea of writing her life story and asked how she would divide it into chapters. She began immediately to tell me about life during the depression in New Jersey. It was a detailed, un-chaptered account of living with in-laws and raising her two sons. The sons soon became the focus of her remarks, the saddest part of which was losing one of them two years earlier. As she talked about this, she sobbed grievously.

Jay: Can I get you something? Can I get you a tissue or something?

Rita: No. I'll be all right. [Pause]

Jay: Is that better? So . . . you lost him, what . . . two years ago?

Rita: I don't believe it's quite two years. I lost my mother, my oldest sister, and my son. All within about a year. [Weeps] I lost my oldest sister. She's only a year and four days older than myself. We were very close. And then my mother. My mother was ninety-seven. And then my mother died in July. The following November my son died.

Jay: Mmm. I'm sorry. That's very difficult.

> *Rita:* You can lose your mother, your sister, but losing my son is so [weeps] . . . well. I'll get a Kleenex. I'm sorry.
>
> *Jay:* No, that's okay. [Comforting Vandenberg] I'm sorry.

We talked about the deaths and eventually returned to her early married life. Again, her sons were prominent.

> *Rita:* I always said I could write a book. But I don't know. Having my babies was very happy. I was very happy with them. They were . . . kept me busy, because they were small. Both of them were small. Then as they grew up, there was no trouble. I didn't have trouble with them. I always can say they were good to me. And this one's still very good to me. He's not well. I wish he would be well. But he was in the marines too long. I said, "Are you sorry you stayed too long." He said, "No, Mom, I'm not." He was in Vietnam twice.
>
> *Jay:* Oh, he was? About my age then.
>
> *Rita:* He was a pilot of the helicopters. Got shot at a few times. So I don't know why he liked that life. That was a worry of mine.

At that point, we began to talk about the present—her life in the nursing home, her room, her roommate, daily living, and her need for privacy. She complained of the constant presence of her roommate's visiting husband. The husband, Vandenberg claimed, had no respect for privacy. He'd turn on the television while Vandenberg napped and barge into the bathroom unannounced, even ignoring a room-occupied sign that the social worker had devised to solve the problem. Yet Vandenberg felt sorry for the roommate because the roommate was helpless and bedridden, worse off than she herself was. Vandenberg complimented the nursing staff, whom she described as very friendly, remarking, "I haven't come across one I disliked at all. They call me Ms. V."

Having few complaints about the quality of care and judging the home superior to any in which she had resided, Vandenberg again spoke of her family, her life rearing two sons without benefit of husband. Mentioning her "dead" husband again, she stopped and backtracked.

> *Rita:* So those were nice times. I had sad times, too, and I'm divorced. I told you my husband's dead. To me he's dead.
>
> *Jay:* You were divorced? How long ago was that?
>
> *Rita:* I was about thirty-seven. He was in the service and he was running with women and drinking. So . . . but I tell people he's really dead to me.

She described her years with him and the very few contacts she has had with him since, mainly through her sons. She was quick to point out that he hadn't been part of her life for years, someone whom she didn't care much to think about. Her thoughts promptly returned to her son's health and her own shrinking future.

I redirected the conversation to the present and her life in the nursing home, aiming to see how that figured in her story.

Jay: Now that you've been here for a few weeks, does it feel like home?
Rita: Yes, very much. I feel as if I'm going to be happy here. I wish I could feel better because my sugar goes up. It's over four hundred. So then they call a doctor and he says to add more insulin. But the nurse who comes and gives it says, "You might end up in the hospital." I say, "Well, I don't want to go in the hospital. This is good enough for me."
Jay: So you say it doesn't quite feel like home yet? You say that it will feel like home? Or what would you say, Mrs. V?
Rita: I think it will. Things are strange yet to me and I don't know many of the women. The ones that I talk to a little bit at the table and that stuff, don't make sense. And people are hard . . . I mean if they're southern, it's hard for me to understand them. [Elaborates] Now when someone talks to me, I face them so I can kind of concentrate if they talk fast. But that happens I guess when you get older.

I asked her how she felt about growing old. As sure as Vandenberg noted that she hoped to eventually make Bayside her home, she remarked that she was ready to die. Her enduring worries about her son's health combined with worry for her own health. The possibility of becoming as helpless as those around her led her to explain:

I don't want to live to be that I can't take care of myself. I don't want to be in a wheelchair. To be helpless—that would be terrible for me. So I'm ready to go anytime. I just feel that there's nothing much ahead of me. My son's responsible for me. He comes and visits me every two weeks. He's coming this Saturday. But he's not well. I'm so worried about him. He teaches school every day and when he comes home he's on the couch. His legs feel terrible. [Elaborates] I always said this old age is for the birds. It isn't for us. [Elaborates] When I see some of these women that can't even remember anything or talk funny, or they're really lost, really lost . . . I don't want to get like that. I see these people here can't even feed themselves. They can't hold their head right. Some of them hold their head all the way back. I don't want to get like that. No, it wouldn't be living. I'd be half dead. But, don't get me wrong. They treat 'em all real well anyway.

For Vandenberg, these residents who were frail and more helpless than she was signaled her future, not the quality of care in the facility.

Six Months Later

Six months later, Vandenberg is reinterviewed by Carol Ronai, my research assistant. The looming end of Vandenberg's life—as a thing now much over—hardly enables her to retell her story. As it does for some other residents, the interview lead-in, centered on life as a whole, too vividly rehearses the central themes of being worried to death and ready to die, even while the margins of the narrative are filled with attempts to appreciate the present situation as homelike.

Carol: I was wanting to talk with you again about your life.
Rita: No. [Weeps]
Carol: No, we're not going to do that.
Rita: No. No. I couldn't. That's too hard. [Weeps]

Ronai tries again, asking Vandenberg to speak of life by starting with when she was born and describing her childhood. Vandenberg readily speaks at length. This time, it isn't life as a whole that comes under consideration, but specific points not necessarily formed as a grand narrative about its entirety. As in the first interview, she talks about her family in Pennsylvania and her children. The conversation soon returns to her present situation and her feelings about living at Bayside.

Carol: So is this like home to you now?
Rita: Yes, a lot like home. A lot of times I wished I was in Pennsylvania cause I had my family up there. But the sister that could have taken me, she passed away. And the others, well, their husbands like trips. They take a lot of trips and I would have been left out.
Carol: Sure.
Rita: And the doctor didn't want me alone. So I wouldn't want to go and interfere with no family life at all.
Carol: What is it about this place that's like home?
Rita: Well, everybody seems nice. Now maybe there's somebody that don't care for you too much, but I never came across somebody like that.

Talk of the happy and sad points of Vandenberg's life eventually leads again to her son's death and, following that, to her own future. Vandenberg recalls her dead son's last words:

You get over it cause you know that it's going to happen some day. And I'm so happy that I helped him. He [the son] called me everyday, and sometimes twice a day, even from the hospital when he was in. [Just before he died], he called and said, "I have something to tell you, but I don't want you to cry Mom." But I did.

Asked what she thinks her daily life will look like a year from now, Vandenberg remarks:

I don't think I'll be around a year from now. . . . No, I really don't 'cause I have some bad days now. I don't tell 'em every time cause, uh, what can they do? . . . But I can feel when my, uh, I get a thing in my heart. I don't know where my heart is anymore because I had an operation on my, uh, breast removed. And I had a hernia operation since I'm down here. I feel as if I'm ready to go. . . . I know it's coming to me . . . the way I feel. So I don't want to live too long.

As the interview winds down, it is evident that Vandenberg has settled her affairs with life. Hers seems at times to be a stoic wait for death, ironically riven with casual, almost lighthearted commentaries about life in the nursing home. Yet, as before, she worries—for her son and over the possibility that she will become incapacitated and helpless. The quality of care and life in the nursing home are incidental to these primary concerns. Toward the end of the interview, asked what her philosophy of life is, Vandenberg sharply juxtaposes worry and an activity of daily living:

One would be not to worry too much. I'd try to, to overcome that. And to eat. I love to eat. One time I was pretty heavy.

REBECCA BOURDEAU

Rebecca Bourdeau, a resident of Florida Manor, is discouraged and, as she reports, "worries about everything." A seventy-six-year-old widowed white female, Bourdeau had a stroke a few years ago and recently suffered a hairline fracture of the pelvis that left her in a great deal of pain. What seemed strange to her about the fracture was that she hadn't fallen. The fracture happened suddenly one night while she was in bed. The unexpected occurrence worried her terribly because it happened despite the care she took to prevent such accidents. She now worried over everything because her expectations about returning home had been dampened repeatedly and unexpectedly, first by a long period of rehabilitation following the stroke and more recently by the pelvic fracture. An overriding worry was that another setback would make a return impossible, causing her profound disappointment.

Bourdeau's worry was different from Vandenberg's. Bourdeau's was focused on the possibility that she might never be able to return home to her thoughtful and caring family. The possibility caused her to even feel she was losing her religious faith. Faith was incapable of stemming the disappointment she was experiencing. Fate, it seemed, was arbitrary and not working in her favor, which did little for her faith. In contrast, more at home in her nursing facility, Vandenberg's worries were for her son's health and the reflection of a possible future self she saw daily in other incapacitated residents. As in Vandenberg's account, the main linkages of Bourdeau's narrative hardly touched on Florida Manor's quality of care.

Bourdeau had been a resident of the Manor for two and a half years when interviewed. Speaking of life for her was an enduring narrative of past, present, and future domesticity. As with Vandenberg, I began by asking her to tell me about her life.

> *Rebecca:* Well, I've had five children. I wasn't married too young. I was twenty-seven when I got married. [Weeps]
> *Jay:* That's okay. It's alright. [Pause] Let's stop a while. [Pause]
> *Rebecca:* I had a good life actually, because I had a wonderful man and he was a thoughtful family man. He took care of his family and never was without work. It was warm and wonderful. He was a good provider. I never went without anything. [Weeps]
>
> We gave our children the best education we could. Most of them went to college at least, you know, part of the time even though they did drop out. But they all have good positions today. So I'm happy about that. I didn't have a very exciting life, but satisfying.

Bourdeau goes on to describe her husband's multiple myeloma, which led to his death four years earlier. She speaks of the fine man he was.

> He was a remarkable man anyway. Not great or anything like that. Never looked for any praise or anything like that, but he was the handiest man you could ever think of. He could do anything. He could, you know, he could do woodwork and he could do plumbing. We had a house that he completely made over. We bought a normal house in Albany, New York, and he completely made it over. Worked all the time. He was what you'd call a "workaholic." Never gave up. Sometimes I feel sorry that he didn't enjoy life more, but that was his life. He had to keep going.

She talks at length of her home, winters in upstate New York, her happiness, and the hardships she and her husband endured. It is a glowing nostalgia. The conversation turns to her move to Florida and her sons' lives, of which she hopes again to be a part.

> Well I still lived there [New York] by myself after he [her husband] died a few years, until this happened to me, until I had a stroke. I was living by myself and I guess it wasn't the best thing in the world. But that was meant to be, too. Now this house that we had built [in Florida], my oldest son and we were shareholders. He had it built for us, but he said, "Now you can live there the rest of your life. It won't make any difference to me." He says that and it's supposed to be his house you know.
>
> But it's not gonna happen that way at all because now my youngest son wants . . . has bought the house. The deal hasn't gone through yet, but he wants to buy the house and have me go back there and live with him, which

I think is great, but I don't know if I'm gonna make it. I'm so awfully disappointed. I just don't feel as though I'm gonna make it because here I had this one setback. [Weeps] Maybe that isn't meant to be either.

I ask her what she means and she explains:

I mean you don't know from one day to the next what's gonna happen. You think, well, this is all planned and everything, but things go wrong and then something else happens to make it different. My middle son, the one who lives in Fort Lauderdale, is supervising a courtroom. He has a good position. And the youngest son works for the telephone company on underground wiring and that. And the older son is in a business partnership with somebody else in the construction business. So he is very well fixed. He has a beautiful home. He has two sons, but he has been unlucky because his wife of thirty-nine years old passed away in March of cancer. So there he is by himself, too. That's what I say about life . . . it's a funny thing. You don't know what's around the corner. [Weeps]

I have two daughters and three sons. Yeah, I have a nice family. It wasn't planned that way, but it's a nice family. [Weeps] I cry a lot.

When she regained her composure, I asked her what made her feel the way she did, which we explained in relation to writing her life story.

Rebecca: I don't know. I get discouraged. That's the story of my life.
Jay: Really? What makes you discouraged, Mrs. B?
Rebecca: Well, I think the sickness that I've had, because I would like to get on with my life and go with one of the children and I can't seem to get it together. I guess otherwise my health is pretty good. I shouldn't worry about it so much.
Jay: Yeah. [Pause] Let me ask you this. If you could, like, write the story of your life, what would the first chapter be about?
Rebecca: I really don't know, except that it would be about my husband and I . . . how we met and what a good life we had and all that. I imagine that's what it would be about.
Jay: What would the second chapter be about?
Rebecca: To tell you the truth I don't know. I guess it would be about our life in New York and maybe moving to Rhode Island and living there a while and then moving to Florida. [Elaborates]
Jay: What about the last chapter? What would you say that'd be about?
Rebecca: As far as I'm concerned, there's no last chapter yet because I think I have more life to live.
Jay: Do you think about the future?
Rebecca: Well, how much future can there be when you're seventy-six years old? How can there be much future? I imagine you probably think the future would be my children—what they're going to think and what they're going to accomplish. [Weeps] Excuse me. I should hope that I would be living with my son somewhere, one of my

> dear boys and that I could enjoy a little bit of life a little . . . proba-
> bly a little more enjoyment with the family and grandchildren. In a
> way it is promising, if I am ever able to go live with one of my boys.
> It looks like it's promising because as far as I know my health is
> good. I've had this setback, but other than that, it's been pretty
> good. I seem to worry a lot these days . . . about everything you
> might say.

Broaching the possibility that she might not be able to return home, I
asked Bourdeau if she felt she could make a home of the nursing facility,
reminding her that she had lived in the facility for about two and a half
years. I wondered whether, if she gave the place a chance, she might get
used to it, explaining that other residents felt it was not such a bad place
to live and had made it their home. Bourdeau responded:

> No. This does not feel like home. This will never be home. I know I have a
> lot of good feelings though, for some of the people that have taken care of
> me because they've been very nice to me. But it's not home. Home is where
> family and children are. That's what I want to get back to.

I asked her if there was anything that could be done to make it more
homelike. She doubted it, adding that no matter how good the quality of
care, the facility could never be home.

> I don't know what we could do to make it more like home. They try to do
> everything to make it . . . I mean they try to make it pleasing for everybody
> . . . the social part and all that. But right now I don't care anything about
> that. It doesn't matter when you don't feel good. It doesn't matter much
> what people are trying to do. I appreciate it, but it'll never be like home.

As we proceeded to discuss the meaning of home, the possibility of
making the Manor her home, and the Manor's quality of care, it was
clear that Bourdeau was set on a life on the outside with her family. The
idea of adjusting to life in the nursing home was out of the question. She
did not so much think of the last two and a half years as a period of
adjustment, but as one of rehabilitation. She repeated her appreciation
for the Manor's quality of care and, indeed, at one point when I asked
her if she considered the time she had spent at the Manor to be part of
her life or separate from it, her voice cracked:

> I imagine it's part of my life. How can I forget those years that I've been here
> and all the people and everything. I can't forget them. Oh gee.

In a way, the quality of care and life at the Manor were the farthest
thing from Bourdeau's mind, even while she felt positively about both.

Mainly, her mind and heart were in another place, led on by a different agenda. It was her role in a family life that preoccupied her, not the role of nursing home resident. The preoccupation, in her words, made her "worry about everything," including the loss of her religious faith, as the following exchange reveals.

Jay: How would you describe yourself as a person?
Rebecca: I don't know. Right now, I'm very discouraged and I'm not a bit upbeat. Maybe I should be. I really get upset about my life when I think of all the things that I could do and what happened to me and here I am. I keep saying that I'm not never gonna get better. You worry about not ever making it . . . dying, you know and not ever seeing your family again. [Weeps] My daughter thinks that's not true at all. She says that I'm gonna get better and not to worry about it. But I worry about a lot of things.
Jay: You do?
Rebecca: Oh yes. I'm a worry-wart. Isn't that awful? I worry about everything . . . worried to death.
Jay: What's the meaning of life to you? Have you ever thought about that?
Rebecca: I don't know. I'm supposed to be a religious person. But I think I'll lose my faith. I'll lose my faith very easily. I should, you know, cling to . . . how I've been brought up and that in a very religious background.
Jay: What happened to change that, Mrs. B?
Rebecca: I guess illness changed it all, because I used to be a very religious person. And of course, there's no religion in this place as far as that goes. I'm Catholic and you never have any services like usually you do, you know. I used to be a person who'd go to church every day and there was a little group of people I was friendly with. We went every day and met. That was a good feeling. When I came here, that all stopped and so I'm kind of lost when I think of religion. Now I've let it all slip by. There was nothing I could do about it. Sometimes I think if there was only a priest who would come in once in a while and all and keep spirits up. There are a few people—laypeople—who come in now and then, but it's not the same. I really think that those people should be commended because of the work that they do. They try to, you know, take the place of a priest or religious and they come and visit.

Still, there was hope for the future. The worry and disappointment that prevailed upon her were experienced in relation to an enduring sense of the possibility of going home. While she was as active as one could be in the nursing home, daily life for Bourdeau was mainly a matter of waiting and, admittedly, worrying. The mixture—being active, waiting, and worrying—was evident in the discussion of a typical day.

Jay: What would you say a typical day is like for you in this place?
Rebecca: Oh, it's awful. Ah, nothing, nothing much. Except that now I go to
          therapy and I've been going to therapy three times a week and,
          other than that, there isn't much. Once in a while there is some-
          thing going on that I take part in. I belong to the sunshine group
          and we try to do things for others.
Jay: What is the sunshine group? It's a club of some kind, isn't it?
Rebecca: Oh, we try to make things for other people like . . . like that board
          out there, you know, the big board [a seasonal display]. It's not
          really much, but it's a little something to do to keep busy.
Jay: And what is the rest of your day like?
Rebecca: That's it. I get up in the morning and have breakfast and then you
          wait until there's something to do. With me, it's therapy a few times
          a week. I try to do some reading, but I can't concentrate on that. For
          a while there I was doing embroidery and that was taking up my
          time. I did quite a bit of that just before Christmas. But I haven't got
          anything planned now. God knows I wouldn't be able to do it
          anyway. So I wait and worry and wait.
Jay: Is time an important thing here? Time?
Rebecca: Time? Well, time is very important to me. Now I watch that clock
          like I was going somewhere all the time. But it drags. It drags. You
          know, when you don't have that much to do, it drags. You're sitting
          there sometimes waiting. Of course since my fracture I've been
          laying in bed and I never in my life have done that . . . lay in bed for
          days on end. I thought that was awful. It's funny. There was a day
          when I would be so happy to lay in bed and take it easy, when the
          children were small and I didn't have the time to do that. But now it
          means nothing.
Jay: What do you think your life'll be like a year from now?
Rebecca: I hope it's pretty much like it is now but living with a relative. You
          know, living with family. That's what I hope it'll be.

ROLAND SNYDER

Roland Snyder is also a resident of Florida Manor. He was interviewed
twice by Carol Ronai, two weeks after admission and six months later.
He died three months after the second interview. Snyder is a seventy-
eight-year-old white male, widowed from his first wife, and divorced
from his second. He has had two heart attacks, colon cancer, a colos-
tomy, and is diabetic.

The narrative horizons of his first and second interviews are different.
In the first interview, talk about life is linked with disillusionment and
worry over death. His children did not see fit to care for him on their
own. He had over the years been such a good provider and is gravely
disappointed that he's had to be placed in a nursing home. Being in the

nursing home signifies the end of what he had believed to be a relationship of mutual care and responsibility, the end of life as he'd known it and thought it would continue to be. Like Vandenberg and Bourdeau, his feelings have little to do with the quality of his care. For Snyder, being at the Manor means that life is over. Just about every mention of earlier life and his family causes him despair. At several points in the first interview he simply states that he wants to die.

The First Interview

The first interview, which is fairly brief overall, is taken up initially by a lengthy description of farming in rural Florida during the depression and World War II, a story of family life, hard work, success, and failure. Every mention of his first wife and their seven children causes him to sob uncontrollably. The account of his wife's cancer and eventual death is especially disturbing. He describes his second marriage, one of convenience, and his eventual divorce.

Later, he expresses his disappointment at having been first placed in a nursing facility where he lived with no "menfolks" for two years before moving to Florida Manor. Snyder tells of feeling that his children had abandoned him.

> I don't know why I hated that place so bad. I had no one. I was by myself. There was no menfolks in there to . . . there was one other man that you could get on a conversation with. There wasn't but three of us in there. There was a bunch of women just like these here, some of 'em in wheelchairs, some of 'em couldn't even get out of bed. I feel like that my kids . . . now I didn't, I don't want to stay with any of 'em now. But I feel like they kinda let me down. I tell you . . . we was a pretty close family. And it was hard on me. [Weeps]

The feeling of disappointment has Snyder thinking of death and occasionally suicide.

> I have wanted to die ever since I went in that home in Summerville. I have thought of takin' my life. Yeah, I told the girls [his daughters] . . . and I'm still not saying that I won't. I don't want to be in the shape that I see these people [residents at Florida Manor] yet. [My life] is nothin' no more. Just nothin'. [Weeps] I just wish I could die today.

For a time, the discussion centers on suicide.

At the end of the interview, there is an exchange about growing old. What it means for Snyder in the context of disappointment is death.

> *Roland:*   I didn't realize that I was as old as I am until about two years ago when I went in that home.

Carol:	What does it mean to be old?
Roland:	I don't know. You're just here and that's all. Ain't nothin' to life. That's the way I look at it.
Carol:	Is there anything you like about being your age?
Roland:	No ma'am. I hate to get older. As long as I'm livin' I know I'm gonna be gettin' older.
Carol:	Do you think about the future?
Roland:	Yes, I do. I know that there's nowhere for me to go. There's here or in another place like it . . .
Carol:	Do you have any plans?
Roland:	No ma'am. I'm nothing now. It's just like I say, I just wished I could go. [Weeps]

Six Months Later

Six months later, Snyder is still disappointed, but not because his children have abandoned him. Talk of life is not as much related to death, as to what he has to put up with. He is not as much profoundly disappointed by life as a whole as he is by what fate has chosen that he forebear. His narrative horizon is daily living in the nursing home. He is angry and annoyed with the quality of care and the quality of his life in general. Complaints about other residents, especially his roommate, consume him. Except for a "nice looking" nurse he's taken a shine to, daily life leaves much to be desired.

The start of the six-month interview is much like the first, a long story of farming, hard work, close family ties, his first wife's cancer, opportunities, and failures. This time he says more about the bad market for yellow squash and zucchini in the years he farmed, among other trials of making it farming. He later speaks of his daughters' visits and, especially, recently seeing a woman friend with whom he once lived intimately. Prompted by interviewer Carol Ronai's question about how he would put his life together in the form of book chapters, he talks about a young Florida Manor nurse who, according to him, lavishes attention on him and gives him at least something to look forward to.

Carol:	It's about six months ago when I interviewed you the first time. Remember you weren't feeling so well then. You were pretty disappointed and discouraged I believe. So now, let me ask you this. Um, let's say we were gonna write a book about your life. Let's just pretend we were gonna do that. I was curious . . . what kind of chapters . . . what would the names of the chapters in your book be? Like what would you call the first chapter?
Roland:	I don't know cause I don't know nothing about writing a book.
Carol:	Oh, that's okay. You can still make up a chapter. Make up chapters. What would it be on? What would you write it on?
Roland:	Well, if it was my life history, it'd be before I ever got married.

Carol: Okay. And then, the second chapter?

Roland: Would be after I married.

Carol: How about the third chapter?

Roland: Well I expect it'd be three or four chapters of me and my first wife, 'cause we lived together forty-something years. I've forgotten now just how long. My memory is not very good now.

Carol: What would the last chapter be on, the last chapter of the book about you? What would that be on?

Roland: You'd be surprised.

Carol: Would I? Okay, what'd it be about?

Roland: A girl that works here.

Carol: A girl that works here. It'd be about her? Tell me about that.

Roland: Well, I don't know much about her, but she just made like she fell head over heels in love with me. And she's not but thirty-two years old. She's a nice looking girl and, uh, she um . . . in other words she waited on me. When I first met her, I was over yonder on the other side [of the nursing home]. Hell, she couldn't wait on me two weeks ago this weekend. She works on the weekends. And, uh . . . but she's going to college, going to nurse's school, trying to get a degree in nursing where she can make more money. She's got three or four kids. I don't know. She told me the other day she didn't have but three. I thought she had five. She brought five to see me. And, uh, I knew one of them wasn't hers—a girl, a little girl. Course, she said that was . . . she was keeping her, but it was her husband's child. And somebody told me that fella she married was just as damn sorry as he can be. Course they not living together now. He's married again. I don't know much more about her.

Carol: So the last chapter would be about her?

Roland: Yeah. But, now I didn't care much about that girl to start with. But she kept on till I got to where I thought a lot of her. And then she done me just like that woman that live with me for six years. She just quit coming to see me. But I think I know why. Cause the other weekend when she waited on me, she says, "Why in the hell did you let them put you in this room with George?" That's the guy who's in the room with me. I says, "Well I didn't know he's like the way he is." So they's good and they's bad, too. At least I looked forward to seeing her.

Underscoring both the good and the bad in life, the conversation develops into a tale of interpersonal attraction disrupted by what life in the nursing home has come to be.

Ronai interrupts to ask Snyder what his roommate is like.

Roland: Oh, goddamn, he's a damn nasty. And he don't care what he says.

Carol: You mean he's mean?

Roland: . . . or who he says it to.

Carol: He's mean?
Roland: And they would bring him in here and put him in bed. Well they got
to clean him up. And, uh, I suspect you seen him coming down
here, out there in the hall walking. He walks on his toes, kind of on
one foot.
Carol: Mmm.
Roland: And, uh, anyway. Yeah, this girl, she asked me the other week
when she waited on me. I haven't seen her since. Now she said
she'd see me this weekend, but she didn't. She worked. They all tell
me that she worked. But I didn't see her. I don't know where she
worked at. Some of them said that she was at Station 1. I don't
know. But not this one. This here is 2 and that's 1 down there.
Carol: But you think she doesn't like to be in here because of George?
Roland: Yeah. And I've been trying to get out of this room ever since. I got
the supervisor to come into my room, Monday a week ago. That was
the day after she left on me.

The rest of the conversation is decidedly nursing home oriented.
Snyder's "typical day" contrasts with Vandenberg's and Bourdeau's. His
is less a matter of waking up, eating, waiting, sleeping, and passing time
than it is a battle with daily living. Describing his remaining wherewithal, Snyder remarks:

When I was younger, I'll say I done anything I wanted to do. In other
words, I was man enough to do it. I'm not bragging. But as far as fighting, I
never did do much of that. Like this here roommate I got, I'm all done
cussing him out and threatening to beat the hell out of him. They all say he
don't know nothing, but he does. He knows, thank God, that I'll get him.
Or he thinks I will. I wouldn't, but he thinks I will.

I slapped this woman this morning on the arm when I was going to lunch.
She was a nitwit and she just run up the side of me [in her wheelchair]. I
didn't know she was coming around me. I didn't even know she was back
there. And she came around me and just run into me and my hand on that
side. She caught it between the wheel of her chair and wheel of mine. And it
did hurt. I cussed her before I could think and I reached over and slapped
the hell out of her.

Snyder no longer despairs of death, which seemingly is kept at bay by
his attempt to bear up in the face of daily intrusions on his life by the
"worst ones," referring to the most incapacitated residents.

I don't look forward to dying, but I don't dread it. Of course, if I live with
him [roommate George] much longer, I might live to dread it. They got all
the worst ones from here to that desk up there. The worst ones is from here
up to there. They moved two here, down here, that was up there somewhere since I been here. And they just holler. I don't know why one of 'em

ain't hollering now. One of 'em is bad about coming in my room. She won't pay you no mind. I go to cussing her and tell her not to come in and she won't pay you no mind. She'll come in and go to the bathroom . . . well I won't get into that. No, I'm not scared of death. I may go to hell if I die, but I'm not afraid like some people. I'm too busy fightin' with 'em to think about it much anyhow.

Still, as Ronai probes at the end of this interview, there is a broader horizon—the context of his life as a whole—one that can never be displaced by the current situation, even while he seems to have "adjusted."

> *Carol:* I was curious. You've been in this place six months now. Do you think you've adjusted to it? You got used to it? You're not used to it?
> *Roland:* Never will.
> *Carol:* Never will. Why?
> *Roland:* It's just too much different . . . what I was used to . . . my life. But I reckon I've adjusted.

* * * * *

All three of the residents in this chapter worried to death or were otherwise gravely disappointed about particular aspects of their lives. The three might seem to present in terms of the public image of the typical nursing home resident—abandoned, depressed, and ill. While, to be sure, all three residents share some of these characteristics, their stories convey complex narrative linkages, few of which connect directly with the quality of care in their facilities. Indeed, even as Roland Snyder becomes engrossed by the quality of his immediate care, particularly his resented placement with roommate George, Snyder ends by telling Ronai that he will never get used to the nursing home under any circumstances because it is too different from his life, linking adjustment to something much broader than daily living in the facility, namely, his life as a whole.

3

Making a New Home

An idyllic image of domesticity communicates carefree childhoods, loving homes, parents who are good providers, happy marriages, long healthy lives, and intergenerational charity. The positive qualities are enticing sources of identity and the whole is a widely shared model for family formation. The qualities and model provide background explanations for why some nursing home residents "worry to death" about their current separation from loved ones or are disappointed that family relations are no longer what they were.

Another domestic image stands in contrast. As scholars of family life are discovering, in reality domestic life conveys both positive and negative qualities (see Skolnick 1983, chap. 4). In this context, we need to recognize that what some residents bring with them to the nursing home are domestic lives ridden with strife—difficult childhoods, poverty, loneliness, marital infidelity, sickness, and death. When these residents look back on life to tell their stories, the present contrasts less negatively with the past. Secure homes and nurturing familylike relations may not be matters so much lost, as possibly gained for the first time in a facility. Such is the domestic horizon of Martha Gilbert's story, a resident who has made a new home for herself at Oakmont, where she now lives. Yet, even for Gilbert, the idyllic image crops up from time to time as she talks about her sons and how they might have treated her, their mother.

New homes are made, too, by those who count wherever they have caring friends and whatever they've gotten used to as home, notwithstanding the family relations they once had or that continue in other locations. To some extent, getting used to something is a matter of relatively short- versus long-term stays. A patient who expects to be hospitalized for a few days is not likely to consider the matter as something that needs getting used to, let alone the possibility that the hospital may become home. Likewise, the nursing home resident who is a short-stayer, spending a few weeks in a facility undergoing physical therapy or convalescing after a period of hospitalization, looks ahead to discharge and a return to his or her former way of life. Long-stayers, however, face the possibility that the nursing facility may be their last home. For some of them, like residents Jane Nesbit and Ruby Coplin, who have faithfully attuned to "making the best of it" most of their lives, with or without the support of religious convictions, a long stay in the nursing facility suggests making a home and life of it.

MARTHA GILBERT

Martha Gilbert has lived at Oakmont for five years when I interview her. She is a seventy-six-year-old widowed white female with congestive heart failure and emphysema. As Gilbert first mentions when I walk slowly with her to the resident lounge near her room, exertion makes her short of breath. I soon learn that illness and exertion are constant narrative linkages in her life story, from her childhood in rural New York State through her move to the South. Hers is a hard and unhappy life from the start, far worse than what her life has become in the nursing home.

Without tears or remorse, Gilbert begins her story by describing childhood:

> I've had a rough life. I had to go to work when I was young. I've been on my own practically since I've been eleven years old. At that age, I was cleaning or . . . I mean I used to go from house to house and do house cleaning. Then when I was big enough where I could really be on my own, I got to be a waitress and I stayed that way even after I married. I did waitress work.
>
> I had two sons. The closest one is in North City [forty miles north of Oakmont] and the other one is in South Carolina and that's about all I can tell you. I mean, I don't have a very interesting life because I had to work all my life. It was a hard life, not a pretty picture. I didn't have girlfriends or went out to parties or anything else because I always had to work.
>
> My parents were very poor. So as soon as I was big enough where I could go out, Mother made me go out to work. I used to go to work after school, work until about nine at night, then come home and do my homework. I got real tired and I think that's one of the reasons I ran my system down. I wasn't able to fight anything, any colds or anything, because every time I got a cold, it would really hit me hard . . . because I was in no condition to fight it. I've had pneumonia three times and that didn't help my lungs any.
>
> The first time that I had pneumonia, I was about eleven years old. I had double pneumonia. I had it real bad. It crippled my system and everything else from the fever. And then I had pneumonia twice after that. I had two boys and they were both caesarean.

I asked about her husband and her life raising the boys. Again, it was the narrative of a rough life and being on her own, made worse by both her husband's and sons' long absences from home because of work.

Well, I'll put it this way. Ever since '72 . . . I lost my husband in '73 . . . I was on my own again. I had to work. And I just, well, the only time that my son, my youngest son would take care of me was when I wasn't able to help myself. Other than that, I was on my own. My son and his wife both worked, so they couldn't take care of me. The reason that I'm in here is because I need twenty-four-hour care and I couldn't get it. I had to come into a nursing home. It was a rough life I had. I've been here about five years now. Before that, I worked when I could. When I couldn't, my son would take care of me until I got better and I'd be on my own again. But, as I said, he and his wife both worked, so they couldn't take care of me. So, I had to paddle the boat by myself.

I was married and lost my husband in '73. I was married to him for twenty years before he died. And both of the boys are on their own. Like I said, one is in North City and the other is in South Carolina. So I don't see much of the children. They both drive trucks—those big trailers, you know. Convoys. And when they go out on the road, they don't come home for a week or ten days. They always go out of the state. They drive anywheres from here to California. Long distance. My husband drove a truck too. After I lost my husband, I was all by myself and didn't have nobody. I never had nothin', really.

Then when I got so sick where they told me I had to have twenty-four-hour care, I lived with my son. It was rough. My daughter-in-law figured that I had to do things for her. Well, you know if you're not well, you have a hard time doing things. I had a hard time just trying to breathe and navigate by myself, let alone work. She just figured that I had to clean house and cook and what have you and I couldn't do everything. I just couldn't. It was too much for me. So I had a chance to talk to my son in private and I told him that I just couldn't take it. The only other solution I had was to go in a nursing home. It was his idea. I think at the time I didn't think too much of it because I was too sick to think. I really had it rough.

I asked Gilbert what the word *home* meant to her, which returned her to childhood and married life.

Not much, because I always had to work. I didn't have much of a home life. It means zip. Even when I had children and they were young, I still had to go out and work. When the boys were little, we had a farm. I'd have to get up at four in the morning to help my husband milk cows and do chores before I would make breakfast. Then I'd have to go ahead and get the children off to school.

Whatever the circumstance—whether Gilbert's childhood, her married life, her life alone following her husband's death, or living with her son—it was rough and unhappy. Whether or not one would judge her responsibilities as particularly onerous for her circumstances, Gilbert's is nonetheless a narrative of hardship, which she eventually contrasts with her life at Oakmont. But the transition to a nursing home life wasn't easy, as the following exchange reveals.

Martha: Anything was better than to put up with it.
Jay: Put up with what? I'm not sure I understand.
Martha: With the life that I was leading.
Jay: Oh, you mean in your son's house?
Martha: Yeah. So when I had a chance to make the move, I just told my son that they had better put me in a nursing home. I couldn't take it.
Jay: Did you have any idea what it would be like before you came to a nursing home?
Martha: No. No, I didn't. I cried. I was in bad shape because I couldn't take it. I just never thought that I would wind up in a nursing home. After I got here and I was here for a while, I found out that it was best for me. But at the beginning I couldn't get it through my head that I had to be in a nursing home.
Jay: What was it like at the beginning, Mrs. G? How did you feel?
Martha: Lonesome. The environment is altogether different, you know. When I came in here, I didn't know a soul. I had to make friends all over again and I didn't feel good and everything. Every little thing that happened just bothered me too much because I was sick and I couldn't take it. Now I'm used to it, I'm well, and it doesn't bother me. But I do have a hard time breathing.

Gilbert's reference to being sick and not being able to take it reflects two important distinctions, made by many residents. One is the difference between being sick and being chronically ill or disabled. When residents say they are sick, they typically refer to acute conditions like having the flu, a bad cold, or being in pain. When they are not sick, they are mainly in "pretty good health," "having a good day," "well," or "feeling okay," even while they may otherwise suffer from chronic conditions like congestive heart failure and cerebral palsy (see Charmaz 1991). In this regard, Gilbert was more sick in her son's home than she is in the nursing home at the time of the interview. Her daughter-in-law made matters worse by expecting Gilbert to do household chores while she was sick, which Gilbert reportedly couldn't take.

The other distinction, not evident in Gilbert's preceding remarks but implied in comments both she and others make about one's quality of life in a nursing home, refers to how being sick as opposed to the quality of care affects the quality of life. Time and again, residents state that it is being sick, sometimes very sick, that makes being in a nursing home "rough" or depressing, not the quality of care as such, even while particular matters of caregiving, such as employee attitudes and the food served, can be sources of considerable irritation.

As long as Gilbert wasn't sick and though she had a hard time breathing, Oakmont was a pretty good life, was now home—and family. We talked about friendship, which in time lapsed into a discussion of domesticity.

Jay: Would you say you had friends here?

Martha: I have a roommate and we've been together five years. So we sort of understand each other and we get along pretty good. But other than that I don't associate too much. I'm more or less on my own, privately. I don't like to . . . I don't like big groups.

Jay: I think I understand. I'm like that myself. What's your roommate's name, Mrs. G?

Martha: She's Sara Sanders. She's been here as long as . . . maybe a couple of months longer than I am, but we've always been together, since we joined up. Even when they moved us from room to room—you know, changing rooms—they always managed to keep the both of us together. They didn't try to separate us. So that makes it nice. They know that we get along very good, so they don't. But other than that, I guess it's just the way I make it. You either try to get along well or you don't and I'm a person who tries to get along. I don't have too many enemies, I don't think.

Jay: Now that you've been here five years, does it feel like home?

Martha: Well so far it does. Five years is a long time. I've readjusted myself. So I think that, God willing and I don't get sick and much worse than I already am, I think I can make it. I know most everybody now. I don't associate too much with them, but I know them. The only thing, the only problem I have, I can't join everything that they have because I can't breathe. I have a hard time breathing and I mean I can't have too much activity because I'm short of breath. So I don't join the crowd too much because I can't breathe.

Jay: When did you start feeling . . . I believe you said earlier that you didn't feel that this was home at first? When did you start feeling it was more like home?

Martha: Well, after I'd been here about six months and they all tried and I know they did—the nurses and the aides. They tried to make me comfortable and they know I have a problem breathing. They understand me now better than they did at the beginning, but until . . . I guess I had to have the feel of it myself. I had a hard time trying to understand because they have their work cut out for them, but I couldn't join everything that they had because of my breathing.

I guess once I began to understand, it started to feel like home. At first, I couldn't get it through my head that I had to put up with it. When I found out that I couldn't be with my son, I couldn't be in his home and I got it through my head that I had to make the best of it, that's when I began to feel a little different. It wasn't all that great there anyway. That's when I began to feel that I really would have to make up my mind that this was my home. But it takes a while. I mean you have to fight and when you get to be my age, it's sort of hard to accept things. Now I guess I learned my lesson and I found out that I either accept it or you don't have anything. You don't have no friends. And the sooner I did that, the better I was and, since then, I've had no problem.

Explaining how Oakmont was now her home, Gilbert compared what she now had or had come to accept with the family life she never had before.

It's part of my life now. It's home. I know I can't depend on my sons. I haven't seen my son from South Carolina in ten years. Not much of a son, huh? He's not one to visit, and Jimmy, my youngest one, he drives those big convoys and he's out on the road. When he comes home, he has one day off and it's sort of hard for him to go ahead and just come home and to visit Mother because there are things that he has to do at home. I couldn't accept that at the beginning either. I figured that, well, he's got a day off, he should come to see me, his mother. But that isn't the way it got to be. I mean I had to accept that he couldn't do it. They, neither one, was ever too homey anyway, I guess. So here I am. It's hard, but after you accept the things you know you can't have, things begin to run a little bit smoother.

But when you look back, I've never had a family life. I always had to work. It was bad, real bad. Even when the kids were small, I had to work. Sara's my family now, my roommate. She's been pretty nice and she's got a daughter that comes in here . . . I mean if I need something, I can't depend on my son to get it for me because if I would say to him that I needed something, he'd probably be six months getting it. Where if I tell Dotty [Sara's daughter] that I need something, I mean she takes my order today and in a week's time when she comes to visit Sara, she brings my stuff that I need.

I encourage Gilbert to tell me about Sara, their relationship, and what that means to Gilbert. As before, she contrastingly links her current "easy living" with the sad points of her earlier life.

Sara's ten years older than I am. She's okay now, but back a while she had a slight stroke and things were a little rough because I couldn't communicate with her. That was about three years ago. But she seems to get better every day and that makes me feel better. Things are easier.

I've never had anything easy happen to me. Now, well, I don't feel very old because I had it so hard when I was younger. Now that I'm older, I think I've got things a little bit easy. If I didn't have such a hard time breathing, I'd be okay. I've never had a very interesting life. I've always had to work so hard and now that I'm seventy-six, I've got it easier now then I've ever had in my life. A lot of people don't think I'm seventy-six because I don't have gray hair. I don't use no dye. [Elaborates]

But like I said, it's easy living now as long as I'm not sick. Everybody says that they can't understand why Sara and I been together for five years and never had words or we haven't changed roommates because it seems like they have a problem with other residents here. They don't get along. They have to change the room or change the resident. I think Sara would do anything for me and one of the things I appreciate is, because I really have a problem with my health and when she knows that I don't feel good, she tries to help me. She's like a nurse. I don't have to depend on the aides or the nurses here because Sara takes care of me more or less. Even though she's older, she's more active than I am because she's never been sick as much as I have.

I didn't always have it as easy. I had a rough married life. You can't try to get along if you're separated like with my husband on the road for a week or ten days. There's no way you can get along like that. You can't tell me that if he's out truckin' away from home that long and he's gonna be by himself, he's not gonna look for companionship. I'd find things in his dirty laundry. So you just have to make the best of it. I loved him but that's not saying he returned the love, because I know that he had other things that occupied him more than me.

My whole life was like that. I've never had a happy life. I mean I couldn't go to this girlfriend and tell her what a good time I had. I couldn't go to another one and say what a beautiful party it was because I've never been to any of them. I could never go anywheres because I didn't have no way of going. [Elaborates] When Easter would come, the other kids used to dye eggs. My mother, she would go ahead and cook onion peels and dye eggs with onion peels and they were all brown. That's the only color we knew. I can't say I had a wonderful time because I didn't have it.

Well, after the rough life that I've lived all my life and then you come along and live in here and you don't have your problems, I means that's easy. If I didn't have such a hard time breathing sometimes, I think I'd be on Easy Street. I have to be careful not to catch a cold because if I do, it hits me much harder than anybody else because my lungs are so bad. Other than that, I'm living on Easy Street, like I said, and this is home.

JANE NESBIT

Jane Nesbit's story is one of lifelong satisfactions, filled with the usual tragedies certainly, but she is still accepting of what God has destined for her, as she remarks. It is not as much a narrative of contrasts, as is Martha Gilbert's portrayal of life before and life on Easy Street. Rather, it is a story of always making the best of what God offers. Nesbit's place in the life of the nursing home reflects her placement in life as a whole. As Nesbit has always done, she continues to make the best of it. At the same time, while hers is a life lived by God's grace, it is not one immersed in "lovin' the Lord," which is the narrative horizon of Chapter 5's residents.

Nesbit is a ninety-two-year-old widowed white female with arteriosclerotic heart disease. She suffers from hypertension, has occasional minor strokes that leave her temporarily dizzy and confused, and is partially blind. She has spent all her life in the South, having moved from Alabama to Florida in 1917. Nesbit also lives at Oakmont, being resident there three and a half years when interviewed.

Nesbit begins her story by briefly describing her childhood and the 1917 move. She then tells of her husband's tragic death, her widowhood, and her final placement at Oakmont.

> I was born in Alabama. Montgomery was the capital and my daddy was a mail carrier. I used to remember going with him. [Elaborates] He died when I was a child and that left me to take care of my mother. She finally died and that left me. [Elaborates] I wished a thousand times that I went on to school then but, back then, you know, I never would go back to school. So I married and had my family and come down from Alabama around in '17 I believe it was, the third day in March. Everything was covered in snow up there and we got down here and everybody is in short sleeves, aplanting. They had cucumbers growing. I got to pick cucumbers that year. I tell you, I've had to do it, though, since I was born. Everything just turned over for me to do because my two sisters married and I was left to do things. But life has been a pleasure to me. Most of my life's been in Florida.
>
> My husband got killed at Dailey's Foundry down here. He and another man were welders and they told them that the gas tanks were all clean. They rolled them out to do and, as soon as they touched the thing with a torch, it went off and killed both of them. Exploded. They said they heard the noise clear up here. And that left me at home with four children. He was killed in '41 and I had to try to get the kids through school, and I did.
>
> My son went in the navy. They talked him into going and told him that would be best for him to go in the navy to where he could help me out. So if it hadn't been for that, I don't know what I'd have done. The girls finished school and I'm thankful for all that.
>
> And then, after all of 'em got married, they didn't want me living by myself, so I lived in the house with my baby daughter. I lived there for about ten years until two of my grandsons graduated. Then we moved to Judson's Lake; stayed down there until I got to where I had to come out here. My daughter fell and fractured her back and she wasn't able to take care of me. So they just put me in here.

As we continue to talk, Nesbit recounts the events surrounding her husband's death at the foundry in 1941. While it is retrospectively conveyed as the tragedy it was for her and the children at the time, there is an aura of destiny about it, filled as it is with signs that his death was imminent. As we will see, a similar aura—of enduring equanimity with self and one's circumstances—conveys the meaning of the present as well. Recalling the death, Nesbit explains:

> When he was killed, that was the most shocking thing that I think that I ever witnessed. We got up and had breakfast. He was a coffee drinker all right, but he hardly ever drank over two cups. That morning he drank coffee and drank coffee. He got up to leave to go to work and one of my girls . . . she was always a tiny little thing . . . we called her "Teeny." He says, "Got to get some sugar off my little woman here." He was chasing that little girl around the table to get sugar off'n her before he went to work. She darted under the table and he couldn't get her. He made like he was going to get her though and havin' fun. [Pause] So he says, "Well I got to go." And he looked at me, turned around and come back and said, "Just another swig of coffee" and said "I got to go." And then he left.
>
> Well, this one that worked with him, his wife says that he said the same thing, like it was meant to be. His wife says he said, "I've got to have another sip of coffee and I've got to go." The same thing.
>
> And when that thing went off, it shook our house. I thought the whole thing was going to fall in. We lived close to the foundry. I knew good and well that somebody was killed or I had an idea that there would be. . . . Blew one of his legs off. They said that his lungs must have been crushed. That was bad, but I guess it was meant to be.

As we talk about destiny and the meaning of life, Nesbit's equanimity, her acceptance of fate, and herself come forth.

Jay: What does your life look like from where you're at now?

Jane: Well, it looks like I'm just ready to go any time. That's the way I feel and I hope it is.

Jay: Uh huh. Can you explain what you mean by that, Mrs. N?

Jane: Well, I've just asked God if there's anything that He's holding me here for. If it's to do something or to say something or whatever it is, I'm willing to do it. If it's to pass on and to go with Him, that's fine too. So I said, "Well, dear Lord, You know what it's about." So I'm willing to try anything. And I'm willing to just give up and say that it's gone.

Jay: Did you ever think back and ask yourself what's, you know . . . how did I come to be what I am?

Jane: Yes, I sure have. And I reckon it just wasn't meant for me to be a big highfalutin person and know-it-all. I'm proud of me like I am. I'm no big talker, nor no highfalutin person, just what God made me and I'm proud of it.

We turn to the present, especially her life in the facility. It is a narrative of participation, home, and family living. Indeed, Oakmont has come to be the home and family she needs to *return* to even when visiting her daughters. While she loves the daughters, Nesbit admits that the time she spends with them can be boring. Still, Oakmont is no bed of roses. Like most things, it too has its good and its bad sides, as she points out.

> Some of the days here is pretty good and some of 'em isn't. Some days we have good days and some days we have bad days. Now today we haven't got help and there's a lot of days that we don't have enough help. Some days we get a good meal and the next day, or three or four days, we won't get nothing hardly. But this is something you have to be satisfied with. That's the ways it is anywhere. I said I thank God that I've got a place that I can come to, to where I'll be taken care of, and not have to depend on my children to do it.
>
> I'm into the Sunshine Club. There's different days that we do things, but on Thursday is the Sunshine Club. We make birthday cards and welcome cards for the new visitors, to give the new peoples they've admitted. We carry 'em a welcome card, introduce ourself, and tell them who we are and what to expect. We want to welcome them here and see that they get good care and to get out and mix and mingle with people to where everybody'll learn you. There's wonderful things that you can do here that you'd be surprised. We make all kinds of stuff. We made pillows and we made quilts. And we've made change purses. We made baskets. I made seven baskets.
>
> Now I'm partially blind. I can't see to do the needlework like I used to. But I glue, put glue on stuff to paste boxes and different things that we fix. So . . .
>
> My daughters, they'll say, "Well, Mama, why don't you lay down and rest? You look like you can't hold your head up." I say, "Well, let me sit up as long as I can." So they know if Mama ever lays down there's something wrong.

At this point, the domestic meaning of visiting her daughters and returning to Oakmont is revealed.

> *Jane:* Visiting my girls means a lot to me. I love to go home down there and I can stay down there for a little while, but then I'm ready to come back up here.
> *Jay:* Home down there is where?
> *Jane:* In [one daughter's nearby town].
> *Jay:* That's near here, isn't it? Yeah. I think I know where that is.
> *Jane:* Or in [another nearby town where a different daughter lives]. Some of my folks are down there. Anywhere that I go, it feels like home. So I'm ready to come back up here.
> *Jay:* Oh, is that right? Why is that?
> *Jane:* I don't know. Just ready to come back. There's a lot of friends here and we get along good. I can only stay a day or two and everybody [at Oakmont] says, "Why do you stay off so long? We missed you so bad."
> *Jay:* The people here say that?

Jane:	Uh huh. "Come back." "Oh, there goes Jane." "She's back." "Why did you stay so long?" I don't know.
Jay:	How does that make you feel?
Jane:	It makes me feel so good to know that they're thinking about me. And Lola . . .
Jay:	Who's that, Mrs. N?
Jane:	Lola Dryden [another resident]. She is around at my door every morning and comes every night. She'll come see how I am. It just kills her for me to be sick. She wants me right with her. I told her, I says, "Old mare ain't what she used to be. I can't get around like I used to no more." Lola thinks that she's old. I said, "Well, honey, you're just starting." I says, "I don't feel like I'm old." And she says, "Oh, you're kidding." And I says, "No." I says, "I don't feel a day older than I did six years ago." In a way I don't.
Jay:	Isn't Lola down the hall from here? She's been here a while too, hasn't she? I don't recall exactly. And you've been here for, let's see, since '87 is it? It's been a while.
Jane:	It just seems like home now.
Jay:	How's that?
Jane:	I reckon it's because I know I'm going to have to stay here. I say that when I go down to my daughters I'm always ready to come back. I get to thinking about coming back before I'm there too long.
Jay:	Is that right? I wonder why.
Jane:	I don't know, but it's just sit there and watch TV or something and nothing to do, kinda bored. Here I'm going back and forth doing things, talking with different people. So it's just different.

As homelike as Oakmont now is for Nesbit, the transition from life on the outside to making a home of the facility was not automatic. As for most, there was a period of adjustment. For some like Nesbit, it eventually proved to be a transition to a new home. As we talk about it, I ask about others' experiences. Nesbit contrasts herself with two residents whose minds she believes to be weaker than hers and who can't seem to accept things as they are.

Jay:	When you first moved into Oakmont, Mrs. N, did you feel it to be like home, as it does now?
Jane:	No.
Jay:	No? What was it like when you first moved in?
Jane:	I don't know. It was kind of dreary, dreary-feeling. Just that I just didn't know how to take it or something. Didn't know why I was put here, why I couldn't be somewhere's else. I don't remember all that much about it. After about a month or two months, the longer I stayed, the more I realized why I was here. Because my daughter couldn't lift me anymore. Dr. Dunne [her personal physician] told her that she's going to have to either put me in here or get somebody to go over to the

house and keep me and lift me. He says that he'd rather I be here in the home where, if anything happens, that somebody'll be there to look after me. So that's why I'm here I guess.

    As I said, about a month after that, I began to go around and meet different people and one or the other. Things just began to fall in place. It didn't take too long at all. It just, I don't know . . . well, you know you're gonna be here and why worry about it, like anything else in life. Take everything as it comes and that's what I looked forward to. It was the Lord give me strength and courage to go on. That He's done. So here I am and this here is my life now.

Jay: Do others feel the same way, do you know?

Jane: I believe some do. I hear talk about it. Not everyone. Now Adele and Sally round here on the same hall that I'm on? Both of them, well . . . I think that my mind is a little stronger than theirs because they do and say things that really don't cross my mind. Like about being here, you know, [they ask] why are they here? They can't understand why they've been put here and who's taking charge of the bill. "Who's paying my bill here?" They ask all kinds of questions. You don't know what to tell them. The government is taking care of us and we draw our checks and our checks go in on this and such. I tried to tell them that, but you can't explain to them in a way.

Jay: Why is that, I wonder?

Jane: I don't know. Their mind is just different or something, weaker. They can't see it like we do or something. Or maybe we see it wrong and they see it right. I don't know.

The interview turns to social relationships. Elaborating upon her relations with those she feels to be familylike brings us back to resident Martha Gilbert, whom we met earlier and who is another member of the Sunshine Club.

> Adele and Sally both hang around and talk whenever they feel like talking, you know. [Elaborates] And there are the ladies that work in the Sunshine group. I can't remember all their names. Let's see. One of 'em's Katherine. She's close. Not all of 'em are in the Sunshine group. [Elaborates] Oh, I forgot Martha Gilbert and Sara Sanders. They were in the group. They've quit. Sara went to the hospital and she hasn't been feeling good. And Martha, she won't go nowhere unless Sara is along.
>
>   But we're all like a bunch of sisters in there, we are. And I have to say that I'm very much at home here. We're close.

RUBY COPLIN

    The circumstances surrounding Ruby Coplin's admission to Fairhaven, the nursing facility in which she makes a new home, differ from

Martha Gilbert's and Jane Nesbit's. An eighty-six-year-old white female, Coplin has an enlarged heart, suffers from hypertension, and is blind from glaucoma. According to Coplin, she sought admission to care for her husband, who was already a resident and afflicted by Alzheimer's disease, even while she required extended care herself following hospitalization for a heart attack. Coplin couldn't bear to feel that her husband was grieving for her alone in a nursing home. Her husband died about a year after she was admitted. Coplin was widowed for approximately one and a half years when interviewed.

Coplin's new home is not just a source of rest, shelter, and sustenance. It is something more than a network of friends and social support. Coplin orients to Fairhaven's residents the way she's oriented to the less fortunate all of her life. If Fairhaven is a nursing facility and is home for Coplin, it also is a place for charity, somewhere to offer kindness and be helpful to those less fortunate: the suffering, the destitute, and the lonely. Having defined her role in life as that of the carer, Coplin is not just another old woman sitting in her room or receiving help. She chooses to continue playing the carer role in the nursing home, even though she herself has grown frail and become totally blind.

Just as Coplin makes a pet project of being the carer, she makes a veritable career of telling her life story. Starting from her childhood in Miami, she offers more detail and speaks at greater length about her life than any other resident in the study. For well over an hour, she describes growing up in South Florida, her early career in retail sales, meeting the future husband who had seen action in World War I, the 1924 economic boom, the depression, and raising two sons, among other life experiences.

We begin at the end of her story, with her admission to Fairhaven. The role of carer is centrally linked to what follows. She calls her husband "Daddy," a name she grew accustomed to using in speaking of him with her sons.

> Dr. Marsh [her personal physician] told Jack and Gordon [her sons], he said, "Now your mother cannot go home. She must go to a convalescent home." Well, it was good for Daddy. He was grieving so that he called me everyday. He didn't know where he was. If I told him, it wouldn't have done him any good anyway; it wouldn't register. He kept wondering why I wouldn't come. See his mind would come and go. [Elaborates] I guess Jack talked to the doctor and Jack says to me, "Mother, I don't want you getting upset but you are going to Daddy's nursing home, but you will only be there until March 10th. I want a room for both of you together."
>
> Well, I took care of Daddy. I felt bad because he grieved so. They [the staff] did very, very little for him. The only time they did anything extra was to put him on Ativan to calm him down because he kept wanting his moth-

er. This all goes with it, you know. [Elaborates] It's a good thing Daddy went first 'cause he could have never lived without me. Never. He would have never made it. [Elaborates] So, anyway, the nurses and all complimented me and commended me for the way I took care of him.

[The night he died], I got up at 12:30 and I knew he was sound asleep and I bathed his feet and put his socks on. And so he was well covered and all. [Elaborates] So I got back in bed. As I said, it was kind of chilly. So I covered up good and dozed off. And when I woke up, Jack's [son] arms were around me and I knew that was it. The curtain was pulled and he had expired just, you know, while I was asleep. I think I fell asleep just before he died. He had a very bad heart. So he had a peaceful death. He went to sleep and what else could I ask for? You know, in that respect, the ending of a beautiful marriage?

If Coplin thought of herself as a carer, she was quick to point out that she was not "doting." Her aim was to care, not to interfere. Her relations with her sons and their families are described accordingly:

We had a good time. We made [laughs] milkshakes! I was over [at Gordon's home] last Sunday for dinner, for three or four hours. Gordon is semiretired now. I've taken care of them and their little ones. But I'm not the interfering kind. I don't dote on people. Never have.

Turning to life at Fairhaven, the theme of caring reemerges. Describing how she helps out, it is evident that she enjoys the role.

I just take each day at a time and do the best I can with it. I love everybody and I try to help those here. I'm being charitable, you might say. I wheel them around. You know, like I have the legs and they have the eyes. This one lady in particular, I kind of look after her. She's very bad with Alzheimer's and I . . . she sits with me now. So I kind of look after her at the table here in the dining room.

When I first came here, I did quite a bit. Like, oh, I did a lot of little things that I could help Susan with in the activity room. Anything they wanted me to do that I was able to do, I'd do, because I didn't lose the sight of this good eye until a year ago last July. The surgery was a failure because I had so much scar tissue.

But I've enjoyed being here. I love it here. It's home to me. And, you know, when you get older, it's kind of nice not having to wash dishes, make beds, or anything like that . . . 'cause I've worked all my life. But I've enjoyed it, you know.

Coplin's role as carer is not as active as it was before her recent total blindness. But she figures ways to be helpful despite the handicap. To her, even the act of attentively listening to others is a form of help. Describing a typical day in her life at Fairhaven, she notes:

Well, I'll tell you, I wake up quite early and get ready for breakfast in the dining room. We come in our robes and nighties and have a nice breakfast. And then if it's not bath day, we go back to our room. And my roommate is precious . . . we have the radio going and we get all of the news of the day. Then we'd usually dress and get ready to go back to the dining room for lunch. In between, you never know what might be going on. But there's not really too much going on in the morning.

There's not much I can do now like doing baskets, you know, crafts and things like that. I can't do much of that now. So, you know . . . but I can listen! [Laughs] We have a lot, well, of different churches come in with children and we will have a songfest. We listen to them and that. And I listen to those that need to share their misery and that's how I help.

When I ask her what she expects daily life to look like a year from now, Coplin keeps her temporal horizons close to the present, as many residents do. In the process, she explains that caring also means not complaining. Coplin's care extends even to the facilities' professional caregivers, helping the helpers, as she puts it.

I don't look that far ahead. I just take each day at a time. I'm hoping I can live to see that great-grandson of mine and have him remember me. He's seventeen months old now and he's doing the polka and trying to say "Nanna," but he gets it mixed up with banana. [Laughs]

I hope to go to heaven, if that's what you mean. [Laughs] I'm not morbid or bitter or nothing. I just take each day at a time and try to enjoy it to the hilt, if you know what I mean. And I try never to complain. I try to be . . . think of who helps to take care of us [the staff], you know. They're human. Some of these people [residents] don't understand. They give them a hard time, you know. I just try to think of others and just take each day at a time and enjoy whatever there is around and try to help those that help us.

Coplin compares residents in her circle of friends, those who are more able than she now is and those who are more helpless. It's a long and detailed narrative of mutual care and support. At one point, Coplin mentions those special to her and recalls having received a surprising compliment from a "nice gentleman" for helping his mother. It seems to cap a life of giving to others in return for what she herself has been blessed.

. . . a very close friend. She's Madeline. Her husband has Alzheimer's and we've become very close friends. Now, well . . . she wasn't bad when I first came in and I am very close to her. I feel that God has put her in my path, you know, to kind of look after. And then there was Mrs. Edison here. She was special. When Ray [Coplin's husband] was alive, we'd wheel her to and from the dining room. He enjoyed that. If she was cold, we'd go get her sweaters. And then she died. When she left, she had a lot of nice things, which I was surprised at. [After she died], I walked in [her room] one day and I didn't know who was there. I could see a bit then. This nice gentleman comes up and says to me, "I want to shake your hand." He said, "Mrs. Coplin, you're the most wonderful person I've ever known!" And I said, "Well, that's a nice compliment. What's this all about?" He said, "The way you were with my mother." She was two doors down from me and I felt like she was my grandmother and I kind of adopted her as my family. I guess it's that I feel I'm so blessed that I want to do for others.

* * * * *

Making a new home presents a narrative horizon that casts the quality of life and the quality of care positively. When home signifies nurturance, friendship, security, and shelter, what could be a more satisfying life than life at home? In this context, Martha Gilbert's earlier "home" experiences are a marked contrast with her current one. For Gilbert, the nursing home links together the domestic life she never had. Jane Nesbit and Ruby Coplin are now at home for other reasons, equally compelling domestically. What is more, as Nesbit suggests, if there is both good and bad in the facility, such is the fate of things anywhere. For Nesbit and Coplin, the nursing home's quality of life is a narrative extension of what life has always been like.

CHAPTER

4

It's Come to This

There are narratives that convey an overriding concern with fate. Some are sad tales of puzzlement over how, after one has lived by the rules or in good stewardship, it is possible that life has come to this: the uselessness of a sedentary existence with no discernible purpose. Residents like Myrtle Johnson look back on their lives—filled with hard work, enjoyment, and kindness toward others—and grimly wonder how God could have planned this for them. Theirs are not so much stories of profound disappointment over physical or mental deterioration or worry for their own or others' well-being, as they are narratives of quandary over the meaning of life in the face of circumstances.

Not all are completely sad. Resident Alice Stern, for one, tells of being placed in a nursing home because her soon-to-be-remarried daughter can't foresee caring for her mother with a new husband around. Stern jokes that her daughter is afraid the mother will sweep the husband off his feet and take him away. At the same time, she wonders how it's come to this: how it is possible that a daughter could ever place her mother in a nursing home. Stern can't fathom how any relative could abandon another one, which to her violates a foundation of family life.

The stories' horizons extend well beyond the local and interpersonal. If it is understood that there are things a nursing home cannot offer, this is overridden by the broader question of life's meaning. If there are complaints about, or an appreciation of, staff members' efforts, these pale against the issue of what people have come to be. In this narrative context, the quality of care, while a concern, hardly bears on the quality of life.

MYRTLE JOHNSON

Myrtle Johnson is a ninety-four-year-old widowed African American woman who has lived at the Westside Nursing Center for a year. She suffers from Parkinson's disease and has difficulty maintaining her balance. According to Johnson, falls have been the bane of her later years, the main reason she was placed in a nursing home. She also is in some pain from arthritis.

Johnson's story links together themes of independence and being helpful to others, which enigmatically contrast with a felt uselessness. Her story begins with the family's move to Jesse James territory near the Fox River in the state of Missouri.

> I was born in Brice County, Illinois, and I lived there until I was eight years old. Then I moved to Missouri. I lived thirty miles from the Fox River. You've heard of the Fox River Outpost? Well, I lived thirty miles from there.
>
> Jesse James was plying up and down that river, you know, at that time. Jesse James just bothered the banks and the trains. He never bothered . . . he would take money from them and he'd, like, pay the widowed woman who needed it. He was shot in St. Joseph, Missouri. He was in his home and he'd gone to straighten a picture—his mother's picture—which was hung up on a wall. They say that Johnny Howard sneaked up and shot him in the back. I've been in the home and I've seen that picture with a bullet hole in it. My brothers live near St. Joe now and they have for years. But Jesse James looked out for the poor people he could help. It was the railroads and the banks he robbed.
>
> The story was . . . and I don't know if it's true or not, but I imagine it was . . . that his mother and his sisters lived over at the edge of Illinois. There was a bunch of confederate reserves from the army who was traveling that way and they raped his sister. That evidently turned Jesse James into . . . he wanted to get back at somebody or something. So he started to rob trains. Really, the people around there never saw any harm in Jesse James because he helped so many people. I don't know. That's about all I can tell you about that.
>
> I was a country girl, always lived in the country. I grew up there. My folks was poor and I began teaching when I was sixteen years old. You could teach if you could get a certificate back then.

Explaining how she came to live in Florida, Johnson compares an earlier useful life with a life now hardly worth living.

> There was one thing my son disliked. There was snow in Missouri. You know how it would snow and we'd brave the snowdrifts. So my son took off for Florida. When my husband's health got pretty bad, my son had us move down here so's he could look after him. We moved into my son's house. My husband passed away and I lived there until I got so's every time I got on my feet I'd fall over. [Pauses and groans from leg ache] So I couldn't stay by myself any longer. My son and his wife worked and, of course, they couldn't be there all the time. So that's my story.
>
> But I worked hard all my life. And I enjoyed life. I'll say that what I enjoyed the most was when I lived on a farm in Missouri. Now that's where I enjoyed myself the most because I was able to get out and do things, you

know, help others. If there's one thing I don't like, it's just sittin'. That's what I have to do now. But then I try to make the best of it. But I would say that when I was able to be up and around and work is when I enjoyed myself the most.

My husband was sick for a number of years, but I took care of him. When I took him to the hospital, I stayed with him night and day. I never left his side. He's been dead now for eleven years. I made the best of what I could do and I'm not dissatisfied with it.

Of course I'm not happy sitting here this way. But then it's part of life and you've got to . . . I will say I've often thought about it, just since I've been passing between the chair and the bed. What use is it?

You know, I can realize why some people commit suicide. They don't have faith. People that have faith in God don't commit suicide. But I can see why when people are in my position and don't have faith in the Lord, they commit suicide. I've thought about that so much. You know, you often say, "Well, why did so-and-so do so-and-so?" Well, if you sit down and study about it, you can figure that out . . . there's nothing . . . But as long as you have faith in the Lord, you are going to go ahead and take what he sends you. But there's times you really wonder.

If in the context of her faith she cannot contemplate suicide for herself in the face of being useless, she still is perplexed that God has let her life come to this. As we discuss fate and destiny, I ask her what her life looks like from where she is now. She ties her answer to a doctor's explanation for her mother's fated death.

Well, life looks to me like a big blob! That's just what it looks like exactly, because what good am I? I've often wondered why the Lord lets me live on, because what good am I to anybody? I'm a burden, you see. Now, my son and his wife, regardless of how busy they are, they come over here once a week and they find me. I can call them anytime, you see. I'm a burden in a way. You see I'm a burden.

I wondered sometimes . . . I reckon it was a doctor who told me one time . . . He had a farm out close to where we lived and people lived on his farm, friends of mine. When my mother passed, I said, "Well, doctor, if I would have had more time, maybe we could have saved her." And he said, "Myrtle, I want to tell you something." He said, "I had stood by the bedside of people that there was no unearthly reason why they should go, but they did. I've seen other people who were literally pulled out of the grave and they lived on." So he said, "You can't tell." He said, "We're put here for a purpose. When our purpose is served, we're taken." So I often think of that and I wonder what purpose a person who sits around like this can be anyway. I think about it all the time. Maybe the Lord knows what it is. So that's what I know to tell you.

Destiny and luck reemerge as we talk about the meaning of home. Furniture evokes home, as do the rhythms of being around a household

and one's "things," as Johnson calls her personal possessions. The Westside existence that is a puzzle because it seems pointless is underscored
by the absence of these concrete reminders of a purpose in life. Describing her furniture as old-fashioned, she nonetheless cherishes it because
of its linkage with a meaningful existence and its related bearing on her
identity. Westside is not so much a home in this respect as a place to
receive care, a place she claims is entirely separate from her life, seemingly adding to the quandary.

> *Jay:*   Now that you've been here for a year, do you feel it is home?
>
> *Myrtle:* No! This will never be home to me. Nothing like this will ever be a
>   home to me. To me it's a place where I get care and I have to stay. In
>   that regard, it's fine.
>
> *Jay:*   What would it have to be like to be more like home?
>
> *Myrtle:* Well, I just don't know what it would have to be like. I guess if I had
>   my things, my furniture and stuff, around me. That would be more
>   like home. Then if I could get up and get around, do things, it would
>   be more like home. You know my furniture? You see, I had it from
>   the time I was married. It was old, but I loved it. Before I had to
>   come here, I lived in my son's house, next door to him. And he has
>   just been cleaning out that house, taking the furniture out of it now.
>   But I lived with that furniture all these years. It was old, but it was
>   dear to me. There wasn't any of it modern.
>
> *Jay:*   Why was it dear to you, Mrs. Johnson?
>
> *Myrtle:* Well, because I lived with it all that time. It just became a part of me,
>   you know. I never was into fancy things. I'm just a common, ordi-
>   nary person. I never . . . I wasn't like a lot of people, you know.
>   When they were young, a lot of girls dressed so fancy and they
>   worried about being in style, but that never worried me. People
>   began to use face . . . makeup, you know, when I was young. Boy, I
>   never did that, but it was quite a thing at that time. But it never
>   appealed to me. [Jokes about being made up]
>
> *Jay:*   That's funny. [We both laugh] And what about this place? You were
>   talking before about your furniture and all and that it couldn't really
>   feel like home. Do you feel that this place is part of your life or
>   separate from it?
>
> *Myrtle:* Oh, it's separate. I don't feel that I'm part of this place at all. My life
>   is entirely separate from this. I look on this as just a place where I've
>   been unlucky enough to have to come. It's just like going into a
>   doctor's office or anything else, you know. I don't feel that I'm a part
>   of it or anything.
>
> *Jay:*   Why is that, I wonder?
>
> *Myrtle:* Well, I don't know. I'm just that way. I just . . . it's just not my way
>   of living and I just . . . I don't know why. I guess I'm peculiar.

Johnson is reminded of her upbringing and compares that with what
children and young people are like nowadays. She contrasts her child-

hood, adulthood, and family relations, among other social indicators of a different period and place—her time and place. Her past gave meaning to life, when in her "common and ordinary" way she understood the purpose of existence. As we again take up the present, Johnson returns to a predominant narrative linkage: the perplexity of "coming to this." As she speaks clearly and unemotionally of the present, she suggests that just continuing to live as she does is a burden.

> I'm a bump on a log. I'm absolutely useless. I'm just sitting here, a menace, just, you might say, worthless. Just sitting here and I have to be cared for. I'm not able to contribute to anything. [Groans from the ache in her legs]
> I hope I don't live the rest of the year out because there's no point in it. There would just be more worry and more trouble on my son and his wife. They never miss [visiting her]. They're just as faithful . . . they come every week no matter how busy they are. If I need them, I can call them and they'll come more often. But things like that are a burden to other people. They have to look after me. Of course, many people are left with their folks never bothering about them. But that's one thing, our family has always been close, what little there is of it. We've always been close.

Elaborating on the meaning of her felt burden to others, she asks rhetorically that no one feel sorrow for her. By and large, she's fine now as far as daily needs and cares are concerned. She is reluctant to bother anyone about such matters, least of all her son and daughter-in-law. If there is sorrow in her life, it soberly relates to the unfulfilled larger project of there being a point to it all. In the following extract, Johnson notes that as concretely minor a matter as getting around in a walker to tend a garden might seem, it can signal purpose and meaning.

> Life don't mean anything now. There's nothing to look forward to. All you've got is your memories to look back on. But as long as you are able to get around and do things, life means you can always find something to do worthwhile, if you want to, if you're able. But when you're not able, of course, it means very little to me.
> Like having to be here. Well, if I was able to get up and around, I'd be in my own home and doing things, you know. After I got so I had to use my walker, why I still got out and around and raised a garden. I could use that walker and put it where I can get a hold of it, you know. And I always was active. But when I fell over backwards, I broke so many bones and, finally, I just had to give it up.
> [When you were able to be up and around], you felt like you were still a human being, you see. But when you're like this, you know that you're . . . it's impossible for you to do anything for anybody. You're just trouble, that's all. You know you are. But when you're at home and able to do for yourself, why there's always . . . that's a different feeling. That makes you feel good.
> It's not being able to get up and do things. I realize I have to get old. I know that. But to me, just sitting down and seeing this or that you'd like to

do and you can't do anything, you know how that is. [Elaborates] This thing about being waited on, I don't like that. I can't say that I dislike it. I just put up with it. That's all I can do.

I don't have any future. I'm just here till the Lord calls me home. I think about it for other people. I think for my son. I often wonder what the future holds for him. I think about that a lot.

ALICE STERN

Alice Stern's narrative has the marks of the lifelong curmudgeon. She not only doesn't understand how it's come to this, but wryly jokes about it and speaks her mind of it as a bane on her existence. As it does for Myrtle Johnson, the existential context of Stern's rootless living preoccupies and puzzles her. This is about the quality of an abandoned and "drifting" life, not the quality of her care.

Stern is an eighty-year-old white widowed female who lives at the Greenfield Nursing Home. She was a heavy smoker and now suffers from emphysema. She can't "hold her water" and, like Myrtle Johnson, falls easily. Before moving into Greenfield, Stern lived in another nursing facility for a few weeks, and prior to that in a board-and-care home for women for a number of years.

Stern is interviewed three times over the course of a year. In the first interview, following her admission to Greenfield, she sounds like the newcomer who nonetheless has lived in congregate care for some time. The second interview, six months later, finds her a bit more settled but still in a quandary over the fate of life. By the third interview, Stern has noticeably declined. She is confused and has difficulty focusing on what is being discussed. But her existential puzzlement holds.

The First Interview

Stern's past centers on three marriages. Early in the interview, she dwells on the death of her first husband from a freak mechanical accident. She speaks of it with some sorrow, but is quick to add that there were two other marriages following that one.

> I married when I was seventeen and my husband had two children, a boy and a girl. He was working on a car and I don't know what year. The car exploded and killed him. [Elaborates] He died during the night. That was very sad. So I married a school friend, I mean a young person we had known. I married him and it didn't last long, for four or five years, and from then on I was just alone. But, the second one, he walked out. He didn't want to be married any longer and he just walked out. [Laughs] So that was the end of that. And I just wandered on. I had a family, my mother and

father. I lived with them in Maryland, just outside DC, you know. I just
went back home in other words and I worked a little bit as a waitress for
some. I never had any real experience. So I dabbled in waitress work here
and there. Then I married Stern, Frank Stern, and we got along fine until
one morning he was dead. He just up and died during the night sometime.

Continuing her story, Stern half-jokingly "wanders" and "drifts"
through life. In time, the words signal a concern for how it's come to
this, in particular how it is that her only living child, a soon-to-be-
remarried daughter, could have thrown her mother out and placed her
in a nursing home. It is all wrong somehow, especially as it seems to
have been prompted by her daughter's forthcoming marriage to a man
who, like the daughter, doesn't want anyone "tied around their neck."
Yet Stern acknowledges the daughter's concern for her mother's well-
being and, in that respect, feels that the daughter is good to her. It is the
life situation her daughter has forced upon her that puzzles Stern, especially as it suggests filial irresponsibility and the resulting loss of a familial anchor.

I lived with my daughter for a while when she decided, well . . . [snidely]
she met this gentleman who was going to marry again. She decided I guess
there wasn't room for Mother. So from then on I got thrown out, lived here
and there, in homes like this, you know, drifted and wandered around. She
just felt, I guess, felt like with a new husband, they didn't want something
tied around their neck. In other words, she wanted me to move. So that's
what happened and I don't think it's right.

I have been in these, one or two of these homes and I am satisfied with
that. I mean most of the ones that's here is in the same boat as I am. So I
can't say too much wrong with it.

That other place [previous nursing home], I didn't live there very long.
When I was there, a woman in a bed next to mine, she had some kind of
hysterical fit. She screamed and my daughter said, "I don't think you're
going to like it here." I would have been in the bed next to this lady that was
throwing the fit. Something happened that day and they moved her out or
something. I was there for a while, but my daughter still didn't feel like I
should stay there. So she got this place for me and she said, "Mom, I am
going to move you over to another place that is better." So this is the place
I've been in. She takes care of things for me like that. So that's good.

But, like I said, I've been driftin'. You wonder how this could happen. You
really do.

Stern recalls the board-and-care home, "Miss Beulah's" it was called,
but returns to the enigma of abandonment.

I did live at this other place called Miss Beulah's. That was the lady's [own-
er's] name. She was a little bit like a mean schoolteacher. She had her rules

and if you stepped your toe over the rules, you were in trouble. It was a home that took in elderly women and I didn't get along . . . my big mouth. These poor old women she had, I think they were dying up there. She had them and they were scared to death of her. I talked back to her and she didn't like that at all. If I saw something that I didn't think was exactly right, I would say something about it, like I always done. I had never been in a place like that, where I had to bow down and hold my mouth shut. So it didn't work out too good there. I just felt like I had as much right as anybody else to talk. I did not get along too good there. The other poor women, they just backed around like they was scared to death of her. I didn't get along too good.

My daughter eventually found this place. She thought I would like it. There wasn't quite as many here or something. She was pretty good to kind of look around for me. [Laughs] I am like a drifting leaf or something. I don't know where the next place will be. But I am satisfied here as far as that goes.

I can't say it's a happy life. Been abandoned, you might say. I have always been in with the family, but now I get the feeling that they do not want to be bothered—excess baggage or something. I don't want to push myself in on them. So they feel like they don't need any extra and I just stay away from them and I am satisfied here. I have no reason not to be, but it is not a home atmosphere at all.

My daughter tells me, "Mama, get out and walk around the yard." Well, I don't feel like it. My legs are not in that good a shape. I had trouble with my legs before I got here, sorta like rheumatism or something. My daughter cannot understand. She says, "Get out and walk around." When I was at another place here, I would go and sit on the porch and I could see the street and the traffic going by. But here I haven't even looked for what the porch looks like. I am satisfied here. I have a TV and I figure, well, I will do that. It is not that I am not satisfied. It's just not much else. It's more or less an old ladies home here for ones that don't have a family and I have to go along with that, you know, like wander on. But I do have a family. I just don't know.

Thinking back on her life, Stern talks about her two sisters, one now dead. The past is linked with the present as she tells of feeling mixed up by a world that's lost its meaning, which for Stern is tied to a life with family. Unable to explain her fate, she wonders why she's being punished.

Now I have one sister left. There was only three girls and this one that's still living is awful good to me. If she thought I needed a dollar or something, she would have it in the mail to me. She is working, making pretty good. She told me that if I needed anything, to let her know. The one I was living with, she passed away. It is a mixed up . . . a mixed up life, you might say. I wonder sometimes why I am being punished. It seems like the good Lord is punishing me for something. Why? I don't know.

I ask Stern how she explains what has happened to her and she continues to be perplexed. She feels she has been shortchanged on what she thought she had bargained for—fair and honest living—conveying to her the incredible injustice of fate.

> I can't explain it. I really can't. Because I honestly . . . I am no angel, but I honestly don't know of a trick or a bad deal that I have ever done to anybody. It would be on my conscience. I couldn't sleep at night if I had done somebody a dirty trick like turning me in for something they had done or done anything against. I couldn't sleep at night. It would keep me awake. I don't know. I can't understand it . . . why I been cheated like this.

This conjures up a litany of enigmas: her feeling of being unwanted, her overly long life, and the untimely death of her younger sister. The death is especially puzzling to her, reflecting what many residents say in this connection, that time of death should accord with birth order.

> I'll tell you, life looks pretty empty. I feel really unwanted. I am trying to overcome that now. For some reason, the good Lord leaves me here. I have almost died from my breath. I have an awful lot of emphysema. I guess a lot of it is from smoking. It almost seems like I have died a couple of times, but I am still left here for some reason. I don't know why, at this age. It is strange, they say, if you are left. I don't know why the younger sister passed. I'm the older one. It would have been better for me to go and for her to stay. It seems like she enjoyed life more than me anyway.
>   She [the younger sister] liked to go away, liked to visit. She always took a chance. I asked her not too long before she died, "Were you ever up in an airplane?" and she said, "Yes." Me, I'm too chicken. You can't get me in an airplane, but her . . . she is a rascal. She took a plane trip back to see her son, by herself. She went out and got on the plane. I wouldn't do that for nothing. I am chicken all the way. But she tickled me. She passed away. Lord, that was a big surprise when she passed away. Wasn't right.

As Stern shares feelings about the unfairness of a life that's come to this, I ask her what she might have done differently if she could have lived her life over again. She remarks:

> I can't imagine what I would do. I have never thought of it that way. I really don't know. I don't know how I could live it different because I got along. I have lost three men and I am still here. My children's daddy was working on a car and it exploded on him. I had told him, "Take that car to the garage." He was putting his hand over the carburetor, making the suction, and it exploded on him. He died that night from the burns. He inhaled the smoke, he said. I really don't know why I am left. What good am I? A shell. An old empty shell sitting around. Just can't explain it.

Stern's sense of fate's just and unjust doings is communicated in the prayers she recalls saying as a child. The prayer reflects the precariousness of parental lives in her generation's childhood.

I come from a big family. When my mother and daddy lived, my prayer
instead of "Now I lay me down to sleep" was "Dear Lord, spare Mother and
Daddy till we are grown." There was lots of dying then. The thought of a
bunch of children being left . . . five, six, seven, whatever . . . to me, that
was a horrible thing. That was the worst thing that could happen to anyone.
So that was my prayer, that the good Lord spare them until we got grown.
And He did. We were all grown, married, and more or less had our own
homes when they passed away. That part was alright. I mean it wasn't
alright. We hated to give them up. I mean we did have our roost kind of set
in. We had homes, most of us were married, and more or less settled.
[Laughs] Of course, it was nice to run home if you had a little argument or
something. [Laughs]

At the end of the interview, we have a lengthy conversation about
aging, illness, and death, which is again punctuated by the puzzlement
evident from the start, particularly the question of why she had to leave
her daughter's home.

Jay: How would you say you feel about growing old?
Alice: Well, I tell you, I don't feel good about it. If I had something more to
         hold onto or a little bit of a steadier place. It is just that I am kind of
         drifting. Will it get worse or better? And why this? How'd it come to
         this?
Jay: Will that get worse or better, Mrs. Stern?
Alice: My living? Will I have a harder time to find a place that I enjoy or like?
         I don't know. It seems to be that it is a kind of worry to me. Like if I
         have to leave here, what's going to be the next place? I am kind of hurt
         at my family. I don't mean to be bragging about myself and my dispo-
         sition or anything, but it seems like I never butted in. In fact, I don't
         know why my daughter wanted me out. I was there, I had a room
         there, and I kept my own room. I didn't cause her any extra work and
         I helped if she was going out or if she was going to be out. [Scoffs] And
         all because this man come along that she met at this singles dance.
Jay: At the singles dance?
Alice: Yes and she is going with him, steady. I out and said to him, "Why did
         you put me out? I wasn't going to interfere with you and her." He just
         nodded. He didn't want to say nothing back. He was afraid I guess I'd
         say more. But I never did find out anything. I don't know.
             Now if my health breaks, what's going to happen to me? You know,
         if I was bedridden? Who knows what's gonna happen. No, I really
         don't know. My future's as blank as a side of a wall. I really don't . . . I
         can't picture anything. I really cannot. It's kind of a worry. Where do
         you go from here? I tell you, the government, I think, is paying for
         this. That is kind of a relief if it is. I hope it is. I am on Medicare and
         this last one, Medicaid, that's sort of like the medicine that wherever
         you live is taken care of. So that's good if it's true. And the daughter's

taking care of this. I mean she got the place and brought me over here and all. I guess if there is any paying to be done, she would tell me about it. But anyway, she is kind of taking care of that, till I die I guess.

Jay: Do you think about death, Mrs. S?

Alice: Yes, I do. I would like to die in my sleep. I think most everybody would. There is many a night when I lay my head on the pillow and say, "Oh, if I could just die tonight, never waking up." I don't know what is ahead of me, but I mean I feel that way.

Jay: Why is that, I wonder?

Alice: Well, I don't have nothing to hold to. I am like . . . I am just drifting, you know, hoping it turns out all right. That isn't any way to live. It isn't fair, you know. It's a kind of shaky setup. How did I get into all this? [Pause] You have to have something to look forward to, some kind of a future to hold onto or something. I don't have nothing . . . [jokingly] an extra change of clothes is about all and they ain't too good.

I don't know. I have to depend on my daughter I guess and she'd rather go to a garage sale than stop by and see her mother. She knows what a dull existence I have here.

Jay: Dull?

Alice: Dull! *Dull* is what I said. I don't expect them to entertain me or anything, but it is just kind of dull. I don't know. It seems to me that if my daughter was in a place like this, that I would drop by or call her or keep in touch with her more. I would want her to know that I know that she is there and if I could do anything. Families just do like that.

Stern is both appreciative and jokingly critical of Greenfield's quality of care, which she extends to institutions in general.

Still, this place is holding me together and it don't seem too bad. I mean I am as well off as these others and they aren't complaining. In fact, I might be a little better off because they don't seem to have much more company than I do or as much.

[Points to her roommate's bed] And that one there, she is not one of these that mixes. She's colored but that doesn't make a difference to me. I mean I am just the same with that. But her family comes and on weeknights they keep me awake for that matter. But I don't say anything about it. I only have one good ear, so I can lay on my good ear and go on to sleep if I want to. Anyway, her company don't bother me except they block the bathroom. I hate to ask them to move. About two of them will be sitting there by the [bathroom] door. If I want to go to the bathroom before I go to bed, I have to move around two of them. They should know that they don't have to be right up against there. [Elaborates]

They [the nurses' aides] know I can be as nice as I am going to be and I can be the other way too. This one comes in here in the middle of the night and turns the light on and asks, "Let me see. Do you want anything?" She is supposed to be looking after you. [Scoffingly] So she comes in and wakes you

up! Like the son-in-law once said about the hospital (he was in the army), he
says that they come in and wake him up from his sleep to give him a sleeping
pill! [Laughs] He would fuss to my daughter. [Elaborates] Bless his heart, he
is gone now. I swear there are a lot of things like that. You can laugh about
some of them. You can get mad about some of them. This one come in and
woke me up and I said, "Can't you find something else to do in the middle of
the night?" I don't think that she has bothered me since then.

I can be grouchy or be the other way. I am a little bit like that. If I get wide
awake in the middle of the night, it is a little bit hard to get back to sleep and
I don't appreciate it. I told one [aide], "Can't you find something else to do
instead of waking me up?" I was fussing and she said, "Oh, I didn't know
you were like that." But I didn't want the argument to go on. I felt like
saying, "Well, you know it now! Remember!" I didn't say it.

Six Months Later

Six months later, Stern has had a birthday and is eighty-one years old.
Her health and mental status remain just about what they were before.
This time she is interviewed by Carol Ronai.

Stern again recalls her life, having married three husbands, all of
whom died. She jokes about sounding, in her own words, "like I'm
killing them off." She continues to mull over how it's come to this. When
Ronai asks about the last chapter of her life story, Stern admits to thinking about suicide because no one wants her. Stern feels that her whole
family is avoiding her, especially the daughter.

I think there's been times in the past year that I've thought of suicide. It
seems the whole family is afraid that I'll want to come and live with them. They
just don't know what to do. They're ducking me like I was a plague.
And I know I don't butt into their business. My daughter, she couldn't be
sweeter now for anything however she tried. But she absolutely asked me to
leave. She said she . . . this man come into her life . . . and she decided, you
know, that she likes him. Gonna get serious. I don't know what they're
waiting for to get married. Don't look like he got much intention. [Laughs]
Maybe she's afraid he'll fall for me and I'll steal him away!

But, anyway, before he comes into the picture, she told me . . . at first she
said, "Well, Mom, you can live here. I've got a three-bedroom house." It
was just her. Her husband was passed away and I thought that, well, this is
home, you know. Then out of the clear blue sky, "Mom, you'll have to
move." And that was because he was coming in. Well, I wasn't going to
bother with him and her. I don't know why. She just wanted me out. She
didn't give me too much of a notice. I said, "Can't we wait till next week?"
She said, "No, I want you to go tonight 'cause I'll change my mind if we
wait."

So now she's doing everything, seems like. Comes by almost everyday
and brings me something. It seems to me like she's thought it over and she

. . . but she's never asked me to come back or anything. I don't think I'd go if she did. But she seems to be very attentive, you know, giving me attention, bringing me something. She's bringing me things to eat—strawberries were the last—and she brings me all kinds of little things: Mickey Mouse and the little doll and the little dogs. She knows I like things like that sitting around. I never got over my childhood, I guess. I think they're so cute but . . .

I don't know. Ask me more questions, baby. I done run out of wind.

Ronai continues and they talk about Stern's past. Ronai asks her whether Greenfield could be home, to which Stern responds no. Stern nonetheless comments on Greenfield's good care compared to other places she's known, the point at which we return to the interview.

I tell ya, I seem kinda different. I talk too much or something. But people seem to like me and I think they're glad to have me here. I don't know, it seems like I've gone and spruced up the ones that wasn't talking and I seem to be well known. I guess when I first came in here, they said, "Have you met so-and-so, Alice?" It seems like, you know, they welcome me. I don't know what more you could do.

But I tell you what I like about it. In this other place—Miss Beulah's—she was kinda strict. If she snapped her fingers, she wanted you to jump, you know. She wanted her rules right to do. Like she wanted you in the bedroom at eight o'clock and she didn't want you back out. And the other place was a bit like that, too. Here, it's a little looser. I do notice the colored girls come in here. There, they were supposed to come in before you went to sleep, you know, and see if everything was all right. Never once came in. Here, a lot of the colored girls come in and ask, "Did you want anything before you go to sleep?" or something like that. That's okay, but not in the middle of the night. So I think that's pretty good. I'm satisfied here, as far as that goes. Can't say much against it.

They talk about Stern's placement at Greenfield, something that Stern again mentions she cannot understand. The quality of Stern's life is informed by linkages to the meaning of family, not by the particular cares of the nursing home. It isn't so much what Stern imagined the quality of care in a nursing home would be before she entered one that gives Stern "chills," as it is the puzzle of how it could have come to this.

Carol: Let me ask you this, Mrs. S. Before you went into a nursing home, what did you think it would be like?
Alice: Well, the thoughts of it would just give me chills, that this could happen.
Carol: What kinds of thoughts did you have about it?
Alice: I felt like it was strangers. The idea of that made me shiver. I felt like

they'd look at you like, you know, "Who is that coming in?" I just didn't want to go. It broke my heart. To think my own family, you know, some of my own—my sister and my daughter—would let me go to face strangers. I remember my daughter after she told me I had to go. She had arranged all this, too. She had arranged . . . her and her daughter . . . what time to pick me up. Her daughter was there, my granddaughter, and my granddaughter kept saying, "Grandma, I told her I'd be there by eight." They had done set it all up. They hadn't talked to me at all. I asked Susan [her daughter] when she was standing there . . . I had a plastic bag of clothes or something, a satchel, maybe a suitcase, and I said, "Susan, couldn't we talk this over next week?" "No, no. I want you to go tonight," she said. And my granddaughter spoke up and said, "Grandma, we better go. I told her I'd have you there by eight o'clock." And I thought, "Well, they've already set it up." That kind of hurt.

Carol: I see what you mean.
Alice: It hurt, 'cause I said . . . I said I would have never sent *my* mother out. I would have got down on my knees and scrubbed floors if I had to, to make a dollar and keep her. I wouldn't never tell her to get out. So that's the difference.

But now Susan just seems like she can't, like she can't do enough for me. I think it's kind of coming back at her, how she didn't . . . And I hope her conscience hurts her a little bit. [Laughs] I got to be nasty, dear Lord.

But I trust in the Lord, I'd say. I'm not too religious. Some of them, I think, take it too far. But I believe I know there is a God in heaven. There's got to be. Things are too unnatural to not be a God in heaven. Oh, I don't know. I can't express myself like if I could.

The conversation returns to Stern's early life. Describing what she was like as a girl, Stern contrasts that with the present, laughs about it, and even remembers the first interview. She half-jokingly recalls her youthful love of clothes as the most important thing in her life at the time. But the persistent quandary of life is paramount.

I was just sorta like a country girl. I never dressed fancy or anything. And I was never fresh around the dances, you know. I didn't go to a dance unless it was more or less a church outing or something. I never run around to dances along the way. I was quiet, I think.

Now I'm just a plain country woman growing old. That's all I know. [Laughs] One man sit in here and asked me questions about me getting old and we got to talkin'. We laughed and cut up. [Jokingly] He said, "Well, how do you feel about your men?" I said, "Well, I ain't chasing no man, or looking for one either." [Laughs] And things like that, you know. But there was some of the same type of questions.

But, I tell ya, it used to be clothes. [Chuckles] I used to love clothes. And now I don't seem to care about anything. Clothes don't matter. That's nothing to me now.

I tell ya, it just looks like, for me, it looks like a struggle. I absolutely . . . I always was a person that liked to know what's coming tomorrow. Ahead, you know. I don't know. Many a night, I laid in my bed and I think what . . . what'll happen to me? I'd rather have, you know, know a little about it. I sure don't. I can't figure what all's happened to my life. That there is the thing.

The Third Interview

A year after the first interview, Stern's recollections are lengthy and detailed, but it is difficult for her to sort her thoughts and express them coherently. She laments her memory loss. She is now on oxygen. The sound of the pump and being "hooked up" crimp the style of an ebullient woman. Yet her curmudgeonly self comes through, as does the narrative puzzle of her life.

Mainly, life's dull, just dull. I just sit there and think and wonder how it all come to this. It's kinda quiet and she [roommate] generally goes back and then I come back over here . . . unless I'm looking for company or something. [Pause] I'm tryin' to remember . . . I come over here and lay down and I may go off to sleep. If I slept a little, in the evening I wouldn't be sleepy. So I might get a dress out or something and, uh, sew a little seam up the side or something like that, or something else. [Labored breathing] Oh, this thing! [The pump] And if there's anything on that TV . . . now there was one program I missed, doggone it, that I especially wanted to watch. I done forgot what it is. If I look back over the program, I'd remember. But I forgot it. What I have to do is write it down. [Chuckles] I got my pad here.

I don't mind it too bad now. They're good to us. But I still don't know what's coming next. [Turns to look at dozing roommate] That poor soul don't do a thing, but she's there and I've got to think about her every time I do anything. I think she's in ga ga land. To tell you the truth, sometimes I don't know myself if I'm still here. You know what I mean? How'd this happen to me? Bein' in this place and all. God only knows.

* * * * *

Myrtle Johnson and Alice Stern both have complaints about daily life in their nursing homes, from the dissatisfaction of "just sittin'" to the thoughtlessness of aides who barge into the room in the middle of the night. The women nonetheless appreciate the fact that they are being cared for. Still, to them, these are matters separate and distinct from the overall meaning of life, which is an enduring issue. It is this larger horizon—the question of why "it's come to this"—that preoccupies them and provides the primary narrative linkages for the quality of their lives. In Johnson's case, it relates to her love of God and in Stern's it bears on her relation to loved ones. As with other similar residents, puzzled as the women are by fate and the overall meaning of life, the quality of their care is a comparatively minor concern.

5

Lovin' the Lord

Horizons of meaning for residents arise from many directions, not the least of which is otherworldly. Whatever the features or qualities of earthly life, they can take on meaning in connection with the life beyond, where as one resident who loves her Lord put it, "They ain't no rushin' and no pushin', just bein'."

According to these residents, longings for the earthly past, wants for the present, and wishes for the future are small favors to relinquish in comparison with what the life beyond will bring. While the cleanliness of one's premises is important, what does it matter that a bed is temporarily soiled when one is confident that "God will provide"? If a nurse's aide has a bad attitude or a roommate incessantly complains about her family, does either have much significance compared with heavenly bliss? Can the pain of bodily ills and the heartaches of personal loss be as important as God's bounty?

The stark contrasts in such questions tell of residents who live in this world but orient to another one. Certainly, in relation to matters of this world, cleanliness, kindness, and daily life satisfaction in the nursing home are desirable. But their place in this world is temporary and hardly matters in the final analysis. In relation to what is said to be important in the end, the negative qualities of care are just irritations, the positive qualities mere comforts. At stake in the end is something grander than daily living, the source of everlasting life—God's kingdom. For these residents, this is the ultimate context for speaking of life, a horizon that makes all matters meaningful, great and small.

To love or serve the Lord is not to ignore the ills and discomforts of daily life, only to think about them as less important in a larger scheme of things. For these residents, their roles in life are, while in this world, shaped by and for the beyond. Those who love the Lord hold to a different world and in that context speak and evaluate life and its immediate conditions.

The interviews conducted with such residents could be boldly framed by otherworldly concerns. At times, no matter how insistently I probed for views of the quality of care, responses were linked with otherworldly meanings, the residents insisting on the relevance of another reality. At these times, residents mainly spoke past my inquiries, with life everlasting or "churchified" being the preferred narrative context.

JULIA McCALL

The first of the two residents discussed in this chapter, Julia McCall, brought me into her narrative more than any other respondent in the study. She not only highlighted her life "working for the Lord," but engaged me in affirming it, taking for granted that I too worked for Him. Time and again, McCall turned responses into questions, rhetorically asking me whether I didn't think or feel the same way, and following that, blessing me for what I said. McCall also was the resident who had lived the longest in her nursing home, being at Westside Care Center for twelve years.

McCall is a ninety-year-old widowed white woman who has gone completely blind in the last few years and suffers from congestive heart failure. No longer able to read the Bible, she is an avid radio listener, spending hours tuned into religious talk shows or services. When I met her, she was holding a radio to her ear, engrossed in the word of God. As we settled down to talking, a long-standing involvement in church life came forth.

Jay: Ms. McCall? Why don't you tell me a little about your life?

Julia: About my life?

Jay: Yeah. Tell me about it.

Julia: Well, you done asked, bless your heart. I was raised in a little place in Georgia called Damen and my granddaddy, my mother's daddy, was from England. Well, them days my granddaddy, he did get killed in a war. He was only twenty-eight years old and he was buried there, I believe in the Arlington Cemetery. My other granddaddy, his name was Joe O'Donald and he owned half of Georgia. He sure did. He had a gold mine. [Elaborates] I bet you heard of that, ain't you? It's close to Clinton, Georgia, and he had a cotton gin. [Elaborates] It took somebody pretty rich to have a cotton gin, didn't it?

Jay: Um hm.

Julia: When he first got his cotton gin, he was 49 and he was in Clinton. I had a pretty good life. My granddaddy liked me. I went to school and lived in a house. He gave my mother a home close to the school. [Elaborates] There's a Methodist, a Baptist church there . . . Clinton Baptist Church. Have you heard of it?

Jay: No, I haven't.

Julia: The school was named Clinton High School in Clinton and I went to school with the preacher Taylor. Gus Taylor was the teacher. He preached at the Baptist church and I went to church there. I was a member of the church there. I was christened when I was a baby. I joined that there church when I was twenty-three. I went to school and that was the only place I went to school. He taught school. [Elaborates] I graduated from high school at fourteen. That was . . . wouldn't you say that was kind of smart?

Jay: That was.

Julia: And I went to singing school in Clinton at the church and I could sing and took music. I could sing ballads. Don't you think that was kind of smart too?

Jay: That certainly was, I'd say.

Julia: Bless your heart. Well, I got married kind of young. I was just sixteen. My husband was a good bit older than me and we lived on a farm. My granddaddy give us the farm, about fifty acres of land and we lived there. But some people got back from that war and couldn't do much of anything after that war.

Jay: This is which war, Ms. McCall?

Julia: President Wilson was president. My brother was in that war. Oh . . . that's right . . . I had three sisters and one brother. They're all dead, been dead a long time. I just kind of lasted.

Jay: You sure did.

Julia: You know I guess it's because I actually had a pretty good life. [Pause] I don't act like I'm grouchy, do I?

Jay: No.

Julia: Bless your heart. I think I've had a pretty good life. I think the Lord's been good to me. I been in church all my life. [Elaborates] I've been in this place for twelve years. That's a long time. I was seventy-nine when I come in here. I didn't think I'd live to see ninety. I've been in pretty good health too. I've just about had every sickness, but I was tough. I got over it, ya know. I've had a lot of pains and sicknesses, but I was pretty tough. I'm still livin', ain't I? The Lord provides, bless Him.

I was raised to be a nice person. I was raised to go to church. Don't you think that's right? Huh?

Jay: Yes, I do.

Julia: I was raised to go to church. Sure was. And I went all the time. Yesterday was Sunday, wasn't it?

Jay: Yes.

Julia: I got my radio that I could get a preacher on. He's a Baptist at the First Baptist Church. Do you go to church?

Jay: I don't go to that one.

Julia: Are you a Baptist?

Jay: No, I'm not.

Julia: What are you?

> *Jay:*   I was Congregationalist once.
> *Julia:* That's kind of like Catholic, ain't it?
> *Jay:*   Well, no, not exactly.
> *Julia:* Well, you know, there ain't much difference in none of them. All
>   working for the Lord, ain't ya?

This last statement—"All working for the Lord, ain't ya?"—highlights the subjective meaning flowing through McCall's narrative. As she returns to her childhood growing up in rural Georgia, she reminds me that, regardless of the religious differences in town, all were working for the Lord. When she describes the many people, good and bad, she has met over the years, she downplays the differences because, in the end, all are God's children and work for the Lord. As she repeatedly draws me into her story, asking me about my life, family, and beliefs, differences once more are erased because we both are working for the Lord.

In the context of working for the Lord, the troubles and troublemakers of life evaporate because they are mere veneers over what, to McCall, are actually good intentions and "sweet" people. For example, while the quality of her care at Westside at times leaves something to be desired, McCall says that she knows in her heart that she's well cared for, especially as the Lord keeps watch over her. The horizon of lovin' the Lord makes everyone her friend—staff, those residents she knows well, and those she doesn't. All are equally valuable in the sight of God, as McCall points out.

> You know, I got a lot of friends. A lot of friends in here I don't know, but I think I have. There's a lot of friends in this place. You see, I can't see. I can hear them mostly. I can tell who it is. I got a lot of people in here that, well, some's can be nasty, but they're still good people. I like my nurses. I like my nurses really good. If it weren't for them, I don't know what I'd do. They're my favorites. They sure are good to me. They're better to me than anybody, even better to me than even my children. But, really, they're all sweet, God bless 'em all. God loves all his children no matter.

As we talk about all her friends, McCall explains that she not only has "sweet" nurses but believes the nurses consider her a favorite resident, which leads to a story about Ann, a nurse who no longer works at Westside but still visits McCall and, according to McCall, will undoubtedly join McCall in heaven.

> I got some sweet nurses . . . I can't remember all of them, but I got about three nurses now. I got two that come at night and I think they're my favorites. I bet I'm their favorite patient. I think the way they act, they like me. If it weren't for them, I'd be, well . . . But I can dress myself. I can do a lot of things by myself.

I think I'm going to heaven from here. The Bible says that heaven's full, don't it? Well, I think He's got a place up there for me, don't you? [I nod]

I have a little friend. She was with me when I first come in here. I wasn't blind then. I done a lot of things, ya know. Her husband was a flyer and she learned to sew and she was doing a lot of things for me. She was working in here. Ann still comes to see me. She belongs to the Grandmothers' Club, kind of, you know. I went to the Grandmothers' Club a long time, as long as I could see. That was a long time, and then I went blind. Ann comes to see me.

So, as I was going to say, just before Christmas, she'd come and she'd sit in the room. Then I told her, I said, "Ann, the Bible says heaven's full up there." But I said, "I think God's got a place for me." I says, "He has," and I says, "I believe I'm going to be up there." And she says, "You know what?" I says, "What?" And she says, "I'm gonna be right up there with you." God bless her. She's got a mother living and a mother-in-law. The mother-in-law is in a nursing home. She's about the same age as me and Ann don't like her. I thought maybe people that Ann sees would be real sweet people, you know. She really likes me.

I ask McCall the question about living over again and doing things differently, which leads to a series of exchanges dotted with comments and questions about hell, heaven, believers, nonbelievers, and everlasting life.

Julia: I don't know. I think I would just live it. I don't think I've had too bad of a life. Do you think if people still hold on to God, do you think they're too bad a person?

Jay: No.

Julia: I don't feel like . . . I don't feel like I'm old. I don't want to go to hell, do you?

Jay: No.

Julia: I wouldn't want to live it over. It might be worse, don't you think so?

Jay: Well, it might be. I guess I never thought of it quite like that.

Julia: I have never had anything that I have really hated. I ain't never really hated nobody, have you? I don't hate people, do you? I'm sorry for them sometimes, aren't you? Like some's—some nurses and old ladies here—got bad attitudes. I'm sorry for them when they don't believe such a thing as God. Have you ever talked to people like that? I've talked to some of them once and I don't think they've got good sense. I don't think they've ever read the Bible. But they all God's children.

You know, as long as I could see, I've been going to church on Sunday. I went a lot since I've been here. I had Spanish people do church. They come in and we was having a little church.

Well, now, I don't have me anything much to look forward to here, but I told you about Ann coming to visit. But as I says, I'm looking to going to heaven and being up there. What are you looking forward to?

Jay: Oh, I don't know. I guess I'm not sure, really.

Julia: Are you looking forward to going to heaven?
Jay: I would think so.
Julia: Bless your heart. I think that's the best thing we can do for us.

I try to turn the conversation to more mundane matters like daily life in the nursing home and McCall's view of the quality of care. She responds, but the matters seem to be the farthest things from her mind. Her remarks are made as if mundane affairs were fleeting concerns, which McCall attributes at one point to forgetfulness.

Jay: Does it feel like home to you here?
Julia: Sure, since I been in here. I have to sleep here. I don't get to go nowhere much anymore. I go all around here. Once in a while . . . I got one daughter . . . she's sick and goes to the hospital and she comes visit sometimes to take me down there [in the sunshine]. And I got the nurses take me down there in the sunshine and all. And we have a nice, sweet time.
Jay: Ms. McCall, do you feel that this place is part of your life?
Julia: Well, I sure do. I been in here a long time. I think this is one of the best nursing homes. I think over all the world, I don't think you'd find a better nursing home like this. Now what do you think about that? I think the Lord blessed me to be in here, don't you?
Jay: Uh huh.
Julia: Do you think this is a pretty nice nursing home? It's a big one. Did you know that the man that gave all this property is from Georgia? Did you know he was from Georgia?
Jay: No, I didn't.
Julia: He sure was. That's where I'm from, like I said. And like I said, they're very sweet to me. I'm going to heaven. Like Ann says, she's going to be up there with me. I think that's kind of sweet of her, don't you?
Jay: Yes, I do.
Julia: She's pretty, too. She's in her forties, like you. Didn't you say that's your age?
Jay: Yes, I believe I did.
Julia: She's got three children. In here I got a lot of other friends, too. God bless 'em. They're all God's children. [Pause] Sometimes I'm getting kind of forgetful, you know. But don't you think I do pretty good for my age?
Jay: [Affectionately] Very good, Ms. McCall, very good.
Julia: [Chiding me] Do you know somebody else that's better than me?
Jay: Oh, I don't know. You're pretty good, I'd say.
Julia: [Laughing] I know you're a sweet person. I know that. I'm gonna tell my daughters about you. I'm gonna tell 'em what a sweet person you is. Bless your heart.
    I try to be a nice person. I try to be a good Christian and I think . . . the Lord has been real sweet to me or I wouldn't feel that way. I have

had a lot of sad things happen to me, but I think the Lord . . . I think we got to look up to Him.

Jay: Tell me about the sad things, won't you?

Julia: Well, losing my husband and my only son and all that was sad. My mother and dad was pretty old when they died, but I think when you lose them when they're young, I think it's kind of . . . it's, you know, you don't ever get over missing them. I try not to be sad. I don't know. Some people just want to be sad. Some do in their beds. I don't like to see the sick people being so sad.

I look to heaven, to go to heaven and be up there with the Lord. The Bible says if we do right, we'll rejoice. Don't you think we'll be happy up there?

Jay: We probably will. [Pause] But what about this place? Tell me about life in this place. How is the care here?

Julia: Well, it's not too bad. There's some pretty nice people in here. I think some don't know much, but they can't help it. I think the nurses and doctors is the most smartest people there is, most of 'em anyhow. I got a sweet doctor. I've had him for over thirteen years.

I was real sick once, real sick. They had put a tube in my hand. I couldn't take it through my mouth. It was poison to take in my mouth. He sat by the bed and held my hand so I wouldn't take it out. I said, "Well, why don't you just let me die?" He said, "I ain't gonna let you die 'cause you're too sweet to die." He'd take care of me during the daytime and the nurse would take care of me at night. I told him I wasn't afraid to die. And he said, "I'm glad to hear that because I don't hardly ever hear it."

No, I'm not afraid to die because I'm going to the right place. I think I'm going to meet my Savior. I tell you, if we don't read the Bible . . . I was trained to read the Bible from the time I started to read. You know, I've read it three times and every time I've found something different. I sure have. I read it right through and I didn't know my name was in the Bible. Did you know my name was in the Bible?

Jay: Is that right?

Julia: Yeah. Julia. J-U-L-I-A. That's what my name is. I didn't know it was in there. I read it through three times. It's in the last chapter of Romans. If you'll look, you'll find it.

And so it went. As McCall recounted her past, it was a life serving the Lord. As she spoke of the present, I prompted her to detail what she felt to be good and bad about it. She returned repeatedly to everlasting life. Needless to say, the future was a time of life closest to her destiny, when she would be in heaven, as she reminded me again and again.

I was hardly a bystander in her narrative. According to McCall, I was to be right up there in heaven with her, as sweet a person as she remarked I was. As she drew me into her narrative with questions of her own, her love of the Lord took control of the interview as much as it conferred a lesser status to the mundane matters of concern to me. The interview became a resource for her own project, which served to remind me that there was more at stake in life than the qualities of earthly living.

MARY CARTER

Mary Carter also loves the Lord. Her brand of love is to serve Him by going to church, cooking, and singing in the choir. From the start, hers is a life, if not actually spent in church, then lived in relation to church activities. Childhood centers on church affairs, adulthood embellishes the connection, and now old age affirms what she always has been, as she puts it, "churchified" through and through.

Carter is an eighty-five-year-old widowed African American woman. She suffers from pulmonary vascular disease, and hypertension, has ulcers on her legs, and is wheelchair-bound. Her husband died in 1962 and she never had children. Her closest relative is a nephew, who visits her regularly at Fairhaven, the nursing home where she lives.

Carter was one of the few respondents in the project to be interviewed four times. The first interview took place a few days after admission. She was discharged three months later and interviewed the second time in her apartment. Six months after the first interview found her returned to Fairhaven, where she was interviewed the third time. A fourth interview was completed in the nursing home a year after the first one.

Not all residents who come to reside in a nursing home, even longstayers, stay there continuously for the rest of their lives. Some, like Carter, enter and depart several times before they stay put. While Carter's first interview was conducted a few days after admission, she had had a six-month stay at Fairhaven the year before. Carter was well acquainted with the nursing home when we first met.

The First Interview

Following introductions and some small talk, I began the first interview by asking Carter to tell me about her life. As Carter preferred, I called her "Miss Mary."

Jay: Miss Mary, why don't you tell me about your life.
Mary: Well, I have ulcers on both of my knees. I had an operation about four years ago on my leg and it formed kind of an infection on the heel. [Elaborates] So that's why I'm out here. They try to keep me off my feet most of all, you know, until I get strong, you know what I mean.
    My life seems to be very happy. I had a good husband. He's dead now. Been dead since 1962. My life has been good.

When I was real young, startin' in '19 I was a cook. I cleaned house and all like that. I enjoyed it very much. I used to wash the clothes for the lady that I was working for in Jacksonville [Florida], and clean the house and take care of her mother. [Elaborates] Yeah, it was a pretty good life.

Jay: If you were to write the story of your life . . . you know put it into chapters . . . what would the first chapter be about?

Mary: Well, I'd have a chapter of religion. I love church. That's most of my chapter. I get up in the morning and lay down at night. The Lord is my shepherd. I shall not want. I lean on the Lord. For one thing, I thank Him for everything 'cause, I tell you, not many people don't live long as I live, I'm telling you. Eighty-five years old is hittin' toward a hundred.

Jay: What would the next chapter of your life be about, Miss Mary?

Mary: Well, I used to sing in the choir, too, at my church and then at Bethel out on Tenth Avenue. I enjoy singing and also, you know, so many different things. I enjoy it 'cause . . . when I get so I can get around, I'm going in the room [in the nursing home] where they have a church on Sunday. I love to sing. And the lady that plays the piano, she love to hear me sing. Sure does. And I sung the song one time, [singing] "Meet me at the river . . . " [sings several verses].

Jay: Oh, that's wonderful! You used to sing that often?

Mary: Yes, I'd sing that here, out in the wheelchair. Uh huh. They love to hear me sing.

I loved the choir in my church and I love the good singing and everything. I love my church. That's the reason why I say, when I get better, I'm gonna connect myself right back to the Main Street Baptist Church.

The goal of getting better leads her to talk about her eating habits, which then prompts her to recall her work as a cook and housekeeper. Mundane as these activities are, she thinks of them as service to the Lord. Carter's is not a life easily divided into otherworldly and earthly affairs. As she speaks of these and other activities, her religion is fully present. Even the matter of arranging her husband's funeral serves the Lord.

Mary: I'll tell you, since I had ulcers, they don't want me to pull too much grease. I mostly cook with butter when I'm home, cook with margarine and things like that. That grease is bad on ulcers, you know what I mean. I used to cook.

Jay: You were a cook?

Mary: I used to cook roast and baked pies and sweet potatoes and cook cracklin' cornbread and pearly rice. Oh, I just cooked a lot of things. I remember the lady that I worked for. She had about seven people coming and I had to fix something right there. I potted a big ol' roast.

Then I put it in the stove and let it bake. And honey, they went for that, honey, I'm telling you. And you'd make gravy, you know, stir a little mix in, you know what I mean. Oh yeah. She enjoyed the cooking. I served the Lord all my life.

I enjoyed all the parts of my life, when I was married and then, since I got single, I enjoyed myself very good. I don't seem to worry about nothing. I have a lot to be thankful for. If it wasn't for the Lord, I don't know what we'd do.

I used to cook for a doctor once out in Jacksonville and wash clothes and clean house and take care of two children and everything. I've had a right good life. That was a pretty happy time. They was good people to me. See, I didn't have to work but Monday through Friday. I didn't have to work Saturday and Sunday and that was beautiful. When I wanted to go to church, I could always go.

I always believe in doin' good by the Lord. When my husband passed, I did him right. We went to the funeral home . . . I wouldn't tell you no story [no lie] . . . Covington Brothers had his body. So we looked at the caskets and the first casket was $200. I said, "I don't want that." The next one was $300 and the next one was $400. I said, "I don't want that." But the $500 one, I got that. I done the best I could. I had my husband put away decent, doin' good by the Lord. And you know, people in church didn't know me and him were married?

Jay: They didn't?

Mary: No, we was separatin' for so long. They had the church decorated so beautiful. I was real happy. And I asked the preacher to please make it short 'cause I got a brother-in-law who has heart trouble. So he didn't preach no longer than forty-five minutes.

But I was closest to my daddy and my mama. They're about the closest. I mean, Jesus is ahead of that and then they behind. But I loved my husband. I tried to stay with him. I sure did.

All I have left is a nephew. He lives on Fourth Street. His name is Robert Brown. He's kind of sickly. He has bad asthma. He come in to see me every week.

We talk about daily life in the nursing home. She compliments the staff and especially the administrator, whom she calls "the manager," for the concern he shows for the residents. She describes at length how the staff serve the Lord in their own right, which, she repeats, she herself has done all her life.

I'm very happy because the manager sees us being taken care of. I'm telling you can tell that. He checks in on you, whether you had your meetin's in the morning and asks did we enjoy our food. We have plenty to eat. And then, when they serve dinner, he walks to the dining room and goes to the kitchen and sees if the people are fed good. I think that's good. And we have a nice colored man at night that helps these girls, the kind that do lifting. Last night, that girl got on her knees and he says, "No, no. I'll lift this side up." So I thought that was very nice. I really did. He say he is used to taking care of old people. They all be servin' Him right.

We all servin' the Lord, really. When I was up on my feet, I was stood there right in the choir. Sometimes when we had to raise money for tour . . . our choirs . . . I would buy vegetables and go down to the dining room and cook them and bake chicken and bake biscuits and all like that. I give service when I was a young woman, I'm telling you, from about twenty-five years old, I give good service. I sure did.

But I think it'll be a good life now. It's pretty good through all my sickness. What I like about all the nurses is that they are good to me, the white and the colored and all. They are really nice to me. They treat me so good. I have a lot to be thankful for.

In sharing thoughts about the nursing facility, the meaning of home for Carter takes a twist that it doesn't have for many others, tied as it is to her long residence in the local black community and especially her active participation in church. Even though Carter is newly admitted to Fairhaven at the time of the interview, her presence is a homecoming because several old church friends who now reside in the nursing home and the new friends she made when she was at Fairhaven the first time around welcome her back into their lives. Also welcoming her are kin who work in the facility as housekeepers. Returning to Fairhaven, Carter brings some of home with her into the facility. Still, at the end of the interview, after several residents and staff members "peep" in on her, a more enduring sense of home prevails—coming home to the Lord.

Mary: [After a brief interruption] You see how they peep in on me when . . . they be doing that all day.

Jay: Is that right?

Mary: Yes, Lord. Now they even . . . a lot of 'em know me, like I told you.

Jay: So coming back here is like . . .

Mary: That's right . . . like comin' home. Comin' home to the Lord. I like to be churchified. That's my life. That's chapter and verse.

In Her Apartment, Four Months Later

Four months after Carter's first interview at Fairhaven, she is back in her apartment, discharged from the nursing home one month earlier. Carol Ronai conducts this and the next two interviews. The second interview is adapted to reflect Carter's new circumstances and I focus here on Carter's comments about home, the nursing facility, aging, and death. Well into the interview, asked to compare living in the apartment, which is subsidized for the elderly, and living at Fairhaven, Carter remarks:

Well, I tell you, I'd rather be on this side. Out there's [Fairhaven] nice, but it is . . . you see, I got my things here. See all these here is mine. I've been here . . . pretty soon it'll be ten years. I come in here when it opened up. And the rents are not bad. It ain't but $112 a month. This is for senior citizens. They built a lot of these.

Mostly, I love church and I love music and that's my hobby. Most I like church cause sometimes I can even sing by myself. We had good church out there [Fairhaven] too.

When I was a little girl, my daddy built us a little kind of pulpit like a preacher, you know, preachin'? And we'd get out there in the playhouse, then we'd . . . the children would come up for preaching and when we'd get through preaching, why, we'd sing. We'd have out our little songbooks, you know, and my daddy said, "Look at my children." Mama . . . with long dresses she didn't care nothing about, put them on us like they was robes, you know. We had a good time, I'm telling you.

I won't recount the details of her life that Carter repeats in the second interview: The years cooking and working as a housekeeper, her marriage and long separation from her husband, her husband's funeral, her church activities. She emphasizes that she hadn't wished to remarry because, according to her, all the men left were dope addicts, noting in the process that dope traffic now makes her wary of the neighborhood. She worries for her nephew, who continues to visit her and who could get mugged anytime.

As Carter speaks of daily life, Ronai takes the opportunity to ask questions about life in general, causing Carter to recall fondly Christmas festivities at Fairhaven.

Carol: If you could live your life over, would you do anything differently?

Mary: Well, honey, I don't really believe I would. I'm very thankful and very fortunate because I know I can't live it over again. See, I'm getting older, honey. I'm not getting younger. You see, I already lived three scores in my life. I'm starting on the fourth score. I'm eighty-five and my nerves ain't bad and I have a lot to be thankful for and my speech ain't bad and I thank the Lord.

Carol: How do you explain what's happened over your life?

Mary: Well, I haven't had no bad life to live. My life is very pleasant and I learned to get along with people, like all of them people out there [Fairhaven]. We all be servin' the Lord.

We had . . . what you call a parade contest of the halls, you know, for Christmas. So Helen [social worker], out at the nursing home . . . she fixed us for her hall. She didn't fix us until, you know . . . Christmas come on, I think, a Monday. So we had a parade, you know, on Friday, on which one had the best hall. So that Friday, she come in there and asked me which dress did I want to wear. I told her I'd wear white. So I had me a new wig on and she cut some paste board and made some wings, you know, and then put that silver thinglike down there on it and tied that to the back of my chair, you know, where it comes down here.

Carol: So you had wings on the back of your chair?

Mary: Uh huh.

Carol: That's fun.

Mary: They called me the engine and then Helen, she put some little dolls on the side of my, you know, dress. Oh, she dressed me up real pretty. She didn't show off her group until they started, you know, the parade of halls. So when it got ready to go down there to see which had the best hall, they had three prizes. We won the first prize! Lord, it was funny to see me with them wings on the back of my chair and I had some gold earrings and they was showing up, you know. I was in the parade before I left to come home. It's like I was in the parade that Friday and next Monday I came home. Lord, that was fun.

At the end of the interview, Ronai and Carter talk briefly about aging, health, and death. Despite her bodily aches and pains, Carter finishes by relishing her Lord, appreciating what her apartment window reveals of His bounty.

Carol: How would you say you feel about growing old?

Mary: Well, I know I'm growing old, honey. I can tell it in my legs. I'm not as strong as I used to be.

Carol: Do you like anything about being your age?

Mary: Yes, I have to be thankful because the Lord gives life to me. He let me live all this many years.

Carol: Do you think about death at all?

Mary: I know I got to die, honey. So there's no use worrying about that. All I just want to be ready when the Lord calls me. 'Cause you know He don't notify you. It's something you got to be ready when He comes. You can't say, "Well, God, I ain't ready yet. I ain't." You can't do that. He give you all these many years to get ready.

I look out this window and look at the vision way over yonder and I say, "Lord, we got a good God. He's good to us. He give us the birds that sing and the trees for the wind and everything. He's good to us."

The Third Interview

Six months after Carter's first interview, she is interviewed a third time, once again at Fairhaven. She has given up the apartment where she lived for a decade, not able to keep up rent payments while in the nursing home. A relative is storing her furniture.

This interview, conducted by Carol Ronai, starts with a discussion of how Fairhaven compares with apartment living. Carter resists the idea that Fairhaven could be home. But as the discussion unfolds and particulars of daily life are considered, Fairhaven is cast in homelike terms and living there, as elsewhere, viewed as part of where her life ultimately "really be"—at home with the Lord.

Carol: You've been here now, off and on, for many months. How is it being here?
Mary: Oh, honey, it's nice. People are so nice to me.
Carol: That's good to hear. Do you like it out here?
Mary: Yes, I like it fine, but I like home the best.
Carol: Why do you like home the best?
Mary: Because that's where I live.
Carol: Uh huh. But could this place ever be home to you?
Mary: It'd be hard for it to be for me, to tell you the truth. I just like the old place . . . 'cause I been there nine, ten years and I haven't missed a week's rent since I been there. I'm more used to bein' in that place. Course, out here is nice too.
Carol: But you don't think it could ever be home?
Mary: Oh no. See, yonder's [her old neighborhood] where my things is at, over yonder.
Carol: If your things were here with you, would it be more like home?
Mary: I don't think so for a while. Maybe I would get used to it, but it would be hard for me. I tell you, when you get used to a place like I did before, honey, been there about goin' on pretty near ten years . . . why you, you miss the place where you at.
         But I got a friend that's got a cousin works out here [Fairhaven] and she's very nice. I got quite a few friends works out here and some cousins in housekeepin'. And I got my nephew; he's forty-three. That's my sister's baby. She's dead now. He comes by every other day. When he come, he don't come with no empty hands neither. He bring in somethin' to eat and he go to the drugstore and get my medicine and things for me. [Elaborates] He does nice things for me, but he's not too well hisself. Whenever he get ready to go, he always kisses Auntie and say, "Auntie, I'm goin'. I'll be back tomorrow." He's so sweet.
Carol: Tell me about a typical day in your life now.
Mary: Well, honey, I'm happy. That's the most of it. I'm lovin' the Lord, like always. I'm not layin' up here worried. I'm really glad to get to see every day. I gets up in the morning and puts this old wheelchair over this side and I go in the bathroom. And I go down the hall to Coffee Club and then I go play bingo.
Carol: You enjoy all that, do you?
Mary: Yes, I sure do, honey. And then I sing. I go down there when they be singin' and playin' the piano. It's a lot of things I like to do.
Carol: Your days here, are they different from your days at home?
Mary: No, they seem to be the same. Not too much different, you know. Well, I know I be growing older 'cause if I live to see the tenth of June,

I'll be eighty-six. So I know I'll be getting old. I'm beatin' on four score and almost six. [Elaborates at length]

Carol: I see what you mean. Let me ask you this, Mary. Is it hard for you to go home and come back in a nursing home and go home again and come back? Is that hard on you?

Mary: No. I done got used to things like that. I've been out here the second and third time already. I'm glad I'm like that, honey.

Carol: How's that, Mary?

Mary: I don't get myself all upset by it. I don't. I can only live one day at a time. That's all. So I'm home now, honey.

Carol: What does home mean to you?

Mary: It mean my whole life. That's what home mean. I done gotten used to bein' here. It's part of my life.

Carol: Some people talk about it as being separate and they get all depressed.

Mary: It ain't separate to me. No way, honey. You know, some people gets old and everything worries 'em. Some people, like a lady over here in that last bed, she's talking about how her children do and they won't come out here and see about her. I say, "Honey, don't worry 'bout them children." The oldest one, he come see her regular, but the other son don't come see her. She be complainin' about that. She just sit up and worry about that. I say, "You gonna stop that worryin'." I say, "You gonna have heart trouble." I say, "You can't live but one day at a time." That's what I told her. That's good advice, ain't it?

Carol: Uh huh.

Mary: Sure do. My life, just like I told you, is singing and prayin' and reading the Bible, you know, and all like that. I like that, servin' the Lord. In the morning, when I get up, I say my prayers, you know, thank the Lord for bein' livin', each and every day of my life. And that's a great release.

Carol: A release?

Mary: It's just, like in the morning you get up with a bad feelin' and you can maybe sing a song or say your prayers and everything else then just goes on. You know our God, He's almighty God. He loves all his children. He don't love one and hate the other. That's where my life really be, always bein', no matter where you is, honey, here or yonder.

Ronai and Carter cover old ground. They discuss Carter's former neighborhood, crime in the vicinity, the quality of care in the nursing home, other residents, daily activities, Carter's past, and her future. For better or worse, the quality of care, the neighborhood, and their differences pale against a horizon of otherworldly concerns. The linkages of serving the Lord overshadow everything. At one point well into the interview, when Ronai asks if Carter had the opportunity to write her life story what the various chapters would be about, Carter explains:

Most any in the Bible is great, I would say. They's my story, honey. I say all the scriptures in the Bible is good. Now I like that Psalm, say "Fret not thyself." Happiness is singin' and prayin' and thankin' the Lord for the good things He is to me, no matter what it's like here, honey, and it ain't bad. I thank God for livin' to eighty-five. They say you can't plan ahead 'cause, you know, sometimes the Lord cuts you off. That's what I heard old folks say. So it ain't good to plan too much, honey.

The Fourth Interview

The fourth and last interview is completed a year after the first one. Carter's daily life at Fairhaven continues to be one of acceptance and happiness. Her life story and its chapters have no meaning separate from biblical chapters and verses, as the following brief exchange illustrates:

Carol: Let's say you were going to write a story about your life, sorta like we did before. What kind of chapters would you have in your book, about your life? Like what would the first chapter be about?

Mary: The first chapter would be, "The Lord is my shepherd, I shall not want." And the other one is, "Jesus wept." Just all of them kind of verses, you know, is in the Bible.

Carol: Those would be in the story of your life?

Mary: Yes, it sure would. I love church. My church is Main Street Baptist Church.

Carol: What would the last chapter in the book about Mary Carter be?

Mary: Well, I used to sing in the choir. [Hums] Never was too quiet. But after I got like this, you know, I couldn't go over there much. Used to sing in them two choirs. We had three choirs. Number 1 and number 2 and number 3. Number 3 is the little children and they could sing, too.

As they discuss daily life, Carter speaks of God's kingdom, something beyond earthly possessions and desires. If she is working toward anything in this life, it is, as she puts it, that "building up there," which gives significance to the "down here." Nothing else matters.

The Lord let me come to this earth buck naked. But long they suffers for clothes and things. When they face the heavenly Savior, all He sees is you. Our whole body go in the earth and only our soul will go on up to heaven, you know. Nothing else matters. That's right. That's the truth.

Yes, honey, I want to go to heaven when I die. I want nothing down here to keep me out of heaven. They say it's a sweet place. You don't have to eat no more. You just drink honey. You eat honey and drink milk. You don't have to eat this food what we eat down here. And the Lord say they done with devils. They [devils] come to the gate and He'll push 'em back. And them that served Him, He'll let them in. So, Lord, I hope I'll be one of the ones, honey. I'm trying to work for that building up there. I go to bed praying and wake up praying, honey. The Lord, I know, has been good to me, as ill as I have been. He's been so wonderful.

* * * * *

In this secular day and age, it may be hard to imagine how the quality of life can be distanced from daily living, other than perhaps among those we label unrealistic or eccentric. Yet there are people, like Julia McCall and Mary Carter, for whom the significances of each day are suffused with meanings separated from earthly affairs. The horizon for their judgments about matters such as the quality of care and the quality of life in a nursing home is outlined in spiritual terms, for which the good and the bad in the final analysis are "all God's children" and the most trivial activity can "serve God's purpose." Such are the narrative linkages of quality for those "lovin' the Lord."

CHAPTER

6

The Vigilant

Not all residents are stoic about or orient otherworldly to the conditions of everyday life in the nursing home. Some are enduringly vigilant for infringements on their personal space by other residents or staff members. For the vigilant, it matters that people keep their places and mind their manners. Their narratives attest to "taking no lip," especially from the disrespectful.

Residents who are believed to know better but who persist in bothering others, are verbally abusive, or otherwise inconsiderate to a roommate should be physically removed from the premises. The resident who knowingly wanders into someone else's room, disturbs belongings, or pilfers cannot be tolerated. Those who don't know better should be kept under tight rein. Public spaces such as hallways, lounges, and the dining room are to be used with due regard for others' privileges and a wariness for hazards. While hallways, for example, are generally wide enough for the passage of wheelchairs in both directions, wheelchairs can be unwieldy. This is understandable and minor accidents can be rectified with an apology. But residents who carelessly careen into others and staff members who overlook the incidents are contemptible.

To the vigilant, nurses and aides should do their jobs with the utmost concern for those served, being kind and considerate in the process. The staff should promptly attend to bodily cares, see to personal needs, quickly respond to requests, and generally keep the premises clean and odor-free. The aide who openly and perfunctorily cleans a resident following a bout of incontinence, ignoring the resident's right to privacy, should not be working with frail, elderly people. Vigilant residents don't expect to be treated royally by staff members, even while some are alleged to desire that, but they clearly and forcefully do demand decency. At times, such residents wonder why they are thought to be demanding.

Vigilance is a narrative horizon girded by lifelong independence and linked to an ethic of distributive justice. A firm standard of fair treatment narratively prevails. Vigilant residents apply it to themselves, and can be excruciatingly circumspect about their own conduct, lest they carelessly overstep its bounds. From these residents, we hear mention of how they scrupulously keep to themselves, how they would never do thus and so to someone else, and what they would not say under any circumstance.

Vigilance and ethic combine to highlight the quality of care. At times, quality of care is so narratively foregrounded that the overall quality of life for these residents centers on matters such as uncooperative roommates, administrative indifference, impertinent aides, even plastic bedsheets. For some, like resident Bea Lindstrom, this is directed outward and angrily or sarcastically conveyed. For others, like resident Betty Randolph, it also is aimed inwardly and is a source of agitation.

BEA LINDSTROM

While there is a sense in which all vigilant residents "take no lip," Bea Lindstrom expresses it vigorously as she informs me and Carol Ronai of how she responds to rude and unfair treatment. Lindstrom is interviewed twice at Bayside Nursing Center, the first time five weeks after her admission and the second time six months later. She is aware of, and is frustrated by, a mild dementia, but still manages to tell it as she sees it.

The First Interview

At the first interview, Lindstrom is a soon-to-be ninety-year-old. A widowed white woman who has had a hip fracture, she spends much of her time in bed. She is a lifelong heavy drinker and smoker, which is an alleged source of her dementia.

As she tells her story, she becomes angry with her forgetfulness, the first hint of her sense of distributive justice, but, in a rare instance, turned on herself. She describes her early years in the Florida panhandle and outlines the rest of her life in terms of her husband's career. Having recently moved into the nursing home from her apartment, she expresses hope of soon returning to the apartment.

> I was born in Pensacola. I just had a normal life. Went to school. That's about it. Of course, I didn't finish school because I met my husband and we got married. But I was never sorry for anything I did.
>
> I tried to teach my children the right thing, you know. I always told them that I wouldn't spank 'em if they told me the truth. But if I caught 'em in a lie, I would . . . they'd have to pay for it. Taught them respect. I never had any trouble with my children. I had two, a boy and a girl. Yeah, my daughter lives in California. My son's in town. She has six children.

Right after we got married, my husband got a job with Pan American Airways, started flying for them. He was almost ready to quit when they were, you know, when we . . . not tables . . . [frustrated]. See how I get? A person shouldn't do that to herself! Ain't right! [Pause] Trouble. That's it. He would always keep from having trouble because he was a captain from almost the time he was hired.

He retired but he's one person that couldn't sit still after flying, you know. So he got into business, mostly making pizzas. And he did do good. He did real good. He was a man that he couldn't ask you to do it unless he did it. So he always tested his pizzas to see how they were. If they'd taste alright to him, he'd put 'em on the market. If not, he didn't. Start again.

So we went to California for a while, started a business, and did wonderful. He did that till we went back to Pensacola. Not Pensacola. Where? [Pause] Damn it! Stop it girl! What is it I want to say? [Pause] Oh . . . it was the northern part of Florida somewhere. So we stayed there until he got . . . He never smoked or drank or done nothing, but he died of cancer of the pancreas. He was fifty-two. I missed him so much. But I guess the Lord has His ways. So I couldn't do much about it.

I had lots of friends. I sold my house, which was quite large, too big for me. So I sold my house and moved into this smaller apartment. And I sorta snapped into it then, you know. If anybody needed any help, like babysitting or anything, I'd do it. I wouldn't charge them. I mean I loved it. I like doing it, being with people. I love that apartment building. I'm going back there and it's not too soon! I'm on the fourth, no, sixth floor.

We discuss life in the apartment just before she entered the nursing facility. Lindstrom recalls the home accident that caused her to be hospitalized and eventually placed at Bayside. She's sarcastically animated as she describes the course of events.

Bea: They have an alarm in the place [her apartment] so that if you get into trouble or one thing or another, you pull a string and it rings this alarm. It comes in the bathroom and in the kitchen. [Pause] No, not in the kitchen, but in the bedroom. But it doesn't come in the kitchen and doesn't come in the dining room. [Frustrated] No, there's no dining room because the dining room and the kitchen are the same.

Jay: Oh, I see, so you can eat in the kitchen.

Bea: Yeah, but that alarm system doesn't work there. It misses you in that space. Well, what happened was that I was going to cook some lunch . . .

Jay: Did you fall in the kitchen?

Bea: Did I fall? Oh did I fall! I broke two bones in my wrist and I broke two in my . . . I call it my belly. In other words, I have been broken up for about two months now. It's gettin' old. I don't like it. I don't like it at all!

Jay: Where did they take you after the fall?

Bea: Well, they took me to Crescent General Hospital first. They x-rayed me and tied me up, bundled me up and everything. After that, they said that I couldn't be left alone. They wanted to know how much beer and whiskey I drank. I said [sarcastically], "What? Can't afford it!" And I said, "Oh, Christmas I might have two or three, maybe more. That's it!"

Jay: Yeah.

Bea: But that's not going to kill anybody. It takes . . . how long does it take 'em to drink it? It don't take me long! Now my husband never did drink. He didn't smoke, but he still died of cancer. So what the hell!

As Lindstrom turns to the nursing home, her temper and vigilance loom forth to eventually present a view of the world's moral order as dog-eat-dog. According to Lindstrom, in this kind of world, fair and equitable treatment is fleeting. Yet she's not about to take it, no matter how difficult, especially not from the so-called colored people who "have a little bit too much to say." Her racism is riven with the desire to maintain personal dignity and interpersonal respect.

Jay: After you were discharged from Crescent General, what happened?

Bea: They sent me here, [whispers] with all the colored people.

Jay: I'm sorry, I can't hear you.

Bea: [Referring to the nursing staff] These colored people, you know . . . I think they have a little too much to say.

Jay: Oh?

Bea: But they don't do to me 'cause I talk back to 'em.

Jay: You do?

Bea: Yeah, I talk back to 'em. You can hear them screaming at these poor people [residents] that are halfway there and halfway gone and it's pitiful! I usually try to stay out of it. I do pretty good. One of them colored aides I had the other day and she started in on me. Yeah, she started in on me. I told her I wasn't gonna take no lip from anyone. I told her I was gonna leave. And she said, "Who would have you? Blah, blah, blah." I said, "You'd be surprised who would have me." So I told her off! And I told some of the people around me that I knew about it, you know. And they must have told her because she put her foul mouth to a close right away.

Jay: She did?

Bea: And she hasn't spoken to me now for two days. I don't care. I have a temper. I have a horrible temper when it comes to things like that. You have to in this world. It's dog eat dog. People will bite your head off if you don't watch it. You got to watch out for number one.

Jay: Uh huh.

Bea: I don't use it often, but don't knock me around. I don't mess with them and they don't mess with me. Just don't fool with me because I'll stick up for myself. Always been like that; always will be.

As Lindstrom talks of other matters, both in and out of the nursing home, she reminds me of her vigilance, the need to guard her personal space, dignity, but, equally important, her aim of not imposing on others. Referring to the many characters, called "cards," who were resident in her apartment building, she comments on how much she "loved" living there. At the same time, she never went too far with them, which she likewise expected in return. If the staff members and residents at Bayside are not characters and don't provide the enjoyment the cards did, the former are nonetheless held to the same moral standard. Referring to the nursing staff, Lindstrom explains:

> Yeah, this place is hell. Hell! 'Course, they got their ways. Like I guess they feel like that they're supposed to do what they're doing, but I think that it's a little bit rough, about orders, you know. They don't have to be that strict. 'Course they don't bother me. I mean they don't really, honestly and truly. I just keep quiet mostly and mind my own business. There's nothing else to do. If you got into it, you'd have to fight them too. As long as they let me be, I go right along. They let me be; I let them be.

The seriously guarded quality of her life doesn't overshadow its funny side. She uses a joking sarcasm to portray both her past and present, even the "hell" she purportedly now withstands. In the current situation, residents and the nursing staff are fumbling characters on a stage, rude and full of foibles. It is a narrative of "stupid" aides and "really out of it" residents who, ridiculous as they might be, had best stay in their place, if "they know what's good for 'em." Mainly, the nursing home experience is a black comedy she tries to watch from a distance, not join. Lindstrom jokes about how she maintains distance, engrossed in the quality of care.

> I wasn't really happy about moving in here. To tell the truth, there are some really nice colored people in here that are very sweet. I tease them a lot. Some of them can take it; some of them can't. They're stupid. So it doesn't take me long to discard the ones that don't like it. I leave them alone. Never play ball and have the ball bounce twice.
> But the worst is how it starts out. Like this morning when I woke up, it was terrible. No bacon with my eggs, coffee was cold, and things like that. Don't know their ass from a hole [frustrated] somewhere. And then she [roommate] has the accident [fecal incontinence] and they come and start cleaning her up 'cause she's got everything messed up. Christ! While I'm eating. It's a joke.
> You have to wait for everything. I've watched them. [Elaborates] It's a real comedy. Then they make you sit, you know. Breakfast, they bring that to you. Then they give you a bath. You've had a bath already, but you take another one. Well, I says like where Clark Gable says, "Frankly, I don't give a damn." Stay clear. You know what I'm talking about? [I nod] But I want to be treated fair and square.
> I don't want to be too friendly with any of them, 'cause they can get right

under your feet, you know what I mean? I just can't help being sympathetic sometimes, but that's when you can get yourself into it. Some of them [residents] are pitiful. But, more or less, I stay to myself. If they got over-friendly, it wouldn't take me long to get rid of it. [Laughing] I play a kind of trick on 'em. I learn their goofy footsteps and things like that and when they come around, I pretend I'm sleeping [feigns snoring], like that. Then they don't bother you. I do the same with them dumb nurses.

Yeah, it's really a joke around here, like a carnival sometimes. You got people here that eat lunch and they got their food up here [points to her hair]. Some of them, you know, go around with their mouths [makes grunting noises]. They can't help it, but they are living here. You got one fellow whose got a pair of shoes and he'll take his chair and rag and a hankie, whatever he's got, and go around and wipe his shoes on it. You should see these clowns. And we got this woman . . . she goes around like she is going to cry and there's a fellow who picks on her. You have to watch him because he knocks her around.

It's a joke, really. You kinda watch it go on but I don't get involved. Best that way. It can be really funny. But, like I said, I don't let any of 'em mess with me, if they know what's good for 'em.

Six Months Later

Ronai reinterviews Lindstrom at Bayside six months later. Much of the discussion is again taken up with Lindstrom's life story—growing up in the Florida panhandle, the husband's career as a pilot, his death, and events in her son's and daughter's lives. The story is brought up to date when Ronai asks Lindstrom what life looks like from where she is at now and to describe a typical day.

Bea: Well, you wanna get it in plain English?
Carol: Plain English.
Bea: Like hell!
Carol: Why do you say that?
Bea: I don't like it here. I hate it. If I could get out tonight, I'd get out. I told one of the girls [aide], I said, "I'm tempted to just get out myself, get a taxi, and go home." She said, "Oh, I wouldn't do that." I said, "Why not?" She says, "They might call the cops for ya." So she scared me there. But that's it, honey. I'm tied down.
Carol: Let me ask you this, Bea. Describe for me a typical day in your life now.
Bea: I barely ever get out of this hole. I'd be so happy if I could. [Pause] I'll tell you how it is. They wake ya up. You run to the john. That's how it is. And then you get dressed and you go, you go for breakfast. It's not too bad, but it's the same thing every morning. No kidding, it is. Scrambled eggs. So you're not interested in that. But, anyway, there's coffee. And that's it. Ain't no home.

Living here is a rough one. Ya got so many bosses here. I don't like bein' bossed. And I don't have anything to be against the blacks, but some of them are a little bit tough. But I hold my own. I don't take it. Always did.

So that's my story. Like I said, this ain't home. It'd never make it. I don't know . . . too many bosses I guess, and the food, well, you know what I mean. They come in at night and want you to go to bed and you're not sleepy. I won't do it! I'm not going to sleep because they want me to. It's my life too! [Pause] I'm a hellcat!

Violations of her independence are as much the expressed cause of Lindstrom's negative feelings as her engrossment with shortcomings in the quality of care. Lindstrom calls Bayside a jail. She resents the condition of her room and shows Ronai how even the bedding is an imposition on her sensibilities. She informs Ronai that happiness is being independent, respecting others' rights as others respect one's own, bringing Lindstrom back to sentiments expressed six months earlier.

Bea: Well I certainly don't claim this here to be part of my life. I don't claim it at all.

Carol: Why do you say it's separate, that it's not part of your life?

Bea: Honey, I just don't like it. If I could do what I wanted to do and go and come when I wanted to. I don't like to be lost, like I can't handle things. Sure, I would do what my husband would ask me to do. And he would do what I asked him to do, but we didn't *tell* one another they *had* to do it. I think that's the way it should be. And, honey, it sure ain't that way here. Every Tom, Dick, and Harry's always interferin' in your stuff.

They brought me in on a slab in this place. If I had known what I know now, honey, they'd never got me one foot in. This doctor here, I don't think he knows his beans.

Like I say, I don't like this place. I want to get out and if I could get out, I'd go. I won't be happy here. I just like . . . I feel like I'm in jail.

Carol: I've heard other people say that.

Bea: Yeah, even the bed. [Strokes her bed] Run your hand over that.

Carol: [Feeling the bedding] Plastic-feeling, not too comfortable.

Bea: [Sarcastically] I'm not gonna pee in a bed!

Carol: I guess some of them do.

Bea: Well, honey, I ain't some of them! They don't remember that, honey. I asked them to take this thing [plastic sheet] out.

Carol: They won't do it?

Bea: They won't do it! And it makes me mad as a hellcat. They got no respect for no one. Ya have to keep an eye on 'em day and night. [Pause] Oh, hell, I'm just getting ugly and decapitated [sic].

Carol: Decapitated?

Bea: Oh, I don't know how to describe it. Like I say, I'm not happy here.

Never will be. You have to keep an eye on 'em all the time. The treatment stinks. I've seen it all. If I could get back down there where I lived, honey, you couldn't drive me out. See, they didn't ask me to come here. They took me from the hospital, see, and they put me on a slab and brought me.

Carol: So, Bea, what's important to you?

Bea: Oh, bein' happy. Doin' what you wanna do. Respect. I've got a mind of all the things I wanna do. That's what I wanna do and I don't like to be told how to do things and things.

A place like this, honey, ain't good for an old lady like me. We don't like no one mussin' with us. We keep to ourselves.

BETTY RANDOLPH

Betty Randolph, another vigilant resident, is a seventy-one-year-old white female who suffers from innumerable problems of aging. Among other things, she has cardiovascular blockage, osteoporosis, arthritis, and has had a hip replacement. Joint degeneration has caused her to have knee and shoulder fusions. She is interviewed twice by Ronai.

Randolph keeps watch for infringements on her dignity. In turn, she is careful not to impose on others, sometimes to a fault. Just as she would expect others to be angry with her if she showed little regard for them as persons, Randolph is not about to take lip from those who are disrespectful to her. Trying as Randolph does to make things right according to her acute sense of fair play, she does not let things get out of hand. All of this admittedly makes her nervous.

For Randolph, the quality of care is a mark of the effectiveness of her personal ethic: Mutual kindness and respect results in good care. She makes certain that she is kind and polite to others, especially staff members, in the hope that, assuming they are equally bound by the same ethic, they will be kind and polite in return. This is highlighted in Randolph's second interview, conducted after Randolph has been discharged from her nursing home and placed in a small board-and-care facility.

The First Interview

Randolph's first interview takes place five months after she is admitted to the Greenfield Home, a skilled-care facility. Before that, she resided for about a year in another nursing home. Randolph begins the interview with a description of her harsh life growing up with alcoholic parents, then spent briefly with a husband, but mainly on her own. As we will learn later in the interview, Randolph is, according to her, a lifelong loner.

My father drank, my mother drank, and I was always left home to take care of my stepsisters and that. Actually, I don't even know who my father was, because my mother had been married three times. So I just don't know.

But the best time in my life is when I got married. My husband was a fine man. I lost him too quick. We were married five years when he walked out and dropped dead. They said he had a coronary and there was nothing they could do for him. He was dead when they got to him.

But if I had the five years that I had with him . . . if I had to do it over, I'd be grateful for every minute of it. He was kind, he was understanding, and my whole life was his. Of course, then we were in Arizona. He wanted to come back, but we didn't want to come back to New York. That's where I was born and raised and he was. But we didn't want to and so we stayed in Orlando. He got a job in the hospital working as an orderly because he had come out of the service and he had been in the service quite a while and he just didn't want to . . . he wasn't the type that could stay home and do nothing. He had to work no matter what it was. So that's when he took the job. We came back [to Florida] in March, I mean, in January and he dropped dead March 12, 1956. It's like I said, he was the best man in the world.

After that, I had a nervous breakdown. Then I was on my own. I came up to the northern part of Florida and I lived there for seventeen years. I worked in a nursing home there and I stayed there, yeah, for seventeen years.

But I've had a hard life. When my mother drank . . . she got married to this man and they both . . . she never drank until she married the third one. Really, they really went at it. I used to have to go out at night in New York City when I was about twelve or thirteen and bring 'em home out of bar-rooms so they wouldn't get arrested. And then I had to be with my two half-sisters to take care of them all day and night. I was a hard life and I very seldom talk about it because it's like I said, a lot of times I think that I could've had a better life, but I didn't.

The conversation turns in various directions. At one point, Randolph angrily comments on the friends she believed she had in one of the places she lived. They were friends until they became unjustifiably cruel to her. As Randolph notes, "Friends can cut your throat." Paraphrasing a common cliche, she adds, "With such friends who needs enemies?" She speaks of the vigilance needed in life when no one, not even friends, can be trusted. Ronai asks Randolph what life looks like from where Randolph is now. Randolph takes the opportunity to describe herself, putting independence and sentiments of distributive justice at center stage.

It's like this. If a year ago anybody told me I'd be in this shape, I'd have said they're crazy. Of course, I'm an independent person. I'm used to doing things for myself. I don't want nobody to wait on me. And this is the way I am. But I can't make people understand that. When you take care of yourself since you've been fifteen years old . . . I've worked and I've never asked anybody for nothing. Even when my husband was living, he knew I was independent. That's the way he did what he had to do; he never told me what to do. [Elaborates] You put yourself in my place, that you're knocked down like this in this place. It's an awful hard way to go for someone like me. It's really hard. It's like I said, a year ago, if anybody told me this would have happened, I couldn't believe it and I wouldn't believe it.

These people here don't understand me. They think I'm throwing a tantrum. It isn't I'm throwin' a tantrum. I'm just taking care of myself and I'm doing it for myself. What's mine's mine and what's theirs is theirs. Fair's fair, I always say.

It was just this morning. I didn't know she was an RN. She was walking around in street clothes and sittin' behind the desk. I didn't know she was an RN and I just said I would not take any medicine from somebody I didn't know. Would I expect any different if I was in her shoes? No. I didn't know she was an RN till they told me. It's because I had that happen to me one time. I was given the wrong medicine one time. So you can see where I'm coming from. You have to be on the lookout all the time. You don't know if she's an RN or not. What she wore behind that desk could have been the secretary there. How did I know?

Linked with Randolph's guardedness is the view that interpersonal respect has "gone to hell in a handbasket." A lengthy exchange with Ronai conveys particulars, as well as Randolph's admitted racism. Randolph speaks of letting Josephine, a "colored" resident, "have it" because neither Josephine nor the "colored girls" on the nursing staff, who allow Josephine to wander about, show respect for others.

Carol: Before you came to live in a nursing home, what did you think it would be like?

Betty: I didn't think it'd be like this. I really didn't. I can't complain much about some of the people here. The dietician, Karen, and the other ones are good to me. The nurses are good to me. There's only, maybe one or two, like the one [resident] out there this morning . . . Boy, I let her have it. I've just had enough of her foolishness and I let her have it. I don't like doing it because it makes me nervous. But, sometimes, I don't know, maybe I'm thinking wrong, but the colored people come in and they take over things. Ya might say the world's gone to hell in a handbasket.

Carol: What do you mean, Mrs. R?

Betty: Well, I just seen that they think they're better than we are, some of them. It's just like that colored woman that I had the fight with this morning—Virginia. I was sitting out there. I got a $900 chair sitting over there [in the corner of Randolph's room] that's mine and she walks around and she's all wet. And she'll walk in here to go sit down in that chair and I don't want her in that chair. I have the right; it's mine. No, but with her I didn't have the right. She said I don't.

Look, I know she don't know any better, but when they see her going in and out of all these rooms, why don't they get up and go get her and take her back to where she belongs? But, no, those colored girls [staff] just sit there and let her do it. Like I went out to the doctor last Tuesday, I come home, and she was in my bed, all wet. Boy did I get the nurse to get her out. She was in my bed and I said to the nurse . . . went down and got the nurse and asked to please come and get her out of my bed. The nurse come up and I said, "I want some clean sheets on my bed. I'm not gonna sleep there." She said, "Oh that won't hurt you." I'm a particular person; that's my problem.

Carol: I guess I wouldn't want to sleep in a bed like that either.

Betty: Even with my clothes, if you go look at my closet over there, I keep all my slacks in one, my skirts in the next, and my jackets in the back. That's the way I've lived. Anybody knows me could tell you that they could walk in my house any time of the day or night and my house was . . . you could eat off the floors.

But this is what bothers me. This one here [Virginia], she roams all day. There's another one that roams that can't . . . he hit me the other day in my knee.

Carol: He hit you?

Betty: He backed his wheelchair up into me. They didn't say anything about it. And they know that was my bad leg that he had hit.

It's like I said. Some of these here, you could bend over backwards, honey, and you couldn't get along with some of these patients. I had one this morning—it really got to me—I was trying to turn my wheelchair out to get to the table. She comes along and says to me, "Get out of my way!" I said, "Wait a minute." I said, "I'm just trying to get to the table." So she yells, "Well get out of my way!" And that's just how a lot of them are here and I'm not about to take that from no one. So I gave it right back to her. [Elaborates]

Randolph worries about having to openly contend with injustice. She initially attributes her feeling to growing old, but then ties it to her ethic of interpersonal respect. In the process, Greenfield's quality of care is cast in terms of the ethical view and its place in Randolph's life noted.

Betty: I guess it's getting old and getting . . . you get agitated about a lot of things maybe when I shouldn't.

Carol: What would be a little thing that you get agitated about that you think you shouldn't?

Betty: Well, I know I shouldn't get agitated about . . . like I said, these two that roam all day. But I told them [the staff] that it's got to be a halt brought to it. They [the two roamers] belong over on Station 2. That's where they should be kept, not roaming around. It makes me nervous to get involved in things like this, but like I said, too, it's only right.

Last year, I was down in [another] nursing home and that is a fabulous nursing home. There were patients there like these that roam, but they were kept over on the other side. They weren't allowed over where the patients could get around and that. They weren't allowed over there in the other patients' rooms. But here, there's no due restriction. They let them do what they want and it's not right.

Carol: And that makes you feel . . .

Betty: Worried. I worry knowing that I have to stay here and have to yell at them about it. That's part of the problem I guess. Not that it's all that bad. It's that I'm the kind of person that stays to herself and doesn't interfere. I'm a loner. A place like this . . . well, it makes a difference for someone like me. You start thinking about the treatment and all, like it's no good if I have to yell all the time.

Six Months Later

Six months later, Randolph has been discharged from Greenfield and lives in a small board-and-care home called Miss Palmer's. Randolph's fastidiousness and acute sense of interpersonal justice continue paramount and are linked with nervousness. At one point, it appears that no congregate living setting, neither a nursing nor a personal care home, could accommodate Randolph's view to life.

Carol: And they call this an adult congregate living facility, kind of board-and-care. How do you feel about being here?

Betty: Well, some ways it's alright and other ways it's not.

Carol: Oh?

Betty: This one down here, the one in the kitchen [Miss Palmer], it seems every time I say something I'm wrong. That I don't understand, because I never had this problem at Greenfield.

Carol: I'm not sure I know what you mean.

Betty: It seems that, you know . . . See I've had a problem with phlebitis over a year now and I don't have any family or anybody to take me anywhere. When I came out of the hospital, the doctor suggested that I should have my blood done every week because I'm on a strong drug, Coumadin, and it's dangerous, so she [Miss Palmer] should take me to the lab. Well she didn't take me yesterday like she said she would. Says she's got other things to do. If I had known she didn't want to take me, I would have called Medicoach and that. But she offered herself to take me. So that's what I expected her to do, or don't offer. Right? A promise is a promise.

It seems that all the time around here, no matter where I turn or something, I'm always wrong. I try not to bother anyone. That's how I am. I do something, I'm wrong. I get jumped on for something and that, and I'm getting a little tired of it now and it makes me nervous.

Carol: Would you rather be back at Greenfield or just out of here?

Betty: Well, I've tried, honey. I try to cope with it because, it's like I said, I
           don't have any family to stick up for me. So maybe the reason why
           they keep at me is because I don't have people to come in to see me.
Carol: Oh I see.
Betty: And they know I don't have anybody. So they figure they can pick at
           me and stuff. There's nobody I can tell.
Carol: That's sad. Have you talked to Miss Palmer about it?
Betty: Doesn't do any good. She won't listen to you. She just has her favor-
           ites. She has about four or five favorites and they can do no wrong.
           But everybody else is wrong.
Carol: You don't have anyone here you're close to?
Betty: No. I don't bother with none of them. I don't bother with none of
           them around here.
Carol: Okay.
Betty: And that one you see walking now [a resident]? She can go around
           and slap everybody and nothing's done about it. She threatened the
           other day to slap me and I said if she hit me, I'd knock her screw off. It
           just seems that it's always something that's wrong. It's not right. I try
           to be fair, really. I want 'em to be fair with me, too. When I said
           something to Miss Palmer this morning coming back from the lab, I
           said, "I'm sorry I caused you so much trouble." I said, "I didn't ask
           you to take me." She said, "Why don't you shut up and stop letting
           little things bother you."

           I've worked all my life. I've taken care of myself. I never thought
           that I'd be in a position like this. If I had known it would come to this,
           I don't know what I'd a done. But when you got to live like this, it's
           not good. Maybe it's really not good nowhere.
Carol: What kinds of things would you want that you're not getting?
Betty: I like to go out. I like to go out even if I don't have the money to go
           shopping. I just like to go shopping. Here, I don't have anybody to
           take me to the stores.

           I like a place where I have my own things, where I can do what I want
           to do and nobody's on me. I get up when I want to. I go to bed when I
           want to and that. I've done that ever since I was fifteen years old.

           My parents died and I had nobody. I had to learn to do it. I had to
           learn to go to work. I can go back to the time that I lived in New York.
           I was born and raised there. When my mother died, I was living in
           Massachusetts. After she passed away, my father passed away. I was
           fifteen years old. What was I going to do? I had to think. So I got a
           furnished room, paid $14 every two weeks for it. I worked in a laun-
           dry putting sheets through the iron for $56 and I paid my room rent
           out of that, bought my clothes, I ate, and I been doing that ever since.

           I can handle money. It's like when I used to live in the apartment, I
           used to buy my groceries. I knew how to handle it because I'd figure
           out that I buy my groceries for the month and you come to my house
           and the freezer would always be full. My icebox was never empty.
           Because I kept a system. I paid my bills first. I paid my rent first, my

light bills first, my water bill, my telephone bill, and after my bills was paid, then I bought my groceries.

I always kept a nice home. Anybody would tell you that. They'd tell you I kept a clean house. I was always cleaning my apartment. Then when I got sick, it seemed everything fell apart. See, I have osteoporosis, which is a bone disease. I have ulcers. I have a bad heart, too. So, like I said, it isn't good for me to be living alone and that. I don't know how much more of this I can take.

I wouldn't live this kind of life if I could help it, nowhere. I'm a person . . . I don't talk much and I don't have much to say to nobody. I've always been a loner and that's the way I've been. And I've been that way since I had to live by myself all my life.

You can see the point where I'm coming from. If I say something, I'm jumped on right away. If I don't talk, I'm mad. If I say something, I'm looking for an argument. So which way do you go? There's no crossroads.

Carol: You're saying it's a no-win situation because of, well, who you are and what others are like.

Betty: Like I said, I've lived all my life as a loner because I've lived alone and I've done what I wanted and I had no bosses. There was nobody to tell me to go to bed at this time or nobody to tell me when I could get up or nobody to tell me what I've got to eat. If I don't want to eat, I'm not going to have someone say that you've got to eat.

People don't realize that when you've come up the hard way, it's really rough. You learn that you have to fight your way to get along in this world. This is about . . . seems about all I've done. I try to get along with people and all I hear is an attitude problem. I've got an attitude problem. If people would try to understand me, it would be different. I don't want to bother them and I don't want 'em on me either. But they don't try to understand me. And it's really hard when you try to make somebody understand you and try to explain, they think you're mad. [They'll say,] "Go sit down!" It's not fair.

* * * * *

For these residents, being independent combines with an ethic of distributive justice to make the quality of care an all-consuming matter. The quality of their lives virtually revolves around the quality of their care. Their narratives are filled with judgments about how staff members should behave but don't and how certain residents should act but rarely do. According to such residents, if the world were fundamentally different or had not "gone to hell," vigilance would not be necessary. As it is in a dog-eat-dog world, being vigilant is the only recourse, the only means of assuring a modicum of respect. Such are the narrative linkages of vigilance, interpersonally difficult at best and anxiety-provoking at worst.

SPECIAL CIRCUMSTANCES

CHAPTER

7

Travelers

We turn now to residents whose special circumstances offer horizons of their own for subjective meaning. The two residents of this chapter— Jake Bellows and Peter Rinehart—were itinerant travelers, one in show business and the other in sales. To paraphrase one of them, they did a "lot of livin'" on the road and have stories to tell about it. For them, home was a place experienced as a break from life on the road. Home was time out from the usual and customary. These men *went home* for vacation; they didn't leave it.

Bellows and Rinehart accept the nursing home as a place offering care, security, and shelter for the weary, who might not otherwise be able to carry on. It isn't home, but under the circumstances the next best thing to it. Indeed, care apparatus and sickness aside, for traveling men like themselves, the nursing home is a kind of hotel, having both the best and worse features of such establishments. As they see it, residents more or less get fed, have a bed to sleep in, and get their cares attended, but understandably not to everyone's satisfaction.

For Bellows and Rinehart, destiny isn't so much puzzling or decried as it is something that, like life on the road, one follows. They refer to fate in phrases such as "c'est la vie," "things just happen," "goin' where the road takes you," "so be it," and "easy come, easy go." While the men describe the many paths their lives took, the so-called ups and downs of the years, and the good and poor choices they made at various turns, they recognize that such matters are part of the design of living. They don't lament fate; it's just there, the essential "road" ahead.

For them, life does come to an end. Ends being what they are, they are filled with bitter, if not sweet, moments. The men don't turn to religion for answers to why things come to this, nor do they pray to God to intervene on their behalf. They are not especially religious and speak with skepticism about those who are. They scoff at the thought that, if there were a God, He or She would deign to indulge the desire for divine intervention to prolong life or make substantial changes in it.

Yet they take pride in the quality of their lives and what they have accomplished, which are not defined by their present circumstances. While it wouldn't be correct to describe them as awed by fate, they appreciate what fate has brought, both the easy triumphs that have come by and the hard lessons they've learned along the way. As Bellows and Rinehart remind us, such is life.

JAKE BELLOWS

Jake Bellows is a seventy-six-year-old widowed white male who has lived six months at the Greenfield Nursing Home. For years, he has been afflicted by what he calls a "vascular condition," which has cost him his left leg. In the last few years he was in and out of the hospital for other health problems. Two sisters, a brother, and a son live some two hours away by car. They visit him regularly, about every month or so, which according to Bellows suits him fine.

Except for service in the army during World War II, Bellows has spent his adult life in show business. He has little formal education, but is proud of being self-taught and having parlayed good writing skills, incentive, and inventiveness into profitable "gigs." More than for any resident interviewed, Bellows's life is a collection of stories, in his case centered on the stage, the experiences of which he enthusiastically recounts. He begins with his education.

> I went to, uh . . . I have a three-year college, what do you call it? [Audibly sorts his thoughts] The equivalency of two years of college. I didn't go to college and I didn't go to high school. I had to stay home, but I taught myself. I learned correspondence courses, stuff like that at home. I learned myself. I taught myself how to become . . . I was a public speaker and writer. [Laughs] So I'm not a stupid bastard, you know. I learned a little bit while I was at it.
>
> Mainly I was into acting and music. I was a musician and master of ceremonies at night clubs and theaters and so forth. And writin' scripts and writin' plays. I've done it all. Everything. I wound up with a little bit of money and I retired and quit. It's all spent and gone now. I'm a veteran.

I ask Bellows about childhood, which turns out to be a version of the story of how he got into show business. The story begins, jokingly, in south Georgia.

> I was born in south Georgia. [Laughing] I couldn't help that. My daddy was a rather successful farmer. I was born on a farm in Nelling County, Georgia. Then we moved to Maple County and he went into public work there. I started school there. In 1924, we moved to Tampa, Florida. Daddy was in

the construction business there as a carpenter, a good one, and he did all right at that.

So I went to school till the fifth grade and quit 'cause there was . . . we had too many kids. I had five sisters and a brother. So I had to, you know . . . my daddy became sick, so I had to help support the kids. So I cut my formal education short and I taught myself. I guess that's how you say it—educated myself by reading books and other people's schoolwork, stuff like that.

To make a long story short, in time that got me into show business. I learned to play the guitar. After that, I remained in strict show business from then on and graduated up the scale to producer and so forth, right on up the scale. I had an act that I did in a night club that was seen all over the country, on the road most of the time. I worked in five pictures and a lot of production, lots of dramatics and stuff like that, all the way up and down. I think that about covers it.

When I ask him what it was like doing that kind of work, he lights up and relishes telling me about his accomplishments and his acquaintances. As he notes how much he once earned, he remarks "easy come, easy go," which is his first mention of a sense of destiny.

I wouldn't do anything else! If I had my life to live over, I'd do the same thing again. Well, I'd try to make it a little more fruitful, you know, moneywise. But I had fun. I loved it. I loved every minute of it and I met some nice people on the way up. It kept me on the way up like I was a star. I never was a real featured star. I was pretty well known, but not great big. I worked in five pictures. [Pauses] Oh, I told you that. So I got up there on a totem pole a little bit. I was pretty well known as an actor on the stage. As a movie actor, I was just mediocre, you know.

I played everywhere. Every city in the union besides Las Vegas. I never played Vegas, but everywhere else. I didn't play Alaska, but I did play Hawaii. I never went to Alaska but I wanted to so bad. The main thing was money. Alaska paid big, big money way back near the depression, I mean near the sixties. I had a chance to go and I coulda got a thousand a week like nothing flat. I was working for $500 up back then. That was big time considering the salaries of some of them was $200, $125, $150. My wife and I worked as an act for almost nine years and we were making upwards of, well, an average of a thousand a week, for about seven years of it traveling all over the United States, everywhere.

We spent as much as we made, of course, but we lived. We lived high on the hog. We spent high on the hog. We'd tell people, "What the hell, why not?" you know. Easy come, easy go.

That's about the size of my career. What else? [Pauses] Let's see. Of course I'm an artist. I paint and of course I'm a writer. I've sold a few things. I've got a lot of manuscripts to prove it . . . I mean rejection slips to prove it. I'm not a very successful writer, but you know how when you write something you know it's good or you wouldn't have written it? Some of the ones that I think are the very best pieces were rejected and didn't sell. Some of the little things I'd write and say to myself, "Oh well, I'll send it in anyway." They'd sell! I can never understand it. Nobody else can. Things just happen, I guess. Some of the greatest writers in the world have written the same thing I'm saying. They couldn't understand why the stuff they thought was so good came back with rejection slips and stuff they didn't think much of sold. C'est la vie.

Life was not all onward and upward for Bellows. He was especially annoyed by rude changes in entertainment. The night club acts in which he worked a good part of his adult life as producer, stand-up comic, or general entertainer, grew into striptease shows. As he looks back, he takes pride in what he accomplished despite the changes. A comedy act he developed is particularly noteworthy, a story in its own right, which turns into yet another story of appreciation for his work.

I was in show business until '72 and I quit. I just got so . . . the nightclub business had run down into striptease joints. That's what it amounted to. I just got sick of them. I wasn't around actors and show people. I was around scum of the earth, low class. I couldn't stand it, so I quit. I sat home and did writing and put in an occasional club date once in a while. But something like that, that's a different thing.

Mainly, I did solo work. I'm an artist. I paint pictures. My impression book isn't here; I wish I had it here to show you. You'd see all the things I've done without me having to talk about it. When I talk about it, it sounds like I'm bragging, but I'm not! I played a lot of gigs, big times. Like one time I did speed painting in oil on stage and talked comedy. Talk was all I was doin'. I could paint a picture in two minutes, two feet by three feet in two minutes. Used great big house painting brushes and the pictures turned out very nice in oil paintings. I just learned how to put the paint where it's supposed to go and make it look good, you know.

At the beginning of the act, I got all my stuff, my equipment and easel there on the stage. I talked to them [the audience] and cracked gags all the time, and the orchestra's sitting there in the background. I'd try to get funny there for a little while and talked to them all to get acquainted, you know. It was a comedy act—the buildup, the preparation to get into the act was comedy. I talked to them to keep 'em laughing. I said, "Now name a song that depicts a scene of some kind of springtime in the Rockies or the moon over Miami or whatever you can think of. Pick a scene of some kind." While the orchestra played the chorus of the song, I painted for them on this canvas. So, like, they named Blue Hawaii or something out there and I'd say, "Okay, boys, play it" and I'd start painting. By the time they played two chords of the song, the picture was done. So I'd turn around, hold it up this way and that way, and I'd get a hell of a hand because it turned out to be a damned good picture.

A lot of 'em seen it all over the country. We played up in Alberta, Canada, and right after that I went into a barber shop and got a haircut, see. This guy kept looking at me and looking at me and said, "I think I know you from someplace. You look so familiar." I said, "Well, I'm an actor. You probably seen me on stage." [He said], "Ah, that's what it is! I saw you working in Miami, Florida." We were conversing back and forth and he said, "I've got something to show you. I want you to come home to dinner with me tonight. Will you go? Are you too busy?" I said, "No, I'm not doing anything." So he called his wife and told her that he was going to bring a guest home, a little surprise. So I knew that he was going to tell his wife that he had Jake Bellows that he saw in Miami. I figured that was it. I walked through the door. I'm cutting the story down so I won't bore you. We walked in his house and there on the wall was one of my canvases I done in an act in Miami! I said, "That was one of my pictures out of the act." That was pretty nice.

Things like that happened to me all up and down the road. I wrote for a lot of people in show business and they've become big stuff, you know, through the years. Some of them have turned out to be drunks and everything else. A few of them made it big.

But it was up and down, goin' where the road takes you. One week here, two weeks there . . . What the hell am I trying to say? A few weeks out of the year, we'd sit there. I'd have three months of excellent work, play the highest-rated night clubs, theaters, or whatever. The rest of the time in plain toilets used for low class. Well, I had to work. I couldn't just quit and sit on my butt just because I didn't want to play that place. I had to play, had to make money, you know. So it's been up and down for me all my life in show business. Most every actor will tell you about the same thing. Such is life.

As we continue to talk about show business, Bellows describes his acquaintance with various celebrities. He takes special pride in having worked with George Burns and Gracie Allen's vaudeville act. But the happiest time of his life was his association with the Marcus show, a touring company. He beams as he recalls those years.

That was the happiest time of my life. It was a big company of sixty people. A.B. Marcus. Man, that was big time. They played all over the world, everywhere. I didn't go with them on all the tours. I didn't go overseas with them at all. I worked with them in the States. But, boy, that was a show! Some of the greatest actors in show business started out in the Marcus show. I didn't start out with them but I was with them for a while. That was the highlight of my show business . . . and, of course, the picture work I did later.

Just as the ups and downs of show business are accepted as part of life, the current situation marking the end of his life is taken as meant to be and accepted. Yet show business is still in his blood.

But it's finished. I don't have anything to look forward to in show business. I'd like to write about it, talk about it, remember a lot of the things about it, but there is nothing to go back to anymore. At my age, I can't. I could do a couple of pictures sitting in a chair. I can work in front of a camera, act, sit in a chair, sort of like seeing a cripple still be a performer that way. But as far as walking onto a stage again and being a comic like I used to be, I can't stand up.

It's the last chapter in the last story. The end of the road. I think that's the way to say it. C'est la vie. So be it. I don't know how else to express it. I'm on my last legs and know it and don't care. I'm an atheist. In other words, I got brains. I have no fear of death. I'm not religious at all. No superstition. I'm happy the way I'm going out. I like to entertain people. If I could find the right kind of situation or audience so I could work without having to walk on stage, I could still do a painting act.

A long and checkered career in show business, especially life on the road, colors Bellows's talk of home, casting his sense of the nursing home's quality of care in related terms. Being on the road nearly fifty weeks a year meant home was less a natural anchor than it was a place to forget show business for a while. Taking a vacation meant *going* home, not getting away from home, as the following extract indicates.

Jay: Let me ask you something a little different. We haven't talked very much about home. What would you say the word *home* means to you, Jake?

Jake: I tell ya, Jay . . . it used to mean, well, it meant I quit for the season. I took a two-week vacation and I went back home to Millsburg. That was home. Otherwise, leave the house locked up, let someone I knew very well take care of it for me, and then we'd hit the road.

Jay: You say *we'd* hit the road?

Jake: I was talking about my wife Rose. When we were doing our mind reading act, a mental act . . . we did a mind reading act together. You've seen those things I imagine?

Jay: Yeah, I've seen a bunch of those. They're funny. [Elaborates] So Rose went with you most of those places?

Jake: Oh yeah. She was one of the greatest acts, mental acts I've ever seen. But the wife turned out to be a drunk and it got worse. I couldn't depend on her. She'd louse up, get drunk and louse up the show. So I finally had to . . . well, she was absolutely finished by the time we tried to get some help. The doctor said she was finished, like a vegetable. Liquor got her, just deteriorated her brain. Then I heard she was dead. I didn't even go to the funeral. I was on the road.

Jay: How long were you married to her?

Jake: Twelve years. No kids by her. I was married five times. The first wife, Edith, was okay. She was the only *lady* I was ever married to. The rest of them were bitches. It's like any other show business.

Jay: So home life stayed pretty much the same over the years?

Jake: Home . . . yeah, it's been about the same. It's a place to go back to and forget show business, forget everything, just sit down and relax and enjoy the distance. Home's about the same now as it's always been.

We talk about the nursing home, which Bellows doesn't feel is quite home. It's not that he wishes to go home because the nursing home is so different as a source of shelter and comfort from the family home in Millsburg. Rather, compared with "home," Bellows feels Greenfield does not provide enough in the way of time to relax, gab, and enjoy the distance, as he had put it, what home did for him two weeks a year. Greenfield is more like a stop along the way. Bellows explains:

When I came here, the bottom dropped out because there are very few people in here besides the help that are intelligent. The rest of them have lost their minds through the years or didn't have it in the first place. Just one of those things, you know. The help here is all right. They are all intelligent people. You can gab with 'em and sorta relax that way. But you don't have much time with people who work. The nurses and the other help, they're busy. Got a hotel to run. They've got something else to do. [Points to another resident] There's old man Dewey. And up here's old man Smith and me. Usually in the daytime when you see one, you see all three of us sittin' there together, all around together, pretty close together, gabbing. These guys . . . just another place down the road, sittin' around and chewin' the fat.

At the end of the interview, Bellows speaks of the course of life in general. He comments on the virtues of smoking marijuana and offers a friendly diatribe against religion. He discloses how, after all is said and done, fate, not this or that decision or condition, made life what it was for him, "always has."

I have never taken a dishonest nickel in my life. I've never been a crook in any form. I've tried to live a good, clean life, which I didn't completely. I smoked pot, which I dearly enjoyed. I'd enjoy it now. If I had some, I'd smoke it now and I don't give a damn who knows it. I like it, I smoke it, and it didn't hurt me none. If I had some, I'd smoke it right here and now. Of course, music has been a big part of my life. Religion is an absolutely disgusting subject to me. I don't even like to discuss it.

Like life's got some purpose or something? Hell! Things just happen. Things that come up in your life happen that way. The way the card bounces. I mean the way the cards fall or whatever the word is. The way the cookie crumbles. Whatever the hell. No, life don't turn out any particular way. Like I'm in this here joint. Life is like unrolling a tape. You don't know what's there until you unroll it. Some people told me that life is already there and you just have to live what it is. As it unrolls, you just live it. As you think back over your life, you didn't exactly plan anything that you did. It just happens that it was convenient to do at the time and you did it. That's the way it was with me. All my life I'd . . . a lot of times I'd plan on doing something and I wanted to do it and that wouldn't turn out at all. I'd do something exactly backwards before I attended to something. Well, maybe not that bad, but relative to it, but not the same thing. So, you can't . . . you don't judge yourself. You just go where life takes you and life does take you. You don't take life anywhere. It takes you.

There's not much to think about. You live your life, do the best you can at the moment. Whatever you do at that particular time is what you have to do. At the moment, it happens you got to do that, not something else. I know that circumstances ruled my life, not exactly what I wanted, but circumstances. Surrounding circumstances forced me to do exactly what I did. Every bit of it. Sometimes I wish I could have done better and made a lot more money than I did. But it didn't work out that way.

PETER RINEHART

Peter Rinehart also spent much of his adult life on the road, mainly selling Oster products. He took his wife along with him, a house trailer hitched to the back of their van. Like Jake Bellows, home for Rinehart was not a home base but time out from the usual and customary.

Fate presents itself clearly in Rinehart's life. At one point in our conversation about his past and his present situation. Rinehart refers to himself as a fatalist, calling attention to the equanimity with which he has experienced life change. To Rinehart, his three-and-a-half years at Bayside Nursing Home wasn't much of a change from what he had gotten used to—a life on the road, occasionally taking a vacation at "home."

Rinehart is a seventy-seven-year-old white widower, paralyzed from the waist down, the result of a fall. The fall features prominently in his story, dividing it into before and after. It presents a further horizon for evaluating the quality of his life. He has chronic pain in his lower back and is completely incontinent. Yet, like other residents who suffer from chronic conditions, except for the lower back pain, he says that he's in good health.

Rinehart is less of a storyteller than Bellows. But, in several exchanges, life on the road is similarly foregrounded.

> Jay: Why don't we talk about your life a bit now? Tell me a bit about it, Pete.
>
> Peter: Well, Jay, I was born in Connecticut and lived there for twenty-one years. Then I went into sales later in life and I was in sales for about twenty-five, thirty years. My wife and I traveled all over the country, in a travel trailer that we . . .
>
> Jay: You had a travel trailer?

Peter: Um hm. And we hauled that with a Ford van . . . not a Ford van. It was a Dodge van. And I was in that until I fell. It was 1971, I think, that I fell but I'm not sure.

Jay: How did that happen?

Peter: We were living in Donner Springs. We had our place there and the reception is bad there for television. So I had a tower put up and I used to go up and adjust it whenever it needed it.

Jay: You had an antenna up in the tower?

Peter: Yup. On top of this tower. And I had been up there before and adjusted it many times. That morning I got up there and finished adjusting it and I threw my tools on the ground. I had a cigarette and was looking around. Then I went to come down and the first step I took down, my foot slipped and the safety belt broke. I came down fifty feet.

Jay: Oh boy, that's a long way.

Peter: I had a spinal injury and they've been fooling around with it ever since. Still haven't been able to get rid of the pain.

Jay: You have pain too?

Peter: Pain continually. And that brings us, probably be about up to date. I've had, I don't know, five or six operations, including a brain tap that didn't work. They don't want to fool around with that anymore 'cause they don't know what it would do now.

Jay: Yeah. So you have chronic pain, Pete? Where exactly? In your lower back?

Peter: In the worst place it could be: right where you sit. So I haven't been able to sit for any length of time at all.

We talk at length about the injury, how it affects him now, and related details of his medical history. Rinehart recalls his work years, which he shares convivially. Curious to see how the recollections would figure into the writing of a life story, I change gears.

Jay: Pete, if you had the chance to write your life story, what would the first chapter be about?

Peter: Oh, I guess after high school, I went into industry and I was there for a while before I went into sales.

Jay: Yeah?

Peter: And, as I said, I've been in sales till the time I fell.

Jay: So the first chapter would be about industry and sales and so on, if you divided up your life?

Peter: Yeah.

Jay: What about the next chapter? What would that be about?

Peter: After I fell?

Jay: After you fell?

Peter: Is that what you want?

Jay: Well, whatever that would be. You'd write about that?

Peter: That's what I'd be doing.

Jay: I see.

Peter: Just laying here. I was up in Jacksonville at a rehab center there for five months and they couldn't do anything. We went as far as we could go. Then I came down here and I've been between here and the hospital ever since.

Jay: What year was it you said you fell? Was it '71? I forgot.

Peter: I think it was 1971. I'm not sure, but I think it was '71.

Jay: So it's been about, almost twenty years?

Peter: Not quite. Let's say eighteen years, something like that I've been laid up here. My wife and I were ready to go on the road within a week after I fell. [Elaborates] Boy time flies, doesn't it? Such is life, I guess.

Jay: What would you say the last chapter of your story would be about?

Peter: The last chapter would be my being here as a patient. And the time I had to go over to the hospital for treatment.

We drift away from the distinct chapters of a story and talk about his two daughters. But this is cut short when he resumes commenting on sales work and life on the road. According to Rinehart, being on the road in the company of his wife was the happiest time of his life.

> The wife came along with me. I was married twice and I have two daughters by my first wife. They're far apart. One's in California and one's in Connecticut. No sons. So, as I said, the wife . . . the second wife . . . she come along with me traveling. Two daughters . . .
>
> My wife and I actually didn't need a home, but we had it. My sales work covered the entire United States and my wife traveled with me. Those were the happiest years of my life. We had to pull the travel trailer with us. I had a trailer behind the van. I didn't want a motor home. The type of work that I was in, I could just go in a place, drop off the trailer, and I'd have transportation and all the merchandise in the van. I sold all kinds of stuff . . . the last, I sold the Oster Commercial Blender and I sold that till I fell. Then I couldn't walk or move. And I can't drive. So here I am.
>
> The wife died in '85. She had cancer. She didn't know she had it until she went for a physical. They found a spot on her lung and they went in . . . they had to take her left lung out. Seemed to be doing well. Then she started getting pains in her stomach and they opened her up and found a cancer between the liver and the pancreas. She only lasted a couple of months after that. Thank God she didn't suffer very much. [Pause] I don't mean she didn't suffer. She didn't suffer too long.
>
> I fell before she knew she had cancer. She'd come over to see me here as often as she could. She was in no condition even then to take care of me. I'm so helpless as far as bowels and urinary tract. I have no control. But they treat me very good here, then and now.

Rinehart tells me that his daughters call him weekly, which pleases him. He talks about them some, endearingly. But it's his traveling years that preoccupy him and provide the central linkages of his narrative. I ask him if he had a chance to live his life over, what he'd do differently. He remarks:

> Go into sales from the start. I'm not patting myself on the back, but another fellow and I had the reputation of being the best in our line in the country. I've always thought since I got into sales that if I've got the ability to sell, I'm not going to work for somebody else. I'll be working for myself, which I was. My wife helped me, of course.
>
> God, the only state we weren't in was Alaska. It was just too cold. Actually, it's useless to go to Alaska anyway on sales. You have to fly all your merchandise in. I'd have to drive all the way to Alaska. It just wouldn't pay to go to Alaska the way things are now.
>
> But between the two of us [he and his wife] . . . the hospitalizations and expenses . . . I got wiped out. We got wiped out entirely. So that's what it is. Like they say, "Easy come, easy go."

A sense of acceptance was apparent. While Rinehart was proud of his accomplishments, looking back he was not remorseful. According to him, life had brought him a good living, happiness, and now took care of him in his later years as best as could be expected.

> I see people that are worse off than I am. I feel sorry for them, but I'm not looking back with remorse. It's something I can't help. It happened and I have to live with it. Life's been happy and pretty good to me otherwise. I made a good living. You take the good with the bad.
>
> When it [the fall] first happened, I hoped that I would be able to get back to normal. Then I hoped to get . . . they got me into a wheelchair. I hoped to be able to stay in a wheelchair, maybe graduate to crutches and that. It never happened that way though. But it didn't make me despondent.
>
> Gradually, I began to know that I would probably never walk again and I've been about the way I have been now for the last couple of years. They brought a specialist in from the University of Pittsburgh and he put a brain tap in the nerve center of my brain. But that didn't work.
>
> I'm hoping to clear up the pain in my back so I can, if nothing else, sit up. But I read a lot and that takes time and they treat me good here. The aides come in and I kid with them and that. The rest of the time is about the same as an average day when you aren't working. Only instead of working now, I read. It's a long weekend, you might say.

We talk about Bayside and Rinehart compares it with a hospital. He says that he understands the reasons why care in a nursing home is sometimes not as good as it might be in a hospital. At the same time, he describes Bayside as, in some ways, the "nearest thing" to home.

> *Jay:* Pete, before you came to live here, did you have any idea what it'd be like?

Peter: Vaguely. I had an idea. My wife and her sister found this one that they thought was the best in town. And that's why I got here. I guess it is the best. It isn't like a hospital.

Jay: Oh? What do you mean?

Peter: Well, in a hospital you just ring and you got service right away. Here, it's not a hospital. You ring for service and they're on a lean budget, so you may get them right away or you may have to wait half an hour. Depends on how busy the aides are. That's part of it and it affects the care we get.

It's not all the aides' fault either. Of course, aides are hard to keep. I see changeover in the help here all the while. Some have been here a long time, but others will come and go. And I imagine . . . I have no basis for saying this, but I think they're probably on a minimum wage. When they get something better, they leave here and go there. That's my opinion, but you can understand that.

Jay: But, otherwise, does it seem homelike to you?

Peter: Home to me was a place like we had planned to retire, where you could retire, do what we wished, do what we wanted, when we wanted, worked part-time if I wanted to, and just enjoy things. But, as I said, you get wiped out fast. Anyway, mostly I wasn't home. So what's the difference, huh?

Jay: I guess not much if you put it that way. What about here?

Peter: Here? Well, it's not home really. But it's the nearest thing to it, I think. As I said, they help here, well, they treat me as a family. You heard me before? The aide that was in here. I kid her quite a bit in the morning. She was doing something . . . I don't know what . . . and I say, "Hey birdbrain, cut that out," funnylike. That aide knew I was kidding. It didn't bother her at all. Yeah, and she can shovel it back to me too. You can do that with people you're close to and know your ways.

I focus on the meaning of home, particularly the question of whether a nursing facility can be home and if having had a life on the road makes a difference in this regard. At first, Rinehart compares life on the road with life "at home."

Like at home even before I fell and before my wife was sick, the travel trailer was like home even though we had another home. She did about the same things she'd do at home, if we were living at home.

It was eight foot wide and twenty-five feet long. Had everything in it that home would. You had your stove, refrigerator, toilet facilities, everything was in it. We did, many times, stay self-contained for over a week, with no electricity or anything else. But we had battery power. We had forty gallons of waste water. So it really wasn't . . . we was glad to be home again, but there wasn't too much difference. The best part of it is that we saw about every place that was worth seeing in the United States. I really enjoyed being on the road. I suppose you might say a life on wheels.

Rinehart explains that while a travel trailer is not exactly home, it makes the transition to a new environment that much easier. As we continue our discussion, it is evident that home to him means familiarity and having a modicum of personal control over daily life more than it means having a home base. In that regard, Bayside doesn't quite feel like home. Still, in the context of a life of travel, Bayside is one more place on the road. As the following extract shows, in that respect, the subjective meaning of being in the nursing home isn't "too much of a changeover."

Jay: I was wondering, Pete, what would it have to be like here for it to be more like home to you?

Peter: Well, at home if I needed something there'd be somebody there to take care of it right away. There'd be people there to . . . people there to cook my meals, to live a normal life. That's the difference between, I think, living home and living in a place like this. It's different. Here, you have a set menu for breakfast, lunch, and dinner. And of course at home you can get up and around, which you can't do the way I am now.

Jay: Yeah. Is it the place itself or the incapacity that makes the difference to you, in terms of your feelings about home? What I mean I guess is, is it the place you're in or is it the incapacity mainly?

Peter: I don't think either, Jay, because, as I said, we traveled all the while. We were only home about a couple a months a year. So actually, that way, it wasn't too much of a changeover coming here.

Jay: Do you think of this place as part of your life or separate from it?

Peter: I think it's part of my life. I've seen people that weren't as well off as I am and some that were very far from what I am. They're very despondent. Can't face it. Well I don't have that feeling. I can adjust very easily. I think part of that is the fact that we traveled so much. You got to meet different people every week. I think that's the main difference. Of course, when you're stationary at home, you had a home. If you want to stay in bed all morning, you stayed in bed all morning.

Yeah, it's part of my life all right. What would I do if this place weren't here? I'd be another place like it, probably not as good as this place. I've adapted myself for quite a while here. I did adapt all right. Like when the aide brought you in, it didn't bother me to have you come in, even though you were a stranger. Not that you're a stranger now. Somebody else might have cringed down a bit, you know, don't want to meet nobody.

In the end, what Rinehart's life has become is not to be lamented as much as accepted because it is part of one's fate. Rinehart explains as he describes himself.

Me, I'm realistic, down-to-earth. I get along with people. That's why I was a success in sales, I imagine. I guess I don't have much of a future now. Not really. But I've taken the attitude, more or less, that this has happened, I'm here, I can't control it. So be it. So why should I be here crying my eyes out, feeling sorry for myself? Right now, until I get able to use my body where I can sit down, I haven't even thought of any plans for the future. Then again, what will be, will be. Maybe I'll never be able to get out of this bed. Who knows?

They had me where I could sit up for about an hour, but I relapsed from that and got where I can't sit. It's a feeling like if you're sitting on a golf ball. That's the kind of pain it is, if you can imagine that, in the worse spot it could be.

I have a lot of free time thinking here sometimes. I told you what I thought about politics and that. I know even though I'm in bed I know that, physically, I'm probably better off than a lot of other people that have nothing wrong with them except old age and they don't accept it. It doesn't bother me, and even though I'm the way I am, I still have, I think, all my brains yet. And I'm not entirely dependent on somebody else. That's a funny thing to say because I can't move out of this bed without help, but otherwise, I think I'm in good health. I feed myself, which a lot of 'em here have to be fed. I can read, which I like to do. If I could sit up, I could write the way I always did, I believe. [Elaborates]

I don't think about death. I've always been a fatalist. I believe when it's time for you to go, you're gonna go. Everyone that saw me after I fell? I didn't know whether they were lying or whether they meant it, but they said I looked so well and behaved the way I did, even after I fell. I don't bother nobody. I try to get along with all of them. I don't think I'm hard to get along with. My philosophy of life . . . as I said, I'm a fatalist. What comes, comes. Like when I fell . . . I didn't want to of course, but it happened and that's that.

Mainly, I pass the time. Time doesn't bother me, really. You got a lot of time here. But, like I said, I like to read and I read mainly mysteries and spy thrillers. I was reading one by a British author, but don't much like those because the British describe too much. Takes 'em a whole page to describe one thing. [Elaborates] If I get tired of reading, I take a nap and if I feel like reading after I take a nap, I will or I might just lay there with my eyes closed, resting, you know, like in your hotel room. Sometimes they'll come in . . . the aide will come in the room or something and . . . it's funny . . . she thinks I'm asleep and I'm not. So that's life for me. Easy come, easy go.

Barring a change, Jay, I'll be just like I am. Hopefully, I'll get to the point where I can sit up. I'm seventy-seven years old. I've had a good life. Down the road, unless things change, I'll probably be about the same as I am now.

* * * * *

One mark of a nursing facility that would seem to affect the quality of life is the extent it is homelike. This typically means things such as an atmosphere of soft, noninstitutional lighting and colors on the walls and being surrounded by one's own furniture. For the residents of this chapter, special circumstances present a different horizon for signaling home. Home is a kind of vacation, as a hotel might accommodate or a long weekend might offer. For these residents, the quality of life is not figured chiefly in terms of care provision or homeyness, but in relation to another place along the road of life that fate has taken them.

CHAPTER

8

Sisters

Residents sometimes say that, besides the pain, suffering, and helplessness, one of the most difficult things about living in a nursing home is "it
cuts you off," meaning that it separates you from the rest of life, from
loved ones, or from home, often forever. The exceptions are those who
make a new home in the facility or who bring loved ones with them, or
those who never had much of a home or family life to begin with, and
those who for one reason or another accept their fate with equanimity.

In this chapter, we meet African American twin sisters Lula Burton
and Lily Robinson. Their special circumstance is that they hardly have
ever been "cut off" from each other and now continue to live together in
the same room at Florida Manor. At the time of their interviews, the
sisters were seventy-four years old and had been in the nursing home
for a year. Before that, for ten years, they shared a house of their own.

A benefit of having family members or significant others coresident in
a nursing home is that a life once shared continues to be a source of
meaning for daily living. Of course, there are familial coresidents, either
or both of whom are demented or otherwise noncommunicative and, as
such, can share little. Communicative family coresidents do not necessarily share good times or look back solely on positive moments from
their pasts. But for coresident family members such as Burton and Robinson, narrative horizons that extend beyond the period of coresidency
provide a ready-made, long-standing familiarity in a living environment
normally said to be devoid of it. Equally important, talk and interaction
are not limited in meaning to short-term exchanges and relevancies, the
bare "how-do-you-do's" of daily living.

This is not to say that the twins or others whom we will meet in the
next few chapters simply transport home with them into their facilities.
Burton and Robinson, for example, know and speak of the difference
between "real" home and the nursing home. They acknowledge the
homelike quality of care, but they also recognize that the quality of their
lives, as they understand it, is linked with sources and commonalities
removed from the present. More important in their special circum-

stance, the sources and commonalities continue to present themselves as the twins share memories, thoughts, and sentiments, highlighted in their mutual use of the pronoun *we* to speak of what they share in life, both past and current.

The primary commonality in the twins' case is "service," what they believe to have been their purpose, not just their lot, in life. They are like Mary Carter of Chapter 5 in this regard. The sisters speak of serving those for whom they worked, mainly cooked for, as a mission beyond the job alone, one that was meant to be. This is no longer realized in the nursing home because of their incapacity, but it continues to be a desire. Its memories make them happy, shared as the "we" who fulfilled their purpose in life. Yet, Robinson especially is wary of the present, particularly the danger of crime, drug abuse, and their impact on the young, whom, were it not for Robinson's incapacity, she would continue serving for their own good.

LULA BURTON

Like her sister Lily and a few other residents interviewed for the study such as Julia McCall and Mary Carter, Lula Burton has spent much of her life in church and "in service." While Burton doesn't express her love of the Lord with the same fervor that McCall and Carter do, nor is she as otherworldly, her lifelong concern for others is suffused with religious meaning.

I interview Burton alone in a lounge located near her room where I wheeled her, as she is confined to a wheelchair. Burton suffers from hypertension and diabetes, which has caused her to have one leg amputated. Her brief life story has a humble beginning in a rural area of north Florida and develops into a narrative of work and devotion to others, much like her twin sister's story. Burton's is not a charmed life but it is filled with simple joys. Notice, at the end of the following extract, she uses the collective pronoun *we* to refer to herself, a repeated form of identity shared with her sister.

> I was raised from childhood with farmers. Then I married a farmer. That was a great deal of my life. I was a farm girl and I married a farmer, but we didn't have any children. And I like . . . Do you wanna know what I like? [I nod] I like fishing, going to school, always loved the school. I'm a good fisherman. Fishing . . . I like fishing. My hobby is fishing. I don't know nothing else, but working on the farm and fishing. I love that.
>
> My occupation was cooking. I like cooking. That's about the size of it. After I married, I adopted a son. He's twenty-nine now. I sent him to school, four years of college. I helped with my nieces and nephews, helped those

boys and girls go to school. That's the only thing I know, helping people. I helped my mother and father to make ends meet, like working on the farm. My father was a great farmer and my husband was a farmer. I'm just a farm girl. Then I started cooking. I cooked at a sorority house out there on sorority row. I cooked six years at one place and I cooked six years at another place. A-E House. I don't know what the initials meant, but it was a house where I cooked. I cooked for some boys right there, too, fraternity boys. That was another place. And I lived on the premises for five years with Mr. Caleb S. Porter. He worked out there at the university. His wife passed; so I had to leave there. I was chief bottle washer there. I did all the cooking and planned the meals. We got along fine until she passed. He thought he'd marry again. I wasn't with him when he married the next time. I didn't work for him anymore.

I was a church member. I sang in a choir. I was secretary for the church for fifteen years. That's the only thing I know that I really done, a lot of service. My childhood . . . I was going to church when I was eleven years old and I still belong to the same church. I just wanna say that I love church and singing in the choir. I was a choir member. I call myself a good member. We were real good members of the church. Our pastor always told that to us, me and Lily, every time he come to visit and he's been there over forty years.

Now what else do you want me to say?

I take the opportunity to present Burton with the idea of writing her life story and ask her what the chapters would be about. She recounts much of what she's already said, this time divided into chapters. Her last chapter is a summary of aspects of her life that continue to be important to her.

The last chapter would be cooking. I was a cook. My last chapter would be . . . I'm trying to think what year I last cooked in. I think about '70, '71, or '72 I spent my last year cooking. And that's all I can write about, cooking. That's my whole life story, cooking. I spent my life doing that. School started about September. So I'd break through the summer, about three months, and then start right back the next month and live as a cook, plan meals, and cook. I loved it. To me, it was more than a job, helpin' others and all.

I could write a chapter about my son. I adopted him and sent him to school. He went to school and he's out now. I adopted him when he was eighteen hours old and I adopted him in 1960. I picked him up in the hospital, the same day. I never met his mother till I got the baby. But she's a sweetheart. Very sweet child. She was a sweet woman. I think she gave him away not because she didn't want him, but because she wasn't able to support him. So my husband and I thought we'd adopt him. He's a dear heart, a very sweet heart. I love him to death I think. I know he loves me 'cause every time he calls, he says, "Mama, I love you." I tell him, "Well, I just want you to know I'm not your mother. I'm just your adopted mother."

He says, "Well, you're the only mother I know and you're still my mama."
So we let it go like that. He's my son and I love him to death. He made
pretty good in college, because he's the manager of this store now in Atlan-
ta. So I know that's something he loves.

   The rest of the chapters, like I says, is church work. That's all I know that I
could say anything about that I really enjoyed and did well was working in
church . . . service. And cooking, the only thing that I know that I would
enjoy doing and I did that. When I had the operation on my leg, that's when
I stopped working. That was in '72. I had my leg amputated. I had to stop
because I couldn't get around.

We talk about the important people in her life: her mother and an
older sister who became like a mother to her after the mother died. The
important people are shared with sister Lily, which is repeated in Lily's
interview.

   My mother was the most important person in my life. I just loved her to
death. She was a sweet person. I had some lovely brothers and I had a
lovely sister. I had a sister who passed in '69. She was older. She was one of
my important friends and dearest sister. I love Lily of course, but Althea [the
older sister] was closer to me than Lily. Lily and I were twins. We was a
twosome, onesome. And Althea was closer because Althea reared us up.
She was our mother and father and brother and sister too. Most important
person I had in my life was her. I had a husband, but she topped everything. Name was Althea Stevens.

   I had four brothers. I had one brother was a sweet brother, sweeter than
any other. His name was Paul Williams. He was living way down south of
here. Every time Lily and I asked for something, he would always send it to
us. He was very kind to us.

   Now Lily and I are the only two in our family. All our family is dead. I
mean brothers and sisters. So it's just Lily and I now. Lily and I are very
close. We've been living together now about ten years, even before we came
here. She and I lived in our home. Then we came out here. Lily is my
closest. My son and I are very close.

The conversation turns to the meaning of home and to why Florida
Manor is not home. According to Burton, the Manor is *like* home, but not
home. Home is conveyed in the terms of her life story, applying the
vocabulary she knows best: Home is where one plans meals and cooks
according to good taste. To that extent, the Manor is not home. While
food preparation and the taste of food is important to many residents,
for the sisters it resonates with a central linkage of their narratives,
adding to its significance and spilling over into the other life connections
of service. As we will learn later, to that extent the Manor is a horizon
that can never include home.

Jay: What does the word *home* mean to you, Ms. B?

Lula: It means a house that you can enjoy yourself in. That's what home is. That's what I call home.

Jay: Now that you've been here for a year, does this feel like home to you?

Lula: It feels like home. The people are nice and I enjoy being here. It's like being home and friends and relatives and things. It's beautiful to be here.

Jay: So it's home.

Lula: No. It's *like* home but it ain't home. It's different, this and home.

Jay: In what way would you say?

Lula: Well at home you can have some of the things you desire yourself, plan yourself. But here we don't plan nothing. We have to do what they say to do. Whatever they give us to eat, we have to eat what they give us. When you're home, you can plan something of your own, plan your meals. Like if you want a special meal, you can have a special meal. But here you can't. A lot of things they cook I don't like, because I always cooked and I've enjoyed my cooking . . . until here. You got to eat what people cook. A lot of people say they are cooks, but they're not really cooks. But other than that, they're very nice people here. This is a nice place to be. When you don't have nowhere else to go, this is a good place to be. They have some nice help here.

Burton talks at length about the Manor, its "nice help," and the attractive facilities. She even describes some of the help as like family to her and to her sister Lily, noting that the help is not actually kin, but that they're very nice and familylike nonetheless. Burton is careful to mark important distinctions: Homelike is not the same as home; familylike is not actually family.

I ask Burton whether having her sister living with her at the Manor makes a difference in what life is like there. As the discussion unfolds, we learn that the quality of care in the nursing home could never produce the quality of life she once knew, no matter how hard "they" try. The home the Manor is, is a home that Burton and her sister Lily together realize in the memories shared in everyday conversation. Even the seemingly irrational possibility of fishing again continues to be meaningful in the context of a life of common experiences.

Jay: Does it make a difference having your sister with you in this place?

Lula: Oh, there's a difference.

Jay: In what way?

Lula: Well, if they would come in maybe sometime and ask me, "Lula, what would you like to have to eat?" or something like that. That'd be one of the main things. And you don't have no one to talk to here. Maybe the nurse when they bring you the meal or something like that, but other than that, you don't have anybody to discuss nothing with. Lily and I talk together, we talk. It's much better to be in the room with her than to be with someone I don't know.

Jay: Why is that?

Lula: Well, because we have things to talk about life and the other person. It would be anything we did together. That means a lot to talk about things you've had dealings with and doing together and enjoying things together . . . talk with that, about that.

Jay: So that helps . . .

Lula: There's nothing they can do here to make me love it any more than they have done. But I'd rather be with . . . even if my son was here, I'd enjoy being with him. He can't get here because he's working and he's got a job and he can't get away.

Jay: How does it help to have Lily here with you?

Lula: It helps me because she can talk with me and I can talk with her. We're company for each other. We talk about what we did when . . . right now if we was able to do it, what we would do, like fishing and different things like that. Other than that, we just have to live up life like that. Fishing we can't do anyway, but we talk about it. She won't be able to go fishing unless she can walk. The doctor had to amputate both her legs. She's diabetic like me.

Jay: So you share things and that . . .

Lula: Well, I 'bout done give my best life out in service. Not just working, but helping others. I have enjoyed life and I'm still enjoying life. I'm not sad. I like my life. I enjoy being friendly to people and amuse people and everything. I learned [taught] those girls in that sorority a lot. They liked when I learned them. And one of the main things is that I like to entertain. That's my life.

Jay :   Do you miss that?

Lula: Oh yes. I miss that, but . . . I like that. That's life to me. I enjoy life because I've been happy and helped others. I enjoy life because I'm pretty healthy. I don't have a lot of pain and aches and things. That's all in my life.

LILY ROBINSON

I interview Burton's sister, Lily Robinson, in the twin's room, with Burton present and sitting in a wheelchair on her side of the room. Robinson stays in bed throughout the interview, as she does most of the day because of her amputations. She feels more comfortable that way. The curtain separating the two sides, which has been drawn for nursing cares, remains closed. Periodically, as Robinson and I talk, Robinson leans over to ask her sister something. Burton readily responds from the other side of the curtain.

Robinson suffers from diabetes and high blood pressure. Like her sister, she has spent her life in service. She not only was a cook and domestic but has devoted herself, as both sisters put it, to "learning others." Robinson is proud of what she taught her friends, especially the young sorority women who eagerly sought her advice over that of the house mother.

We begin with Robinson's life story.

> Well, I don't have much history in my life. It's hard work. I lived on a farm and I was about four miles from town. I had to walk to school. [Elaborates] After growing up, I married and lived on a farm. Then I decided I would try to cook. My mother taught me a lot about cooking. [Elaborates] And then I went out to cook in the neighborhood. I cooked one place here twenty-three years. I consider myself a pretty good cook. I cooked at that one sorority at the university for twenty-three years. After I left there, I haven't worked anymore. I worked in Daytona Beach in a hotel and in St. Augustine I worked in a hotel. I cooked there for four or five years. I haven't done anything but cook. That's all I did all my life. And 'I guess that's about it. I've taken care of children in my home for a while, maybe a year or two for the summer. I worked at a foster home for children for about two years taking care of children. And I . . . after that, I left the sorority because I became ill and I've been kinda down ever since then. I haven't been any good no more. I worked there until I couldn't work anymore. Then I began going to the doctor and I knew then that I was a diabetic. Actually, I worked a long time before I knew I was a diabetic. All at once I broke down. My legs broke down. They had to take them off and that's about it.
>
> I raised one child, raised one girl. Then I adopted her when she was about five months old. I raised her and she started school. Then she had this little girl right here [points to a framed photograph of the granddaughter on her dresser] and I adopted her too. So I don't have any children of my own. I only have two adopted children. That little girl [in the photograph] is ten years old. I had adopted her mother a long time ago and raised her. [Elaborates] Her mother says that she didn't . . . she wasn't married and she got this child and she wanted to give it away. I told her to give it to me. So I adopted her and so she's with me now.
>
> I guess that's about it. I don't know of anything else. Just hard work, that's all, and service. And I'm a Christian. I belong to the Baptist church and I've given my life for the Lord and that's about it . . . service for the Lord. I don't know of anything else. And now I'm in here with these people. I don't know how long I'll be here. But they're all very nice to us. [Nods toward her sister on the other side of the curtain] We're treated nice here.

Continuing to look back on her life, Robinson speaks of youthful desires and what she might have become. The emphasis is less on the actual job than on the service she might have been to others.

> I mostly loved people, loved to get along with people. That's my whole desire was in life, was to treat people as I wish to be treated and to live that

way, live the way that people would love me. And that's about it. I liked the outdoor life. I liked fishing and things like that, picnics and so on.

I tell ya, I'd love to have been a . . . things I loved to have been when I was growing up, when I was younger. I'd love to have been a schoolteacher so I could teach people something. Oh, I don't know, just learn them the way to live if I could, to the best of my ability. But that's the only thing that I desire, that I didn't get to be a teacher. 'Cause it seemed like I could tell young people what to do. That's about all I had on my mind that I didn't do and I never will do it I guess 'cause I'm too old now.

I know when I was working . . . I was working with young girls. They always came to me for . . . I had ideas, things they wanted to know about. They wouldn't go to the house mother. They'd come to me. So I said, "Why do you all come to me?" They say, "Lily, you always know things." I said, "Well, the reason I know about young people is I was young once myself and I think about telling you all the things that I was used to, how my mother raised me." They said, "Well, we enjoy your talks." That made me feel good. That's about all I can say.

Lula and I both worked in those sororities. But I worked longer than Lula did. We was in different ones, different sororities. I worked at Chi Omega and she worked at Alpha Delta. I think that was it. [Turns toward her sister] Lula? Was it Alpha Delta? [Lula answers yes] Alpha Delta. That was a girl's sorority. We wasn't far apart. She was on one corner and I was on another. We could walk where we worked with each other and things like that. But I worked there, planned my meals. I did my ordering. I did it all, but I enjoyed it.

Robinson recalls her parents, especially her mother and older sister. As twin sister Lula remarked in her interview, Robinson explains that both the mother and older sister were mothers to the twins. Robinson speaks of accepting the sorrow of their deaths, but it is overshadowed by her emphasis on living and service "to make others happy."

The most important one was my mother. That's the only one I can say. Since my mother I haven't really had any important . . . my sister, my oldest sister, she was important 'cause she was just like a mother to us. Other than that, I think that's about all. The only somebody now is my sister. The one right there. That's the closest person I am to now. I don't have anybody closer to me than she is, although my daughter is close to me. But she's not as close to me as my Lula. My sister and I have been so close together and been together all our lives.

I've always been a happy person. I've never had extremely happy things in my life, just from day-to-day things happened. But nothing extremely happy. When I had depression, I never was sad. I'd never dwell on that. I dwelled on being happy and trying to make others happy. So I've always been happy. I've had some sadness in my life. My parents and all passed away. My sisters and brothers. That was pretty sad, but I never dwelled on it because I knew that those days would be. I knew they must go and leave or if I left them. That's why I just accepted it and tried to serve others. Service was the main thing.

Responding to the question about what life now looks like, Robinson conveys her sense of the relation between her incapacity, hope for the future, and living in a nursing home. In the context of her incapacity and being dependent, life is hopeless because she is a burden and can't be of service. According to Robinson, this has little to do with the nursing home. Robinson accepts God's plans for her and looks ahead to salvation. In relation to the possibility of going home, however, there is hope that she again can be of service, especially to her adopted granddaughter.

Jay: What does life look like from you're at now, Ms. R?

Lily: Well, I say it's hopeless, to me. I'm just in other people's way here. I'm no good.

Jay: Being in someone's way—that makes a difference?

Lily: Yes, it do.

Jay: Would you explain that a little more?

Lily: Well, when you can't do anything for yourself, I think you're in other folks' way. If I was up and doing for myself and others, I would enjoy living, but I don't enjoy it.

Jay: So would you say it's the place you're at or you . . . ?

Lily: No, it's not the place. It's just the shape I'm in. That's what I'm talking about. The place is very good to me. But I'm so helpless. I can't do anything for myself. When you're used to doing for yourself . . . and when you get down and can't do nothing unless somebody come and do it for you, that's pretty sad.

Jay: If you could live your life over, what would you do differently?

Lily: I don't know what I would do differently. I don't because I had a good life. Although I worked hard, I had a good life.

Jay: What would you say are the ingredients of a good life? What does it mean to have a good life?

Lily: What I mean is that I enjoyed life. I never had a whole lots, but I've had a comfortable life. What I mean by that is that I was never on the hands of other people. I've always worked and what I wanted mostly I always got at the time. And I think when a person gets the things they want and need in life, that's a good life.

Jay: How would you explain what's happened to you over the course of your life?

Lily: That's hard 'cause I've tried to work it out, but I couldn't really work it out. I wonder sometimes, why this? But God alone knows why this happened to me. So I just accept it as my share and be with Him in time.

But if there would be anything that, if somebody needed help and I could be of service, I would do that. I love to help people. That's my desire, was to take care of people. But I got so helpless that I couldn't help myself. The joy of my life would maybe now be to make somebody happy. That's what I want. I'd like that very much, to make someone happy. The one thing I would like would be somebody to remember me by and say, "Well, Lily did thus and thus before her last day and she seemed happy doing that." That's the thing I know.

I wish I could get out and visit people and talk to friends, have them in sometimes and make a nice dinner for them. And talk about old times and things like that. That'd make me happy. I hope I'll be able to do that one day, hold my own and have a place, and I can have my little girl back with me.

Jay: You had her with you at home for a while?

Lily: I raised her. They just took her from me last year, just before I came here. She went in a foster home. It's been about two months since I seen her. I'm the only mama she has.

Robinson's sentiments about home parallel and elaborate her sister's. While Florida Manor is homelike, it can never be home. The nursing home's quality of care is, simply, nice and "sweet," but never to be taken as part of life. Home belongs to life, the nursing home to a different, more limited domain of experience, the domain of the patient, not the whole person. In regard to the possibility of going home, Robinson points out that as for herself and her sister, they will never "give up," even as they are helpless, because ultimately home is with her Lord in a life everlasting.

Jay: Do you feel this place is part of your life or separate from it?

Lily: Well, I should consider it now as part of my life 'cause I'm here, just 'cause I'm here. But I never will accept it as a . . . really a life for my life. It seem like I'm just visiting here, but not really a part of my life.

The girls here, they're nice to us, kinda like family to us. There's one or two here that's very sweet and they're like family, not kin, but like family. But other than that, I'm more just like a patient is what I am, someone they have to wait on. You don't be your ol' self here.

Jay: When people go to the hospital, of course, they're patients. But I wonder if it's different here being a patient?

Lily: I think they all seem about just alike. I stayed in the hospital quite a long time when they amputated my legs and the nurses are very friendly, but it's not like home. No place, no hospital, no nursing home is like your own home. Not to me. So I don't think it's like . . . They're friendly, but . . . Peace of mind I think at home makes you different. You run your home. These people here run the nursing home. At home, you're the overseer. You take care of everything and I think that's more like a whole being. Here you're just a part. When you're home, you're whole. You're a whole person. You're taking care of everything and everything comes to you by your means and it makes you feel more at home.

Jay: Do you think it's possible to have a life in a place like this?

Lily: No. I wouldn't want to stay here all my life. I just wouldn't. I wouldn't wish that on anybody. I just come for the rest and somebody to take care of you. Then the family of somebody comes and takes care of you. I think that'll be better. We're not going to, Lula and me, give up to live here. Of course, a lot of people do.

Jay: A lot of people do what, did you say? Did you say, "give up"?

Lily: Yes, they gives up and lives here.

Jay: What does that mean, to "give up"? What does that mean to you, Ms. R?

Lily: I will say give up everything. There's no desire for anything. That's why when somebody gives up just something, you're satisfied, not happy. You just satisfied. It's not the matter of being happy; you're satisfied. I made myself satisfied here. That's all. Nothing with happy. I'm just here. I'm not happy or unhappy. I'm satisfied.

What I'm sayin' is that they come and do us . . . I pray and ask the Lord to take care of me and the people that take care of me, and they do their best. I'm not sick. I'm just helpless, but I'm not sick. And I'm thankful that I'm not sick. And that's a blessing. So many people here that are sick. And I'm thankful that I'm not sick. I get up everyday and I don't feel bad. I get up everyday and I sit up all day long.

I'm just a helpless person. That's all I can say. I'm helpless, but I still have lots to be thankful for. I don't say I'm not. I'm thankful that I'm not in a worse shape than I am. There's many people worse off than I am. So I have so much to be thankful for. I can't go anywhere, but I can sit up and I can be taken all over this place, go to church down there [the activity room] to hear the preacher and singing and what not. I get joy out of staying here, but I don't have a future. The only future I have lies in my end, when I pray and ask the Lord to make me ready, make me ready to have a happy day. That day I'm looking forward to and I'm certainly looking forward to it. I have been admitted to the kingdom and going home to life everlastin'.

Jay: Do you think about death, Ms. R?

Lily: No, I don't think about it. I know it's coming, but I don't think about it because it's not for me to think about. I think that's left for the higher above. I'm here, but I don't think about death because I know it's sure. It's coming for sure. I just want a resting place when I die. I don't wanna be in torment. I want it to be in a resting place.

Since I been here, people do die. I know if I could have kept my mother with me forever and ever, I would've kept her. But she died and left me. I know that I must die. So when everybody I see, people are dying. I know that that day will come. I read in this Bible about death. Death is sure. That's why I know it's coming.

I just look forward to not being here and try to meet each day with a smile. That's the only thing I look forward to. I look forward to getting

out of this place one day. I do wanna get out of here. I don't know if I
will, but I'm looking forward to get out of here one day. That'll make
me happy.

Short of going to heaven, the idea of someday leaving Florida Manor
causes Robinson to speak about home and the possibility of again caring
for her adopted granddaughter. As she describes the unfortunate events
involving her daughter that led to the adoption of the granddaughter,
Robinson laments the selfishness of the so-called young race. The young
race cares little about anyone but themselves and certainly not older
people. To Robinson, it is a generation that has lost the value of prayer
and, especially, service. At the same time, Robinson, with her sister,
finds solace in memories of a different era and purpose, one committed
to others in service and to the Lord.

Lily: It'd make me happy to have my little girl come back to me and stay
with me. Just to hear her voice in the house would make me happy.
Jay: So you had her in the house with you until she was about eight years
old? Is that right?
Lily: Oh, I had her in the house with me until . . . let's see. I came out here
in '89. I came out here in '88. She just left me the first of '88. [Turns in
the direction her sister is seated] Wasn't it, Lula? When did she leave?
Lula: She left around, about the last of '88.
Lily: She left me just before I came out here. I remember calling her and
telling her I was coming out here. And she said, "Mama, I won't see
you no more." I said, "Oh, yes you will."
    I don't think there's much joy in growing old. There's so many
things you can't do, things you like to do. I think you send good
people away when you grow old and you can't do nothing for yourself. One thing people get tired of it when you get old. They don't
want to wait on you. Most people don't like to wait on old people.
They don't have time to talk with you. Maybe a few years ago, it was
. . . years ago people would take time out and talk with you. But now
they're going so fast, they don't have time to talk to one another. And
old people don't have anybody to talk to no how, except Lula and me,
we have each other.
Jay: So you think it's made a difference in that times have changed.
Lily: Oh yes, lots of things changed over time. When I was a child, I loved
old people. I loved to be around old people. I loved to talk to them. I
loved to see what I could do, what I could do for them. But it's so sad
now because people don't have time to do anything for you now.
Everything somebody would do for you now they want a lot of pay for
it. Used to be people didn't want that. People would do it out of the
kindness of their heart.

Jay: Do you think families have changed a lot?

Lily: Yes, families have changed lots. It's not the love in the family that used to be in the family. People used to love their family. Children loved their parents, but they don't anymore. I've experienced that in my own life.

I never was a rowdy person but I liked to go to church and I like to participate in church. I was singing in the choir and all those things I miss. I like to go and visit people. I belonged to a lot of clubs. But I don't have that now. A day come and a day go.

I got a joy out of going to church. I'd cook and take meals. We had some . . . some Sundays we'd have homecoming [at the sorority] and things like that and I'd cook food and take out. Then I'd have our pastor and his wife out to our place for dinners, several times. Well I just loved to take care of the people. I like that. Lula and I got a joy out of doing for other people.

Lula: [From the other side of the room] Sure do.

Lily: Old people can't do the things they used to do and they kind of dread it in a sense. Some people are happier in their old age than they were when they were younger. But I don't care how happy you were, when you get older, you're not the same. You don't get the joy out of life when you get older as you had in middle age. You can't do nothing for nobody else hardly. You got to look for someone else to do something for you. That's kind of hard. You got to wait for someone to do for you when you're used to doing for other people. It makes you happy doing for others and you can't when you get old like this. When people get old and they have to wait on someone else to do things for them, that's takes a lot from 'em.

Jay: What would it be like in old age if you could do things?

Lily: Well, if you could do things and get out and help people, you'd be happier. That's what I know. Get out and try to learn the young people what . . . try to learn them and help them.

I think the young people need more help now than they ever did in life. They're going on this ol' crack and stuff and it's ruining the nation. That's one of the worst things that ever happened. I don't know where it started at. But everybody, all the children . . . what's it gonna be? What's the next nation gonna be like when everybody's turned to crack and drugs and all that stuff. It's bad. It's really bad. I feel sorry for the young race. They're not happy unless they're with that ol' crack or something.

One thing I say, they need to pray more. That's one thing. People need to pray more. A lot of people are not prayin'. They just living each day as it comes and that's it. They don't never take time to thank God for them from one day to the other. They don't thank Him for getting the food. They don't thank . . . a lot of people don't say "thank God" for nothing. That's the thing's destroying the world. Everybody is looking for a dollar. And that's bad. Money is the root of all evil. And it really has taken its toll since that stuff come out.

Jay: You mean since . . . ?

Lily: Since crack and whatever it is, drugs and all that stuff. The dollar bill is all a person want. And that's bad. People are afraid to stand in the store. They're afraid of everything, even in their home. It's really terrible. And I feel sorry for the young race. The parents have done everything to bring them up and since they brought them up, they done turned from their parents. Children have really gone away from their parents. Only thing they want is to get these old drugs and go somewhere to have a good time and that's bad. That ol' crack got my daughter like that.

When I was young, people used to bootleggin,' moonshinin,' making it in the woods out there. Crack's about the same thing. They had wars in the woods. Went to war against each other about that ol' moonshine and stuff and this war now's against people with drugs. They killing one another about that. It's just . . .

Prayer would change things. They need to pray more. I just don't know what it is. I know it's sin. Sin is taking over. The government, the high officials are selling this old crack. They got to make a dollar. They making more than they'll ever spend and they still grasping after money. They say that money's the root of all evil and it's ruining all the children.

It's disturbing, very disturbing. I wish, just wish there's something I could do to change the children, the young race. They have enough in this world to be grateful for. This world has plenty of pleasures and stuff. Why should they go to that crack? I know my days are over but I worry about the young generation. I've had a good life, but I think seriously about what the children are coming to; it makes me sad that I can't learn them. [Turns toward her sister] Don't it, Lula?

Lula: Sure do.

* * * * *

A lifelong conversation can be a valuable resource in the context of nursing home living. Over and over again, shared narrative linkages reclaim the distant and the near past and call out the future for purposes of considering the present. In various and particular ways, the quality of life for the residents of this chapter is conjured up in and through overlapping experiences. The nursing home is a place not only to appreciate the quality of care but to recall childhood on the farm, having fished together, having cooked professionally across the street from one another, having raised adopted children, having lost legs, and most of all having served others and God in common.

CHAPTER

9

Spouses

Like coresident sisters, spouses who share rooms or otherwise find themselves living in the same nursing home bring the horizons of their formerly linked lives with them into the facility. For spouses the horizons are expressly those of marriage, financial support, household management, and relations with children. The horizons of the last chapter's twin sisters approximate this in their having virtually grown up as one and, later in life, having shared the same household for ten years before entering Florida Manor. They were unusual siblings in this regard.

Yet there is a difference. The narratives of this chapter show that in addition to familial sentiments, life together is linked with emotional love. When spouses Jane and Tom Malinger and Sue and Don Hughes speak of what they have meant and continue to mean to each other, they not only convey mutual responsibility and cherished routines but sentiments of physical attraction. The difference comes in talk and interaction cross-cut by affirmations of desire. While husband and wife help and look out for each other, share tastes, and teasingly confirm common preferences, they also express affections different from sisterly or brotherly love.

There are coresident spouses, of course, just as there are coresident sisters, brothers, and others with significantly linked lives, whose narrative horizons are less sanguine. Such horizons provide negative resources for talk and interaction, which arguably is more advantageous than having no communicative resources at all. Sisters who hated each other are placed in the same nursing home because families find that more convenient than placing them in separate facilities. Spouses who lived together as strangers most of their married lives or who continually hurt each other emotionally or physically may find themselves under the same roof and again daily contending with their animosities. These experiences aren't represented here because there were no such cases in the nursing homes contacted who were competent enough to tell their stories. However, such cases are important to keep in mind as we hear the contrasting, positive narratives of the spouses in this chapter.

In the years ahead, there may be coresidents who will openly speak of life as gay and lesbian couples, and will have grown old and frail together. They are still rare voices in nursing homes, but they may become more commonplace as a publicly recognized generation of such couples or marriages, as the case might be, comes of age. They will add their voices to the narrative linkages of quality of life and care in nursing homes. This also is important to keep in mind, for spousal horizons can appear in nontraditional forms of long-standing attachment and attraction, adding to the special circumstances from which residents speak of life.

JANE AND TOM MALINGER

Like Sue and Don Hughes, Jane and Tom Malinger are interviewed as a couple. At the time of their interview, Jane and Tom Malinger have been living together for a year at Fairhaven Nursing Home. Their standard double room is packed with household items. Besides the usual hospital beds, nightstands, and tray tables, there is a portable television set, radio, microwave oven, refrigerator, dresser, and smaller objects such as stacks of magazines and framed photographs. Many are the familiar items of a household. Yet, for the Malingers, more important than household items, what makes the room home is that they reside in it together, a key linkage in their interview.

Jane Malinger is a seventy-six-year-old white female who suffers from diabetes and has had a leg amputation. She has been unsteady on her feet, is subject to falling, and remains in a wheelchair. Her husband, Tom, an eighty-two-year-old white male, has cardiac failure, has had several heart attacks, and is in constant pain from inoperable pinched nerves in his back. He is ambulatory.

Tom is alone in the room at the start of the interview. He describes his "short and sweet" life.

> I was born in Turner Hill, New York, and I went to St. Paul's Academy. From St. Paul's I went into Marian College. Then I studied to be a physical therapist at a school in New York. I left that and went into respiratory therapy, which was a bit easier work. But I liked it more anyway; I had better contact with the patients.
>
> I wound up here on account of my back and my legs. I'm inoperable. They can't operate on my back. There's nothing they can do for me. So I just have to put up with it. I'm in a good deal of pain right now. That's it. Short and sweet.

At that point, Jane wheels into the room. From then on, much of the interview is a conversation between the three of us. We share details of Tom's career in respiratory therapy and move on to his first and now second marriage. Jane's own first marriage was a success and ended when her husband died. They had had four children. According to Tom, his first marriage was a disaster and resulted in divorce. He never had children of his own. At the time of the interview, Tom and Jane have been married for twelve "gloriously happy" years.

Prompted by questions about what life now is like, the couple discusses daily living at Fairhaven and the meaning of family and home. Home is connoted less by location than by living together. According to Tom, wherever Jane is, is home, the implication being that Fairhaven is now home. This serves to explain how they both came to reside in the facility.

Tom: I've got nobody else outside of my wife. I've got a younger brother still living some place. I don't know if he's living or dead. We just lost track of each other. I've tried to locate him, but he hasn't been in the same city where I tried to contact him.

Jay: What about now? Tell me a bit about life now.

Tom: Right now, it's pretty good.

Jay: Could you tell me a bit more about it?

Tom: Well, I get medical care now and my medicine. I don't have to worry about a place to stay, my food, or anything else. It's all provided for me. I don't think I could wish for more than that at my age.

Jay: What's a typical day like for you?

Tom: In my life now? Oh brother! It's all the same. Isn't it?

Jane: I'd say.

Tom: You go to bed. You get up. You eat. And you go back to bed. We get out once in a while. It's hard to get out. We don't have a car. She's got one leg and it's hard for her to travel around and get in and out of a van. She lost her leg here [the nursing home]. She stepped on something in the bathroom, in the shower room. She's got diabetes and she got blood poisoning. So they had to amputate. They amputated twice, once below and once above the knee. Outside of that, it's just a question of eat, sleep, eat, sleep, and play bingo on Saturday. That's about it.

Jane: You do the same all the time. I'd say it's very monotonous.

Tom: You can repeat that again. It's the old sleep-and-eat routine . . . but it's home.

Jay: What does "home" mean to you?

Tom: Home? Well, Jay, a place where my wife and I could have a place together. Wherever she's at is home for me. But I didn't want to break up the house until I knew she was settled and . . .

Jay: How long have you been here then?

Jane: Over a year.

Jay: You came together?

Tom: No.

Jane: I came and then he came a month later. He wanted me to see how I'd like it.

Tom: I didn't want to break up the house until I knew she was settled and liked where she was. So I wouldn't move for a month. Then after that, I sold everything out and moved here.

Jay: How did you decide that? I mean how did you feel when you were making that decision?

Tom: The only thing that went through my mind was that I wanted to be with her wherever she was. I don't want to be alone. What was good for her, I figured was good enough for me. But I waited to make sure that she became acclimated to the place and was sure she was going to stay. There was no sense of me going and then turning around and having to leave and start a new life again, another apartment or another home or something else. I figured I'd make sure she liked it. So I came.

She was here a month ahead of me. I missed her. It wasn't home when she was out of the house. I mean if she was there, it would have been fine. I had a good home when she was there. We took turns cooking and baking. I don't feel . . .

Jane: I wouldn't want to be here alone either. I think I'd feel more institutionalized than I would otherwise, I mean if I was alone here.

Jay: You don't feel what, Tom?

Tom: With her I don't feel that way. I feel, well, we've got a home here; we're together. I mean at my age, going on eighty-three, I'm not asking much more than that . . . just to be together with her and love her up. Where she is, is fine with me. You know how it is. Ya got a lot to share, yap about, and all.

While Fairhaven is now home, it has its disadvantages. As the next extract shows, Tom and Jane feel sorry for, but also are irritated by, the presence of the demented. And as others do, Tom and Jane complain about the food. Still, as Jane remarks, "We try to make it a good life." Here and throughout the interview, Tom and Jane seem to be saying that, despite the disadvantages, home is now and their life together is secure for the time being. At the very least, Jane says that she knows this in her mind, if not always in her heart. Both accept the realities of their situations and are grateful that their special circumstance—being together as husband and wife—make it better than it otherwise might be, this quality of their lives overshadowing the qualities of care.

Tom: This is home now. They have very nice people here. We're together. Ninety percent of them [residents] are very compatible. Wouldn't you say that?

Jane: I would, except the ones that are around the other end.

Tom: Yeah. That's a different section altogether, the other end.

Jane: They have . . . what is that . . . Alzheimer's disease.

Tom: God, I wish they'd find a cure for that.

Jane: They can't remember things. You can't talk to them because they don't know what you're talking about. It can be annoying. But there are some here that have their senses. They do talk. They are friendly.

Tom: Yes, on this end.

Jane: On this end, there are very nice people here. And you try to get along, you know, try to be compatible. At least we've got each other for now . . . [endearingly] that big hunk over there.

Tom: I wouldn't be here alone. I wouldn't have come. I would have taken a room some place as long as I was able to take care of myself.

Jane: Like he said, at least in the apartment, we did our cooking and I baked. The food could be better here. But we helped each other. But then I was prone to falling a lot. I fractured three bones up here in my left side. I was always falling. Then he had the heart attack and we couldn't help each other as much as we did before.

So a daughter of mine came down and they knew what the setup was, you know, me falling and all of them worried about it and worried about his heart attack and we couldn't help each other. She started looking around. She suggested a home of some kind, where we could be taken care of. If I did fall, at least I was at some place where we could be taken care of. So this daughter went around looking at different places and we decided on this place.

Like he said, I came here and I stayed a month and it was okay. The only thing I'm against and still am is their food, their eating habits. But, like everything else, you make the best of it, you accept it, and that's all. I mean this is the place when you get old and you have to be someplace where you can be taken care of. So you take the bad with the good. We get our medication. We have a nurse on duty twenty-four hours a day. My doctor comes every twenty-eight days. If I need him before that, the nurse calls him and he comes. So I mean, actually, we have everything. They have a beautiful garden and all outside, where you can sit under an umbrella or just go out and sit. And like he said, we have bingo once a week. And I have PT [physical therapy]. When I put my prosthesis on, I go in there and I walk around and that. We get out once in a while. We have friends here that will take us out to dinner to Red Lobster or one of those places which we like very much to go. And we have each other. So, all in all, I mean we try to make it a good life.

Up here [points to her head], I know it's home. Where else am I going to go? My children are scattered all over Maryland and North Carolina.

Tom: We wouldn't live there anyway.

Jane: And I wouldn't live with them. They'd have to take care of me and all that. It's a big job. My one daughter . . . before she moved to Maryland, she suggested taking a larger home, one that had a smaller home next to it, so that I could have my own place. We were against it because, you know, you get set in your ways and you don't like to be obligated to anybody. You like to be by yourself and be independent.

Tom: We're better off here by ourselves.

Jane: Eventually, we'd have to come to something like this anyway, because, after all, you don't want to depend upon your children to do for you. They have enough taking care of their own needs. So here we are and this is home. We know that.

Tom: Yes, until the black man comes along and takes us away.

Jane: A who man?

Tom: A guy with a Black Maria. The hearse.

Jane: Oh . . . well, here we are anyway.

       I was alone a month and I didn't like it no how. I was in with another woman and I was looking forward to him coming. They set us up in this room and it's fine. At least we're together.

Tom: Yep, that's the main thing.

Jane: That's right, you rascal. [Squeezes Tom's arm] So this is home.

Jay: In your mind, what makes a home?

Jane: A home is a husband and love and understanding and just doing for one another. Love of course . . . you've got that more than being just friends. Keeps us going. It counts for a lot.

       I help him as much as I can. Like you see he helped me when I was in the bathroom. I can't always manipulate with one leg. So I have to have help. At least he helps me. The girls [aides] can't come in always. They don't answer the [call] light when I put it on. So he helps me. If it wasn't for him, I don't know where I'd be. So he's a lot of help. And we have a lot of love for each other, like I said, and we need each other. I wouldn't want to be here without him, like he wouldn't want to be here without me. So that's it.

       But, like I said, if I could only do the cooking myself, I'd get in that kitchen and show them how to cook. I suggested that each resident get a chance in the kitchen . . . one day in the kitchen. Then maybe we'd get some decent meals.

Tom: [Chuckling] They've got a chicken farm on that side [of the nursing home] and a rice paddy on this side. Chicken and rice, everyday. [All laugh]

Jane: It seems that we have a lot of chicken and a lot of rice. You get tired of that after a while.

Tom: We send out and get dinners once in a while, have dinner delivered to us.

Jane: We send out . . . what's the name of that place?

Tom: Lorenzo's.

Jane: Lorenzo's. He likes sausage and peppers. So he gets a submarine and we cut it in half and each has half, and diet Coke or something like that.

Tom: Neither one of us could eat one of those alone.

Jay: Those are big. I don't think I could finish one of those.

Jane: Too big! And sometimes I get an order of spaghetti or something like that. We'll get something else or whatever.

Tom: We've got a microwave and a refrigerator. So we're not going hungry.

Jane: So that's our life. It's our life, period. I mean, where else can we go? We wouldn't go with any one of the children. We can't get an apartment. So once we're out of here, that's it.

Tom: I figure we're a family ourselves, the two of us. Of course, we have our children.

Jane: I had a nice family. I had five children. I lost a daughter in Texas and I have four now. They all took to Tom. They all met him and like him.

Tom: They think the world of me.

Jane: We have a full life, no matter.

Daily, yet minor annoyances are discussed, as are their room's conveniences. Jane repeats the many ways in which Tom helps her—in the bathroom, in the dining room, as she puts it, "just everywhere." Tom tells of the handiness of having a microwave and refrigerator. He's especially fond of salami, which he stores in the refrigerator and snacks on at all hours.

Jane: There're little things like you'd expect that can be annoying. [Elaborates] Things like that. I'll keep the door [of the room] closed all the way because people come by in wheelchairs and look in.

Tom: You'd be surprised. They'll stop and gawk at you. They'll turn around, come right up to the door, and stare right into the room.

Jay: Is that right?

Jane: So we keep it closed and keep the curtain open a little so's we can get some light from that there window. During the night, it's dark, but you do get some light from the outside. If we need anybody, we just press the button over there and the light goes on. Eventually, somebody comes in to see what we need.

Tom: They're not too bad with that, just the times when they're short-handed, they're busy. I've been out in the hall and I've seen these lights lit up all along the hallway like a Christmas tree. Four or five lights at once. You wonder how they can take care of them all at once.

Jane: They have different lights. In the bathroom it's a light that flickers. This light here is just one light that stays on. So they know what that is. If you're in the bathroom and you have the light on, they know you have to have somebody quick. Sometimes I go in myself and I fall. That's why my PT therapist said, "Don't go in the bathroom alone. Don't get off the chair alone. Especially, once you're on the commode, don't get off by yourself."

Tom: I'm here to help you, baby.

Jane: Yes, I know, dear. [Blows him a kiss] He helps me, just everywhere. At least we have each other. We yap about stuff we used to do and things like that. That keeps you going. So we have it made as far as that goes. He helps me quite a bit.

Tom: We have a friend . . . his son has multiple sclerosis and we've gotten to know him real well. So when he visits, he says if we need anything, write it down and he'll get it for us. He's taken us shopping too. We got little cans of stew, spaghetti, hash, and things like that. I can warm it up in the microwave. I have permission to use the microwave. So I can warm it up in there.

Jane: He got two pounds of salami and bread, pickles, olives, and different things.

Tom: The salami kid!

Jane: [Laughing] Yeah. The minute he gets the salami, he's always . . .

Jay: Nibbling away, huh?

Jane: He's what they call a "nosher."

Tom: I love salami.

Jane: He doesn't look it, but he does alright. Except he doesn't eat his meals and that's bad. But he eats what we have in the refrigerator and that makes up for it.

Tom: I'll never starve.

Jane: You sure won't. But I'd sure miss him and his salami.

This soon leads to an affirmation of love, which they describe retrospectively as their having been drawn by fate from their youths. Theirs is an attraction deeper than friendship, something that Tom says gives him "goose bumps." This is their special circumstance, the horizon from which they speak of life.

Tom: [To me] Do you know that all our life we lived a few blocks from each other when we lived in New York?

Jane: But we didn't know one another.

Tom: We shopped at the same stores all our life. I played basketball and she came to the basketball games.

Jane: We went to the same restaurants. We went to the same hotel dancing. We shopped at the same A&P, but we never bumped into each other. I never knew him.

Tom: All our life we were close together, like we were meant to meet someday and here we are finally.

Jane: When he first saw me, he said to himself, "I have to meet that woman." And he did. We met in May and he asked me to marry him in June and July we got married. Twelve gloriously happy years.

Tom: I couldn't let you get away from me, like all those years.

Jane: You couldn't, huh? Why not?

Tom: You still give me goose bumps.

Jane: I still give you goose bumps. That's a good sign if you still get goose bumps!

SUE AND DON HUGHES

Sue and Don Hughes are interviewed by Carol Ronai five weeks after they are admitted to Westside Care Center. Sue Hughes is an eighty-one-year-old white woman with congestive heart failure, chronic back pain, and arthritis that confines her to a wheelchair. Don Hughes is white, eighty-eight years old, and suffers from prostate cancer and heart failure. Don is legally blind but ambulatory. It is their first and only marriage, which has lasted for sixty-three years.

Like the Malingers, the Hugheses live in a standard double room, but without comparable household conveniences. Of course, they are relative newcomers to the facility. It is possible that in time the room may resemble the Malingers' and perhaps in the same way represent home. It is clear from the couple's remarks about what makes a home that such conveniences, personal items, and other concrete markers of one's former life would make a difference. They resent what they perceive as the facility's resistance to the personalization of their premises.

The couple has a negative view of Westside's quality of care. Some of this refers to what they believe are improvable qualities. Some stems from what they admit no institution can do, namely, personalize care so that each and every resident's needs and desires are uniquely met. Sue and Don lament having been placed in the home, but at the same time realize that they could not have continued to make it on their own. Aching to realize domestic intimacy in the context of the nursing home, they confront dead ends at every turn. As their judgments are linked with all of these sources, it is difficult to sort out how Westside's quality of care by itself relates to the couple's sense of the quality of their lives.

As sad as their lives seem to be, the couple has a light-hearted, teasing relationship. They delight and respond with good-humored sarcasm to each other's opinions and sentiments. They even joke about their current situation. This, too, complicates the quality of their lives, just as it enriches their narrative. It is evident at the very start of the interview as Don tells "his" life story, unwittingly ignoring what Sue insists is her part in it, even while she initially helps him along in the account.

Carol: [To Don] I was hoping you'd tell me about your life.
Don: I was a hobo!
Carol: You were a hobo.
Sue: [To Don] Why don't you tell her where you born.
Don: I was born in Minnesota and I left Minnesota when I was 16 years old.
Sue: Go on. So why did you leave?
Don: Just to bum, see the country. So we went, another boy and myself, we went out west on the Northern Pacific Railroad. We was supposed to help put in signal posts. We worked there for a while and then went to Sheridan, Wyoming, and went from there up into the mountains. After that, we came home riding the rails.

I stayed home for a couple a years and then a buddy of mine says, "Let's go to Florida." At that time, I says, "No." I knew a girl and her father was moving to California and he asked me if I'd drive his Ford there and I said, "Sure." So a buddy and me drove out to California, but when we got to the desert, the car broke down. We fixed it and drove to Sacramento. [Elaborates] We stayed up there for about three months. We moved around and worked in a mine. It was hard work and we finally opened up this old mine and went down in it. After that, we built a two-story garage for a Chinaman. He got all the lumber and bricks from the old California state capitol because they were building a new one.

Just about that time they had hoof-and-mouth disease in California and it was terrible. [Elaborates] So we come back to Minnesota. I stayed home for about a year. I was working on a farm for a rich gentleman. Anyway, he was going to sell the place out to Ford Motor Company and he did. So the superintendent of the farm asked me to take some of the registered Jersey cows up into Massachusetts where he lived. He couldn't find nobody to ride the box car and so I said that I'd do it. It was a fairly nice journey. [Elaborates] So I stayed there for a couple of months. Hunting season in Minnesota was open the fifteenth of September and I wanted to get home. The superintendent gave me the money and I went, took the train home, went hunting, and so on.

That January, my buddy called and says, "Let's go to Florida." That time I says, "Fine." So we left the seventh of January and it was fifteen below in Eau Claire, Wisconsin. We were supposed to sleep in the car. Well, it was pretty cold, but we finally got down into Florida. He had been in the army and the government was allocating homestead exemptions in Florida at the time. He thought he might want one. We looked all over and there was nothing but swampland where we looked. So I came to this part of Florida here and we both were working. That's where I met my wife and that's the end of my life story.

Sue: [Sarcastically] Why don't you tell her that we got married in the meantime? I'm part of it, too, you know.

As Don continues, Sue teasingly insists that the story be based on their life together. While his version initially dwelled on work experiences, the story now includes marriage, house, home, and family living. The nursing home part of their story will be similar. For example, each will differentially collaborate in formulating an answer to the question of why the facility is not home. We return to the interview as Don ends a lengthy description of his many years working as a mason contractor in Milwaukee.

Carol: Was this after the depression?
Don: The depression was . . .
Sue: It was just over.
Don: I walked ten miles to work for ten cents an hour. But you know I had a

family and I wasn't lazy. But, anyway, after I worked for this fella, we had a big snow storm, eighteen inches of snow in Milwaukee, and it tied up everything for four days. [Elaborates] So we decided to come back to Florida. Of course, I went into business for myself and built a couple of churches and other buildings. [Elaborates] We enjoyed life. She had penicillin poisoning a couple of times. When I retired, I thought we had money to last.

Sue: You forgot to tell her one thing, that we built our own home stick by stick and every nail.

Don: Yeah. Anyway, our money didn't last. I got so's I couldn't work too much anymore and she got sick two or three more times.

Sue: [Chuckling] Just listen to him. In the meantime we had three more children. [Sarcastically] Remember that?

Don: Yeah, in the meantime we had three more children. But that's all. That's it.

Sue: [Laughing] That's it? You're joking.

Don: [Chuckling] This much I can tell ya. We've been married sixty-three years and enjoyed every bit of it. We worked together and never left. For instance, she had a bunch of girlfriends and she never went out at night. And I had boyfriends and I wouldn't go out at night. If we went to any place, we went together.

Sue: We traveled together. We went all over the country together. We didn't have such a bad life. We loved to camp. We loved to fish. We loved to do all kinds of outdoor sports. We like baseball, football. Name it. And we did all the things together. We never went to one place and let the other fella go another place.

The conversation turns to economic hard times, the money they thought was adequate for their retirement years, and the rude awakening that frailty and sickness brought along. Yet, as Don notes, aside from this, theirs was a "perfect marriage." Nursing home placement, however, soured this, even beyond the hardships of the depression, according to Sue.

Don: But inflation come along and, uh, I don't know if you know about it, but it was tough. I don't mind telling you that we had our home and over $50,000 and I thought, well, we can live on that. But with inflation and the way we was used to living, it just went.

Sue: And sickness. My sickness alone has cost us a fortune.

Don: Well, you wasn't sick any more than I was.

Sue: Yeah, but yours was little compared to mine. I was sick from so far back, it wasn't funny.

Don: I had a prostate operation and I had an operation on my heel. I fell off a ladder and broke it. I had an operation for kidney stones . . .

Sue: And on his eyes.

Don: She finally ended up in here and I'm trying to get up to the idea of being up here with her and accept the idea that I can't stay at home. But, other than that, we had a perfect marriage. And we're still in love, let's put it that way. We gab, too. So that helps pass the time. And that's the story.

Sue: We had a lot of fun together—the traveling, the fact that we had four nice kids, fourteen grandchildren, and twenty-four great-grand-children. There's a bunch of us.

Carol: That does sound perfect.

Don: Until we came up here. They don't do anything for you. You ask them to do something and they ignore you like a dirty shirt.

Sue: No, they say, "In a minute." Yeah, this is different. Before this, we had the life of Riley.

Don: [To Sue] After the depression don't forget.

Sue: Yeah, well, living through the depression wasn't bad. We had something to eat. We had a place to sleep. It wasn't the pleasantest in the world, but we were happy. We had fun. We loved to play cards together. We did all kinds of things together. What more could you want? Right now, if you were to compare everything with what we had during the depression, I don't know . . . I believe I'd take the depression.

Don: Yeah.

Sue: At least we were free to come and go.

The nursing home's quality of care and the quality of life are discussed. The depression continues to be used as a negative baseline for placing the home's quality of life lower. The Hugheses are disappointed and angry that Westside does not offer a better living environment. At times, their view, especially Sue's, of what would be desirable comes close to being a description of the Malingers' living situation at Fairhaven, which has the conveniences of home right in their room. At other times, complaints about the quality of care are about institutional living in general, not Westside in particular. This extends to the ailments that caused them to be placed in a nursing home in the first place.

As the following extended extract suggests, quality of life for Don more nearly references freedom to come and go, while for Sue it falls in the area of household conveniences, reflecting both earlier life experiences and their differential concerns with family living and home life. It would seem that the difference is as much historical as it is individual in that the Hugheses' is still a generation of couples in which men worked outside the home and women tended the household and saw to the family. Future generations of nursing home residents are likely to show less clear-cut differences in narrative linkages between spouses.

A further complication comes in what initially appears to be a racist attitude toward the nursing staff. According to Don and Sue, the black nurses and aides don't much care about the residents. But we also are told that the staff is "there to making a living," which underscores the fact that institutional caregiving is as much a job as it involves caring, race notwithstanding. Indeed, we soon learn that black staff members can be especially caring, enhancing the quality of daily life in the facility.

We return to a discussion prompted by questions about the typical day of the nursing home resident and about everyday life a year from now.

Carol: Describe to me a typical day in your life now.

Don: Oh, boy. I go to bed with the chickens and get up with the chickens. That's about the only thing. There's nothing to do. We get television . . . This is not for us. We're not used to something like this. We're not used to being cooped up.

Sue: We're not used to eating somebody else's food. We like our own.

Don: I never . . . she had surgery on her back.

Sue: My spine.

Don: Four years ago. It's going on four years and four months. It didn't prove successful. She's been practically an invalid all that time. In the meantime, she got arthritis in both hips and so on. We were home. I done the cooking and that ain't my cup of tea, but I done the best I could. When it comes to salting something, I couldn't see how much salt I put in because I was declared legally blind. We got along fine, but we kept getting worse and getting sick and going to the hospital.

Sue: I was allergic to everything. And I was in intensive care. Believe it or not, I swallowed all of my teeth.

Carol: Oh for goodness sakes.

Don: They just fell out, broke off. Yeah, that happened.

Carol: What do you think life will look like a year from now?

Don: I don't think I'll be here. I don't think she will be either. Because I have a rapid heartbeat and when that comes, it's bad. And she had cardiac, allergies, and back trouble and so on. So I don't think we will live . . . especially if we're up here [in the nursing home]. If we could be home together, which the kids don't want us to do, I think it might last a little longer, but I doubt it. I'm living on borrowed time.

Carol: You say that so fearlessly.

Don: Oh, it don't scare me. I know I'm living on borrowed time.

Sue: Listen, if you have lived as long as we have and had as much fun as we've had, death you know is coming.

Don: Well, it's like I said. We've had a wonderful marriage and death doesn't bother me at all. I don't know if it bothers her.

Sue: No, it doesn't.

Don: It don't bother me. So I'm ready to go. We got our cemetery lots out there in Clarkston and . . .

Sue: We don't owe anybody anything. [Pause] But we'd be happier if we could be out at home.

Don: But they [the children] won't let us out. My son says, "No, you got no business out there."

Sue: We can't afford to have somebody to stay with us. So we can't be at home.

Carol: What does the word *home* mean to you?

Don: Everything in the world. Her home is our home and [sings] be it ever so humble, there's no place like home.

Carol: Is this at all like home?

Don: No. No way. This is just like a prison.

Carol: What could they do to make it seem more like home?

Sue: Put a little icebox over there so's we could have some Coke. If that isn't silly, but it would help. You could put Coke in there. You could put fruit juice, tomato juice. We're used to having that at home. If they'd allow us to have . . . well, they're just small iceboxes, refrigerators . . . right there in that space.

Don: They told us this morning that the state wouldn't allow it. So I told my son not to get it.

Sue: I think it's stupid.

Don: Well, really, I tell ya, the way I look at it, this is . . . a place like this is nothing but a place to die. Everybody's in a wheelchair. So you can understand my position. If I was home, it'd be a whole lot better . . . and she was with me.

    I didn't like the idea of coming here, but our son, he put in a lot of time and a lot of work to finding this for us and we didn't want to disappoint him. He said that he couldn't see us everyday either because he lives down in Norris.

Sue: I resent what they [nursing home staff] pulled on us last week.

Don: You ask the nurse for something and she says, "Maybe we'll call the doctor." They don't call them. I asked the next day, "Did you call the doctor?" She says, "We couldn't get him." Well, I know they could if they tried, but they just don't take the time to do it.

Sue: We're not allowed to use the phone. You got to go and ask for permission. Another thing I resent when we came in here was the first week we came in here, they came and gathered all our clothes.

Don: Yeah, they took them down and washed them and we never got half of them back.

Sue: No, they didn't wash them. They took them down and sterilized them. They stripped us and put a hospital gown on. He sat five solid hours in a chair with no clothes on. He couldn't even get in his bed. It wasn't made. They sterilized the bed.

    And that's not the worst part of it. They took our clothes out of the closet. They took them downstairs and they put 'em in three bags. I saw them when they did it and marked the bags "Hughes." I'm not going to wear them damn things like that.

Don: Don't get yourself worked up. Take it easy now. It's not *that* important.

Sue: They were satin. They're gone. And they've marked everything. They got no business taking our stuff and marking them up like that.

If they could tape them, I'd go along with that. Put it inside the collar or sew it in. If they had given me the tabs, I would have written on them and sewed it in. But you can look at them [her clothing]. They're up there. If I was to replace those housecoats today, they would cost me $50 a piece.

Don: And this morning I asked for towels and they didn't get them. When I asked them at noon, they still hadn't got them. So the nurse went out and got them.

Sue: I asked her for two cups of hot water . . .

Don: . . . and she hasn't got it yet. I tell you, to be honest with you, it's a prison. It's just a place to come up here and die, by the looks of all the patients.

Sue: It's changed our way of living.

Don: It's free living but I don't like that at all. I never was used to something like that and never will be. Even when I was on the bum, it was a whole lot better than it is here.

Sue: You know, I wouldn't mind them cleaning my stuff if I thought it was necessary. But why did they have to mark the stuff up like that on the corner and let it sit there hour after hour. They ruined our clothes. My pillowcases too; I had them all embroidered. And there were two satin housecoats I'll never get replaced.

Don: It's bad. All those people in wheelchairs. I hate to knock the place, but you ask some of these black ladies [aides] for something and they ignore you like a dirty shirt. And there's very few white people on the floor.

Sue: There are some real nice ones here. Don't misunderstand us.

Carol: Do you see that as part of the problem, the race thing?

Sue: No.

Don: No, no. I was always a champion of the black man, but in the last ten years I've changed my mind.

Sue: The best friend we ever had was a black, but that isn't it. It's the fact that they just don't care here. They're here to make a living. I know that. You know it too. If somebody don't call their crane, then they just don't do it, regardless. The best one is Sylvia and she's black.

Don: Yeah, but that little girl that's on . . . Saturdays I believe . . . she helps.

Sue: I think she's a nurse's aide. She's black and better than the white ones. They can be when they try . . . and that can help.

Don: Well, anyway, Sue hadn't had a BM movement for four days and she's [the aide] the only one that would help. She told the rest of those nurses, white and black, "We'll see about it. We'll call the doctor." Another day goes by and Sue hasn't had a BM. But this little girl, she really helped out, didn't she?

Sue: Yes, she did. It was kind of ridiculous the way it happened anyhow. She actually had to pull it out by hand. Well, I had gone seven days.

Don: These places are all alike
Sue: You're right about that.

As the interview winds down, the mood lightens. Don and Sue tease each other, conjuring up their respective foibles and confirming their mutual affection. In this framework, quality of care is marginal to the "sassiness" they call out in each other. Now they are not as much nursing home residents attuned to caregiving as they are the Don and Sue they have delighted in over the years.

Don: I'm a hellcat.
Sue: [Sarcastically] You can complain, but you ain't no hellcat. He's lying in his teeth.
Carol: What do you mean by being a hellcat, Don?
Don: Well, I loved to chase around. I wasn't a woman chaser, but I just loved to go, be on the go.
Sue: [Scoffing] I couldn't prove he wasn't a woman chaser.
Don: [Chuckling] I was a no-good bum.
Sue: He's no bum. We're just as close as we were before and I love him. He's the only thing that makes this place tolerable. But he gets sassy sometimes and I have to knock him down a peg or two, but other than that, we still have fun together. He plays cribbage and cheats, but we still manage to get by. We gab and blab, about the old days, you know. That keeps us goin'.
Don: But this isn't the place for us. That's all I can say. It's too much like prison. If I didn't have her, I'd go crazy and so would she. [Elaborates] At least we have each other.
Sue: I know, dear. We've had a good life, but now we're bitching like the devil. [Chuckling] I hope *that* isn't on the tape.
Carol: Well, it is.
Don: [To Sue, sarcastically] You mean to say you're not "itching" now?
Sue: [Chuckling] I didn't say "itching." I said "bitching." We still manage to giggle.

* * * * *

Once again, we hear complex narrative linkages being made between shared meaning and the qualities of care and life. The marriages that are a couple's special circumstance are a horizon that can, in the Malingers' case, retroactively extend the meaning of the statement "as long as we are together" into early life. According to the Malingers, being together in their room, intimately living out their days in the nursing home, is a relationship with very old roots. The Hugheses narratively link the qualities of care and life in their facility with their room's lack of domestic amenities and the shoddy staff treatment, but still manage to joke about their respective complaints. The couple resents, but understands the reason why they have had to be placed in a nursing home. Positive, negative, and even humorous linkages make it impossible to understand the subjective quality of their current lives in terms of better/worse, either/or, more/less, and similar binary descriptors typical of conventional assessment.

10

Disabled

Three elderly white women with long-standing disabilities present another special circumstance. One of them, Grace Wheeler, now seventy years old, has been afflicted since birth by spastic paralysis, a form of cerebral palsy. The second woman, Opal Peters, who is seventy-six years old, has been disabled by rheumatoid arthritis for thirty-five years and is unable to walk. Celia Turner, the third woman, is sixty-four years old, has had multiple sclerosis for forty years, and sits in a wheelchair when she's not in bed.

The women have brought their experience with disability with them into the facilities where they now live. Disability is a central horizon of their everyday lives, significantly mediating the subjective meaning of being a nursing home resident. For Grace Wheeler, the meaning of being a nursing home resident is articulated in linkages with the security of supportive and caring parents and siblings, who in Wheeler's view made it possible for her to live a normal life except for her disability. She speaks of the future in similar terms, looking ahead to, and yet being worried about continued security. Opal Peters views herself as on a mission for the handicapped. Peters hosts a radio program called "Perspectives of the Handicapped," the purpose of which is to inform listeners that one can "fight" a disability, not let it win, and make contributions to life. Celia Turner likewise has a mission, partly informed by a lifetime of writing and similarly rooted in the need to show that even frail nursing home residents can realize new meanings, "reinventing" themselves in the process.

While, for these women, nursing homes have both their good and bad points, which affect the quality of care, the homes are viewed mainly as a base of support for other concerns. The facilities enable them to attend to lifelong interests and long-standing goals. It is not so much the quality of care that is at stake for them in discussions of institutional living, as it is the ability to carry on as before, for which the facilities seem to provide adequately.

GRACE WHEELER

Grace Wheeler's paralysis usually keeps her sitting awkwardly in a wheelchair. During the interview, she was lying in bed because she had hurt her back from the strain caused by the coughing of a cold. According to Wheeler, her muscles tighten excessively at times and this puts pressure on her spine, which is worsened by coughing. Wheeler never married, was raised in a rural area of Ohio, and was family tutored.

Wheeler's mother, Lucy, is ninety-three years old, widowed, and shares her daughter's room in the nursing home. Lucy suffers from high blood pressure and emphysema. No longer able to care for daughter Grace on her own, Lucy nonetheless continues to do "little things" for her, such as getting Grace a glass of water and soothingly wiping her face with a damp cloth.

I interview mother and daughter together in their room at Bayside, the facility in which they've lived for a year and a half. Grace's life story is a narrative of happy times spent in the company of friends and family members. When Grace recounts the sacrifices her disability caused, she is remorseful, as if to tell me that while she cheerfully made the best of her handicap, she does recognize what she missed in life. The support of family members and the security of home are narrative linkages throughout.

     Jay: Why don't we start by your telling me about your life?
   Grace: Well that was quite a many years ago. I was born in Brinton Station, Ohio.
   Lucy: She was a seven-month baby.
   Grace: I was a seven-month baby. That's what it was. Anyway, my childhood, I guess, was as happy as it could be under the circumstances . . . I had two younger sisters that played with me a lot and an older brother that took care of me like a girl. He was wonderful. They've all been wonderful.
   Lucy: They taught her . . .
   Grace: And they taught me as well as my mom and dad. And then when radio and television came to the farm, why I learned from them. I loved the quiz shows.
   Lucy: She types with a stick in her mouth.
   Grace: I type with a stick in my mouth. I paint with a brush in my mouth. I turn pages of the book . . . I read with a stick in my mouth. And I've been to Oregon, on a trip with my sisters. That was quite a flight. I flew over there in . . . what was it . . . 1952.
   Lucy: I don't remember.
   Grace: I think it was 1952. And then we left the farm and moved to Wooster, Ohio.

Lucy: Down where Wooster College is.

Grace: Yeah. And I'm a great [Cleveland] Indians fan, too! I love baseball and I love the Indians. For football, I love the Miami Dolphins.

Jay: So you're a real sports fan.

Grace: Yes.

Lucy: Yes, she is. That television's on . . .

Grace: I love it!

Lucy: That television's all sports to her.

Grace: Well, sports and shows. [Giggling] I love animal shows, too. I love animals.

Lucy: Game shows.

Grace: Game shows, animal shows, detective stories. I like to read detective stories. My favorite author is John D. McDonald.

Jay: That sounds enjoyable. [Pause] You were telling me about Ohio before . . .

Grace: Well, after I grew up, then the rest of the family . . . It was just Mom and Dad 'cause the rest of the family moved out and got work, got jobs. They got married. We moved down to Fort Lauderdale [Florida] and Mom and Dad bought a little home for us. When we couldn't handle it any longer, why we moved in with my sister and brother-in-law. They were wonderful to us.

And I've had a lot of friends. I make friends easy. And I love to be with people. I love people.

Jay: Yes, I can see that.

Grace: And I really like my sense of humor. If it weren't for my sense of humor, I don't think I could get through this life.

So, as I was telling you, we moved into with them, with my sister and brother-in-law.

Lucy: No, we didn't move in with them. We moved in the cottage behind their house.

Grace: [To Lucy] No, no, no, Mother! I'm talking about Jack and Kitty.

Lucy: Oh, Jack and Kitty.

Grace: That was after Daddy couldn't do it anymore. Jack and Kitty gave us three of their rooms for our own place, like our own place. We ate, we took meals with them, but we had our own quarters. See, my daddy had to have his left leg amputated. So we moved in there with them. And then we lived there until my sister passed away. So then we moved in with my brother and his wife. From there, we moved up to South Carolina with my youngest brother and his wife. He had a little cottage back there, a two-bedroom cottage that we lived in, my mother and I. Dad had passed by then. We didn't care too much for it there because it was . . . [chuckles] it was out in the boonies. And then we moved in here. We came here. We thought this was the best place for us.

Lucy: Two years in June.

Grace: Now nobody has to worry about us too much and we are well taken care of here and, well, I like to be, as I said, I like to be with people. Mother doesn't too much. She stays and does what she can for me. She can't do too much for me yet. Does little things for me like give me a drink or, you know, things like that. [Pause]

Jay: Grace, if you were given a chance to write the story of your life, what would the chapters be about? Let's say the first chapter . . . what would that be about?

Lucy: Growing up.

Grace: Well, I'd have to think about it. [Pause] The first chapter . . . the first thing I remember real distinctly is parading around the . . . riding with my mother and my grandmother up to the next town to get some feed ground.

Jay: Some what?

Grace: Some feed ground for the animals.

Lucy: Grain ground for feed.

Jay: What about the second chapter?

Grace: My teenage years, I guess. That wasn't very funny, seeing all the other girls going out and having fun and I couldn't do it. But we had some good friends anyway. They would take me riding, roll me down the streets in my wheelchair. We had a lot of fun that way. And I guess the next chapter would be Florida.

Jay: What about the last chapter?

Grace: I don't know what the last chapter will be.

Lucy: The last chapter would be here.

Grace: Yeah, here so far. They've been wonderful till I hurt my back. I don't know how I did it.

Lucy: You know how you did it.

Grace: When I get tightened up real tight, my muscles have spasms. When they tighten up, it hurts my right hip so bad that I can't sit up in my chair. I had an awful cough, too, and that made it worse. I like to be up. I don't like to be in bed. When I get rid of this back problem, it'll be back to normal. I can get up and type and read and enjoy myself again. I've gotten over the cold pretty well but it did get me down a bit.

We discuss her recent convalescence and talk about sports, especially baseball and football, which are Grace's passions. She laughs and jokes about certain television programs, everyday matters that strike her as funny, and the hilarious things that other residents and the staff do. Her humor is contagious; I find myself laughing with her.

At one point, as Grace explains how fond she is of singing, I ask her what she would have done differently if given the opportunity to live her life over again. Looking back in those terms, she considers how things might have been had it not been for her paralysis. She recalls her hopes, several dashed. She would have liked to become a singer. Yet she is thankful for the support that made possible what she was able to realize.

Grace: What would I do differently? Let's see. I'd get a good education. I always thought I could . . . before when I was younger. I could carry a tune and I thought I would like to be a singer. But, you know, in time you know you can't. I always wanted to be a mother, get married, and have children. I love children. [Pause] Just have a normal life I guess, well, maybe different than I did have. Oh, I think I'd be living in Oregon instead of Florida. I like Oregon better than I do Florida, but Florida was the best choice.

Lucy: We wasn't there long. You don't know whether you liked it or not.

Grace: I did, Mother! I loved Oregon. I didn't want to come home. But, Mother and I are inseparable. Aren't we, Mother? [Chuckles] Inseparable and insufferable, too.

Lucy: I've been her hands and her feet.

Grace: Mother is very, very important to me. My whole family has been really. Some friends, too. Jim Malloy was wonderful. Right, Mother? [Lucy nods] And Pete Sikorski taught me to paint.

Lucy: The man was a painter and taught her to paint. You know, how to mix the colors around and all that. She's done all these paintings. [Points around the room]

Grace: Yesterday, I was typing . . . at the new typewriter. I'm going to type today when I get up . . . type a note. I'll do it this afternoon. [Pause] No, I won't do it this afternoon either 'cause I'll have the Browns to watch play ball. The Cleveland Browns; they're in the playoffs. I love television. I'll go down and have breakfast with my mom and then we'll come back here and watch television. In the afternoon, I watch TV all the time because I watch soap operas. I've got three of them: *Days of Our Lives, Another World,* and *Guiding Light.* Then I watch Oprah or I watch Geraldo or one of the others.

As we talk, Grace begins to look ahead. She expresses worry over her security and remarks that supportive family members have passed from her life. She worries especially about how much longer her mother will be with her. It is in the context of continued support and security that the nursing home takes on its meaning, a place where she hopes to remain living in the way she has become accustomed. As Grace mentions at one point, as old as she is, she knows no other way.

Grace: If I'm still here, I hope I'll be doing just about the same thing I'm doing now, only with a better back I hope. [Looks at her mother] I don't know how long my mother's got to stay with me. She's been a lot of security for me, love . . . the whole family has, really. Right now, I'm all right. We're at home here.

Lucy: Anywhere's home when we're together and have a roof over our
          head and eat. We used up all our resources taking care of her. I had to
          have help to take care of her, which is . . . used up everything. So
          we're here, to be taken care of. I don't know how long. They're good
          to us. We're taken good care of and people are nice. The nurses are
          nice.

Grace: The aides are very nice.

Jay: What makes this feel like home to you?

Grace: Security, especially knowing that maybe soon no one will be around
          to take care of me, except this place will be here.

Lucy: They know that after I'm gone nobody will take care of her. So if she
          feels like this is her home, she needs to feel like she likes it here.

Grace: So this is my life now. But I still have a good sense of humor and I like
          a good laugh. I like to give somebody a good laugh. And I have a
          temper, too.

Lucy: She's a little more independent than she used to be. She used to
          depend on all of us for help for what she needed. Gettin' so's she's
          kind of being a little independent now. Tells me what to do.

Grace: Well, I've been told to watch out for my mother.

Lucy: Yes. She was . . . she led a normal life just like anybody would,
          except for she has to sit in a wheelchair all her life. But we all helped
          her one way or another.

Grace: The way I see it, you've got to make the best of what you got . . .
          doing the best you can with what you have to do it with. You know
          what I mean?

Jay: I think so.

Grace: And I had my mouth and I used it. [Laughs] In more ways than one.
          [We all laugh] Sometimes it gets me in trouble. Sometimes you can
          find my feet in it.
              My condition is funny, too. I used to take this thing here [support-
          ive bandage] and throw it around and around and if Mother didn't
          duck, it'd hit her in the head. Or I'd trip her up with my feet. [Chuck-
          ling] Just spastic, you know. I have a weird sense of humor.

Lucy: She's been that way and pretty healthy all her life. She's had a normal
          life as far as that's concerned . . . except for her condition. Even now
          that she's older, she's pretty much the same.

Jay: Is there anything you dislike about your age, Grace?

Grace: No, because I don't know any other way.

OPAL PETERS

Opal Peters has been at the Oakmont Nursing Home for four years
and lived at several other homes before that. Her disabling arthritis
relates to a different way of speaking of life. Peters is an admitted
fighter, who relentlessly acts against her disability to prove that life goes

on despite the handicap. She brings the fight into Oakmont, where she continues to broadcast her weekly radio show. For Peters, the nursing home represents one more link in a long chain of insults to her independence, which she weekly exhorts those similarly afflicted to struggle against.

Carol Ronai conducts the interview, which, among other things, features Peters's parents' missionary activity in China. In the following extract, Peters recalls her early years, the sister whom her mother favored, Peters's ambition to be a singer, and her developing arthritis. In later extracts, the parents' mission will be linked with Peters's own struggle.

I was born in New York City in 1914 and Mom and Dad at that time were in the dry cleaning and laundry business. They had returned from China where Mother and Dad met and were married. Mother was from Norway and Dad was from Hungary, but they were both born in New York City and they both went to China with separate groups, missionary groups. They met out there, and married out there.

My sister was born out there in Jungdeng Fu, just as some Chinese bandits were trying to kill off all the missionaries and Americans that they called "foreign devils." And so my parents ran across Northern Siberia over to Norway where Mother was from and got sanctuary there. Then they sailed over to New York on a boat and I was born a year and a half later after my sister. A year and a half after me, my brother was born in the same hospital and the same room, but not the same bed.

When I was about six months old, my auntie came from Norway after her mother died. Auntie lived with us and she was our grandma. She did all our sewing and cooking and cleaning and everything while Mom and Dad were doing their missionary work.

Well, in nineteen-something (I can't remember the year) we all sailed to China and while we were over there, Mother did the business work in the mission house and Daddy went out and did the preaching. Then, after the First World War, he was called over to France to clean up after the war. They had imported a bunch of Chinese coolies and Daddy could speak the language. So he was sent over there under the YMCA and I was, I guess, about five or six when we came back to New York.

Then Daddy came back from that and in 1925 he and Mother heard about Florida and the big boom. So, leaving us with Auntie, they all came down to Miami and they fell in love with it. Mother came back and sold the house lock, stock, and barrel and everybody moved to Florida. I've been here off and on ever since. Miami's been my home for sixty years. I remember when it was a nice little resort town. It's different and everybody thinks it's "Miami Vice." But I still remember Miami nice.

I got married when I was quite young because my mother doted on my sister and my sister went away to four Bible colleges during the depression under Mother's sponsorship. There wasn't enough money left for me. So when I was young, about eighteen, I got married and then I started having my children. So I couldn't do what I wanted to do with a career, like singing, which was my wish. I had taken lessons. [Elaborates] So when I got married and the children came, they were all a handful and then later on, their father (their biological father) just left and I married again. My second husband adopted the children and gave them his name. During the Second World War, he had a contract to drive these trucks and things for the government. He couldn't get the help he wanted because all the good guys were in the service. They were either too young or too old. So I was it. I had to help and we took the children right with us and traveled the road.

Then I started to contract rheumatoid arthritis, first in the left knee. We were taking a trip to California and I started to limp before we even got there. In Phoenix, Arizona, I went to a doctor and he said you've got rheumatoid arthritis, which I didn't know beans about and my family didn't either. But we soon found out and over a period of about thirty-five years, it's been up and down. I've had seven operations, an artificial knee, a fused right leg, and things like that that are not easy to live with. And so I've been in nursing homes up and down. I had my own home for a while in Miami and sold that because I couldn't do the yard work and so forth anymore. So, after my husband died, why now I'm here and I've gone from one nursing home to another.

Ronai prompts Peters to continue with her narrative by asking about the chapters of Peters's life story. It is now more decidedly a story of Peters's struggle against arthritis, its ostensible source in the hard work she did in her husband's trucking business, and advice to others based on her experience.

Carol: Let me ask you this. If you were writing a story of your life, what chapters would you have in your book. Like what would the first chapter be about?

Opal: Fighting arthritis.

Carol: Fighting arthritis? That'd be the first chapter in your book? Okay. What would the next one be about?

Opal: How to handle it. How the family can handle it and what is arthritis and what makes it do like it does and a lot of medical questions that I've asked doctors over the years and they have given me answers to. I was too late to prevent it because of the work I did. I'd say how people can prevent it by not overdoing like I did working in my husband's business.

Carol: Other chapters?

Opal: Well, other chapters would be, as you realize it's getting worse, you have to see the limitations coming on . . . to accept them. Don't run away from them. The limitations are what are hard to take, especially when you've been able to do everything. Not let the family get a feeling of guilt that they have to do it. And not letting the children overdo and do what they can't do but try to help anyway. My mission was to prevent them from getting what you've got and so forth and so on.

Carol: What about the last chapter?

Opal: The last chapter? Well, I think it's not a terminal disease. You can never get better but it doesn't happen like cancer in a hurry. So just make your years as enjoyable as you can. Fight it! I have my radio program, "Perspectives of the Handicapped," which I take an interest in and I love to do and think it's keeping me going. I've been doing that now since '72, off and on. So the last chapter is living with it and doing the best you can. Don't give up. Whatever you do, don't give up.

Carol: I'm curious. I've asked some other people the question, you know, about chapters and most of them started out with things like their childhood. I noticed you went right to the arthritis. Why do you think you did that?

Opal: Because I've lived with it a long time and I'm so familiar with it. I know what it could do to you if you let it, which I did for a while because I didn't know how to fight it. It affects how you see your whole life, straight through. Also because I think other people should be acquainted with it.

Carol: So it's been a huge thing in your life?

Opal: Oh yes! There have been times that I've had to cater to it. Just lie there and feel your bones disintegrate and you can't do anything about it. You lay there and cry and cry and cry. You don't want to put that on other people because it's not their fault. But I didn't let it win. That's my mission in life.

Ronai and Peters discuss the ups and downs of the disability, how it affected Peters's family life, and the various goals she had set for herself, all of which her handicap hampered in some way. According to Peters, her religion sustained her and now, supporting her mission, allows her to help others who are similarly afflicted. At one point, following Peters's remarks on the power of prayer and faith, Ronai asks Peters what part God plays in her life. Peters's response appropriates to her mission related images from her parents' missionary activity.

Carol: So God plays a big part in your life?

Opal: Definitely! I think that stems from my childhood. I was raised in the church. We used to go to church three times a week and twice on Sunday. We went to every Wednesday night service and I went to choir practice. My parents were missionaries and that was part of everything. It was just part of growing up.

Carol: What does all of that mean to you?

Opal: It means to me that when I need Him and even when I don't, I find myself singing hymns to Him. It's sort of a way of thanking Him for being with me and keeping me strong for what I have to do with the [radio] program and all, like it did for my parents when I was a child, it helped them in their missionary work. I hope I don't disturb my roommate but I just sing along and every Sunday I have church on the TV from 8 A.M. or from 7:30 until noontime. That's the way I spend my Sundays. I can't go to church; so it comes to me.

Carol: What does life look like from where you're at now?

Opal: I think that God has been with me and seen me through an awful lot and helped me get out on top of the last . . . because the radio program has meant so much to me. He gave me that talent where I can talk to people, try to help those that listen in, if possible.

Ronai and Peters discuss possible sponsorship for the radio program. Peters had been asked by the local radio station to get a sponsor to help with production costs. She is worried that lack of support might mean the end of the program, but also knows that she can depend on the faith that has sustained her, just as it sustained her parents.

The discussion turns to daily living at Oakmont. Peters has been resident in a number of nursing home over the years, either postoperatively or because of her arthritis-related dependency. While in Peters's opinion, Oakmont is among the better homes she's been in, none has been of central concern to her, displacing her mission in life. Peters's responses suggest that Oakmont, under the circumstances, is something to be adjusted to as a way of getting on with living, which in Peters's case is her mission.

Carol: You've lived here since September '88. Is this home?

Opal: Right now, it's all I can call home. I have a room. Didn't think I'd ever be reduced to that.

Carol: Does it feel like home?

Opal: I guess it's all I can expect. As I said, you learn to accept. It doesn't make that much difference anyhow. I've got to do what I've got to do, no matter where I am. I've thought if I won the lottery I would buy a van with a hydraulic lift and I would have somebody capable to help me up and down. [Elaborates] And I would continue with my program, but I would have it spread all over Florida. I would try to get it syndicated, something like the "Oprah Winfrey Show." I would gear it only to the needs and activities of the handicapped and try to get some kind of a transportation system so we're not prisoners in our own homes. That's the way I felt when I had my own home and I couldn't get anywhere. Then they started transportation in Miami, which was a real blessing.

Carol: Do you feel that living here is part of your life or separate from it?

Opal: Oh, it's part of it. I've learned to accept it. They do things their way and I just accept it. I remember a long time ago, Tip O'Neill, who used to be speaker of the house in Washington for years . . . he made a wise statement one time. He said that to get along, go along. I never forgot it. I had to learn to just go along.

But not for things that count! You know there have been a lot of cutbacks by the government for the handicapped and for the senior citizen. A lot of cutbacks! We don't have the help we need and some of the food, I've noticed, isn't what it should be. That shouldn't be. Instead of sending the money across the waters or up in the air, we should do something for our own, the people that put the money there. We paid for it all these years. So what are they doing with it? Pardon me for getting on the soapbox. Gotta spread the word.

CELIA TURNER

Celia Turner is fairly young as far as nursing home residents go, being sixty-four at the time Carol Ronai interviews her. Turner has been a resident at Greenfield Nursing Center for six years, since the facility opened in 1984. Born and raised in Florida, Turner formed her career as a playwright and magazine writer in New York City. She moved about the country from south to north and back again. As she became increasingly incapacitated by her multiple sclerosis and unwilling to have family members care for her, she settled in a Florida nursing home.

The self-realization of the writing process is a central narrative linkage. It is the means by which she casts her identity earlier in life, continues to define who she is, and now searches for who she can be as a woman and as a handicapped nursing home resident. Her story is imbued with the meaning of writing, as the following extract begins to show. In the last paragraph, there are hints of self-realization.

I was born here on March 8, 1928. My great-grandparents were one of the first doctor couples I guess in this country, certainly in town. My mother was a third-grade teacher and was one of the first members of the textbook committee of Florida. My father was a postal servant then. They were very active in community affairs.

I graduated from [the local] high school and went immediately to Columbia University. I had a fellowship and I went to New York with a one-way coach ticket on the train and $25 cash. My mother says that she still gets nightmares thinking about it. New York in those days was not quite as scary as it is now. That's where I met my husband.

I hit New York just at the right time because they were really trying to develop new talent. I had some plays done off Broadway and really was on that track when I had multiple sclerosis. That kind of slowed me down a bit. But the lovely thing is that a good friend became a nanny to our children. I would go to work and then come home and be there. I've always had pride in work. So I worked all the time. I guess you would say that I was sort of a nonstop writer.

Ask my kids, I was a nonstop mother, too. The kids all turned out great.

One of them, my oldest daughter, sort of followed in my footsteps, if that's the word. I had worked at *Cosmopolitan Magazine* and, a generation later, she did too. She's now the editor of her own publications in Chicago. I had five kids in all.

I worked at *Mademoiselle*. That's where my first job was. Then I worked at *Good Housekeeping* and *Cosmo*. The last was *Bride's Magazine*, where I expanded my horizons from fashion to homemaking.

Talking about myself, I think the most flattering thing I can say about myself . . . oh, I can tell you what I'm gonna have on my gravestone! Really, that's important. It was something one of my kids said, Dennis. He was taking the trash out at night, you know, putting it out on the curb and he went out and then came running back in with his eyes wide like that. He said, "Come on, Mom! Let's go take out the garbage and look at the stars." So that's going to be on my gravestone: She's going to take out the garbage and look at the stars.

Turner talks about her five children, their schooling, careers, and their own families. She's proud of them, repeating earlier remarks about the daughter who followed in her footsteps. Turner describes in greater detail the onset of her multiple sclerosis, how she managed motherhood, and developed a writing career in the process. Bringing her life story up to date, she recounts current writing projects, suddenly speaking of the potential of writing for the self.

Now it's writing, writing, writing, writing. I've got something out in two magazines now. I've published articles . . . you know I'm very ambitious. At this point, I've written five, actually six, plays. I have one, which is about a dying man. Another one, *End Time*, is about nursing home relationships, between people who work in a nursing home. I'm now working on a diary called . . . oh, I forgot to tell you that I did a cookbook, a bride's magazine cookbook. [Elaborates]

But the older I get and this handicap gets me, the more writing makes me what I am. Through writing, you make yourself up, write yourself down . . . we invent ourselves that way. Of course, the older we get, the more we have to invent. I wanted to write a book and it's going to be called *Making Myself Up and Writing Myself Down*. That's one title; the alternative title is *Entitled*, which is also a play on words. What I'm excited about is that it's a kind of self-revelation. It's very exciting. I'm on the cutting edge . . . or on the crushing edge of being able.

[Shows Ronai a magazine article] I was fascinated to find this article, which is about the way older women in this women's writing workshop wrote about life and about themselves and, in their way, put differences and similarities together to relearn who they were. I hope I can give a little something to everybody else by writing that way. I can't put my finger on it. I've begun to mysteriously come together as I read and think about what I've written about myself. I feel more useful than I have in a long time because, like perhaps I'll work on this way of writing. You know, you're inventing yourself, you're new again even if you're old.

I'm a bit of a maniac. I don't know how much of this is the old Presbyterian still wanting to make a contribution or it's a way of still finding new meaning, that you're not just used up. I don't really know what it is, but I would like to write something that would help someone besides myself to realize that.

Ronai asks Turner about the quality of daily life at Greenfield. Turner looks to her writing for the answer, her way of laying claim to what a long line of southern women before her has accomplished and that now serves to develop her own identity despite the odds. She speaks relatedly of the concrete shape of her immediate environment, particularly the appearance of her room, casting her mission accordingly, as virtually "rippling" through, time and again, what she is and intends to be, despite her MS (multiple sclerosis).

I've tailored my life here to fit what I'm about. I come from a long line of southern women—I guess you'd call them "thriving women"—who pretty much made their mark on life, regardless. You should hear my children tell it, about my life here. The minute they saw my room, they said, "Mom, your room always looks the same no matter where you are." And they don't mean that it's cluttered. They mean that I have things that I love around me, that I have them arranged in a protective way so that I can sort of nestle in them and nest them. Back there by that wall is . . . the bookcase . . . well, the books. The phone is reachable and the typewriter and the computer are here. Everything sort of works for me, all around me, where I write myself.

It's been that way all along, typical of me at any age. It represents the way I see life, like dropping a pebble in the water and the ripples go round and round. Or you drop a planet in the sky and the gases go around. Well, I'm very good at ripples and gases. I don't tend to go backwards and forwards much in time. I kind of ripple. I mean that I kind of drop that stone there and let the ripples go where they go, which makes me the stone, I guess.

I'm trying very hard to make myself understand the occurrences . . . of MS. [Elaborates] It gets in the way but it's also a background thing, the MS, that I work around, that's not going to keep me from doing what I have to do. [Pause] But I love the tactile business of hitting the keys on a typewriter or computer. I know it's there and it comes out through that. So it's all here, all around me. Wherever I am is where I live . . . I mean it's my room, my home . . . my MS. I really think this is really all I need. I've got space enough for me.

There is a long digression away from matters of daily living, to the collages and poetry that Turner has placed around her room. Turner describes the collages as "self-serving," not completely artistic, explaining that they are her way of arranging on paper, with images and poems, the way she feels about herself and life. The collages concretely renew her awareness that she is ageless, not a useless thing that has ended but one who capably continues to make meaning.

Something in the room causes Turner to giggle as she refers to the way Julia Child, the famous television cook, charmingly fumbles through food preparation and still manages to triumph in the end. The lesson is in the whole, not its parts. It is a whole whose parts, linked together creatively, can invent meaning time and again. Turner offers these final comments.

> Life is a huge and wonderful question. Me, I'm hokey, kind of a word person. I seize on what I need. So the meaning of life is looking for more little words in that great big world. I don't know how I can . . . I put everything in writerly terms. I'm sorry.
>
> One needs to grow. You have to find something, even here. You know you have the seed and you need to look around somewhere to grow up through the ground. It must hurt like you know what, to pop open. But everybody, I'm convinced, has a way that they can grow up. For me, it's through writing and everything around.
>
> I'm aware that potential in a lot of cases isn't really great. But there are people out there doing things that, every so often, I get glimpses of. I realize that what's important to me is not really the most important thing to them. There are people doing crafts. There are people playing cards. That represents to me some of the things that people can do to grow.
>
> But I can only give you subjective answers. Basically I'm egocentric and my main thing is always gonna be to try to do it my way, the way I know, to write myself.

* * * * *

For all three residents of this chapter, being disabled looms prominently in their narratives, further diversifying how the past is linked with the present and future. For Grace Wheeler, disability is a horizon that has organized the meaning of her life from the start, even while she had what is said to be a "normal" upbringing. Now in a nursing home, the quality of care is a concern that questionably links with the security family members had provided. Opal Peters's mission further articulates the horizon. For Peters, the nursing home is mainly a place to engage a life goal, which is to speak for and on behalf of the handicapped. In the context of the mission, the nursing home, notably its homeyness, "doesn't make that much difference anyhow." Celia Turner's narrative linkages center on writing, making it possible for her to invent herself in a world contained by her own immediate surroundings. All told, the special circumstance of these disabled women link the qualities of care and life in ways unaccountable by conventional assessment.

CHAPTER

11

Knowledgeable

Karen Gray, a divorced white woman now confined to a wheelchair from multiple sclerosis, spent ten years of her career as a nurse being what she calls a state "surveyor," inspecting nursing homes, hospitals, and home health agencies for quality of care. She also participated in the certification process. In addition, Gray worked professionally as a public health nurse and nurse educator. Her former husband, a doctor whom she helped through medical school, was in private practice until a stroke forced him to retire.

Gray began to have symptoms of multiple sclerosis when she was twenty-five years old and pregnant with her first child. Now aged fifty-five and our youngest respondent, the last few years of her life have left her so disabled from MS that she has been, as Gray puts it, "floating around in nursing homes." One of the homes was a facility where her own father convalesced and eventually died. As she points out, that home was "as good as any other for me," the only difference being that her father was resident there, which, she adds, "really didn't make that much difference, except that I could look in on him every so often."

Gray's special circumstance is that she is knowledgeable about nursing homes in a way most residents are not. Her adult working life dealt with matters of primary concern to this book. She not only has considered the quality of care as a professional, but has lived the subject matter of her professional considerations, personally experiencing nursing home living.

Gray is interviewed twice by Carol Ronai, the first time as a resident of Fairhaven Nursing Home, where she has lived for two months, and the second time six months later in the apartment to which she has been discharged. Her narrative shows her views of nursing home life to be mediated by two related horizons of meaning—professional and personal—which affect her judgments about all nursing homes' quality of care. As Gray puts it, when she wears her "professional hat," she orients to nursing home living in terms of state and federal "regs" (regulations), straightforwardly and unemotionally. Wearing this hat, Fairhaven for her is more nearly a health care facility than a home and leaves much to be desired. Wearing her "personal hat," Fairhaven represents a daily living environment, something narratively linked with home. When Gray is interviewed in the apartment and is asked to compare apartment living with Fairhaven, the quality of life for her in the apartment pales in comparison. While the quality of care at Fairhaven left much to be desired when she resided there, six months later Gray says that life in the nursing home "wasn't all that bad." The two hats' perspectives highlight the complex ways in which horizons of meaning can link quality of care with quality of life.

THE FIRST INTERVIEW

Initially, Gray's story is a litany of straightforward opinions, which we learn in a later extract is her way of speaking while wearing a professional hat. As many do, she organizes the story chronologically, although Gray will remark in the second interview that she might have preferred to have organized her story thematically.

I'll try to sort of pull it together and try to do it sort of chronologically. I was born January 15, 1935, in Massachusetts in an upper-middle-class household that I detested thoroughly. I went to an assortment of schools. I started out in public school. I was diagnosed as having rheumatic fever, but I don't know if this is really, truly true. My parents ran me into a really weird, private situation. It [the school] was sort of a little concentration camp for several years. I came out of that and I was in public school for a couple of years. My parents didn't think that the people I was running around with were appropriate. So I ended up in one of the best girl's schools in the East, where I did grade eight through twelve. I was reasonably miserable. But I had a love of horses that was always with me. Oh golly.

When I was eighteen, we had a college decision to make. I was turned down at Duke. I was accepted at Middlebury. And out of total desperation, I got accepted at the University of Mississippi. My father was Mississippian; my mother was from Kansas. She floated around. So I moved down to Mississippi at eighteen, married some of the local talent in '55. I ended up in nursing school the summer of '59. Then I was pregnant with my child and was diagnosed with MS, you know, big deal. I worked while I was in school. I supported, basically, my husband Jake, and I had a fairly decent allowance. I sent half to him; he was busy flunking out of medical school on a fairly repetitive basis. He finally went through and it was in his senior year that our son Jim was born. I laid out for a little while and then went back to work.

Later on, Jake started to get funny on me. I was doing public health nursing at that point. He was making fairly good money, but he decided he wanted to do his internship in a residency in Richmond, Virginia, because one of his friends went there. So he took off, actually on our anniversary, and left me with two kids. After a while, I followed him. We eventually got settled. [Elaborates] I was teaching nursing after a while, med-surg. Then Jake decided he wanted to go into private practice. So we moved back to Mississippi and I had probably one of the worst periods of depression in my whole life because all my friends at this point were in Virginia.

So here I am with two kids, no job, confined to a house, and not adjusting. I got a little obstinate and decided I was going to go back to work. Jake went a little crazy with that. I got hired as the director of nursing services at a nice little hospital. It was the sixties and you didn't need a 100 percent education to do stuff back then. I worked there roughly ten years. They had a change of administration, some serious politics, and I ended up not working there. So I went to work for the State of Mississippi and surveyed nursing homes, hospitals, and home health agencies, just about everything that moved. I worked with that agency for as long as I could continue to work with the MS.

The kids had done relatively normal things. By the time I quit, they were both married. But my daughter Lynne was soon divorced and, later on, Jim got divorced. My husband was playing around with my friend that worked in his office and she decided she wanted the goose that laid the golden egg. So she got him, which sort of devastated me. I was surprised (a) that he was screwing around and (b) that he would divorce me. But it was the way things worked out. It was all right because—I'm not a nice person—see, he had a light stroke and isn't practicing medicine. His wife has two jobs. So I don't really feel bad, although I hurt at times.

There was an old fellow that was extremely kind to me, a World War II vet and below-the-elbow amputee. Jerry was sort of my feet and I was his hands. We lived together from '78 until a few years ago. That relationship went down the drain. He had sleep apnea and I was not sleeping well. Then he had some sort of cerebral changes. He was sexually oriented before, but he got extremely inquisitive about my body. We'd been living together and that's all right. But when you get to the point where you're sitting on the commode and somebody is enjoying watching you, it's not any fun. So I backed out of that one, using my illness as an excuse, and I've been floating around in nursing homes, basically, ever since.

Ronai asks Gray about the chapters of her story. As Gray proceeds to answer, the main linkages of a life narrative are conveyed: her "cruddy" childhood, her love of horses and other animals, nursing and nursing homes, and MS.

The first chapter would probably be about my cruddy childhood. I have spent some serious psychology time at the psychologist over the last six months roughly, trying to sort it out. As she [the psychologist] says—and I agree with it—she says that basically my parents should have never multiplied. They were not loving, caring, feeling people. I was basically a status symbol. Everybody had two cars, one child, a dog, and, you know, a living room, a parlor, a kitchen, three bedrooms, two baths, you know, and I was part of the inventory. I didn't like it. I didn't like it as a child and I resent it now. I perceive them being very egocentric and self-centered. At the expense of an only child, who had basically no peer group because they were older parents, I was jerked around between schools. I felt very much like a pawn and I was resentful of it. [Elaborates]

Let's see. I'd probably have a chapter about . . . do a horse and a dog one. I would definitely do a nursing home one. I am thinking very seriously of getting myself a word processor and doing an interesting analysis of nursing homes. I've surveyed them. I've lived in four or five. I'm acquainted with the federal regs and I'm acquainted with state regs in two states fairly thoroughly and I'm working on my third one. I think I would spend some serious nursing home time.

The last chapter is a hard one. If we're doing it chronologically, we're gonna have to deal with terminal things. We know how MS ends. It is not a great disease and it might be about MS. If I was gonna write it now, I would probably do that.

She discusses the history of her MS, how she dealt with it as she followed her husband's career from Mississippi to Virginia and back, and the kinds of sacrifices she made because of the affliction and the moves. It's an admittedly sad tale of truncated opportunities, which Gray continues to tell while wearing her professional hat, that is, in a straightforward, mainly unemotional manner. In an extract from an exchange following the discussion, Gray's manner becomes focal as she describes how she's made important decisions in her life, hedging on her professional self.

Karen: I very hardheadedly decided that I was not going to live in Massachusetts, but I ended up a nursing major instead of something else. I had to deal with it when Jake started sleeping with what's-her-name, or maybe when we lost the ability to talk to each other. I've always had a certain amount of paranoia, and he himself was not without problems, but I think had I not been set up . . . well, maybe not . . . my mother possessed me. I was an object and I was set up for Jake, because he was in charge. I think that had I had the wisdom . . . the wherewithal . . . to fall in love with somebody who would not fall into the control game, you know, that things might have been different.

Carol: You seem assertive to me. You don't seem like someone who would find herself in that fix.

Karen: I'm assertive about some things and not in others. I can . . . I think that, basically, professionally I am assertive, when I have my professional hat on. But when I get down to personal stuff, my personal hat . . .

Carol: Relationships?

Karen: Relationships. I have trouble doing that. I think I'm doing a professional thing with you right now and the stuff we talked about earlier.

Carol: Okay.

Karen: This is a person that can talk to you straight, basically. I think that if we got down to the "me" sort of stuff, I would be sitting here being embarrassed or getting real mushy. You know, I can totally back off into myself and I'm not doing this like that. I don't think that this is one of your goals.

They move on to discuss nursing homes in general and Fairhaven in particular. At first, Gray chooses to convey her thoughts and feelings about Fairhaven while wearing her professional hat. Gray judges Fairhaven to be worse as a nursing facility than many, but at certain points it isn't clear whether, professionally speaking, she is perhaps defending Fairhaven or describing nursing homes in general. This will be cast differently six months later when she thinks back on the Fairhaven experience from the vantage point of the isolation of apartment living. The discussion is prompted by a mention of the lack of a support system, the result of a recent disagreement with her daughter Lynne.

Karen: So I'm a bit miffed at Lynne and she's not too happy with me right now. So I've got less of a support system than I thought I had.

Carol: You mean from the point of view of living in this place?

Karen: Oh golly. I seriously avoid this place as much as I can.

Carol: But you live here.

Karen: Yeah. I go ahead and have breakfast in my room. I have got a pretty vigorous bowel control program. I take care of that, basically take a professional orientation. I find a book and go out and sit here or outside or, you know, spend some serious time scattered here and there.

Carol: Yeah. I noticed that you've had some sun on your chest. So I figured you'd been out.

Karen: Right, right. I'm basically a real kind of pale sort of person. But I've taken some serious outdoor time up here and at the last facility. The noise and confusion disturb me. The lack of privacy . . . not physical privacy . . . but quiet and not being able to go off and sit down and talk with somebody for thirty or forty minutes. [Nods toward her roommate's side of the room] I mean, you know, it is her room, too, but I've been using it. I just haven't had to use it when she did before. The lack of a place to go; that's a problem. But we're getting into the warmer weather cycle and I'm gonna have to find a place to sit where I can stand it.

Carol: What do you think your life will look like a year from now?

Karen: I hope I've got better digs. I don't think I'll be marketable. MS is sort of slow unfortunately, or fortunately, and I imagine that physically I'll be about where I am now, you know, unless something really disastrous comes around. I think I'm sort of stuck in this time warp for a while.

Carol: Before you came to live here, what'd you think it would be like?

Karen: Well, professionally, I knew what it was gonna be like. I mean I had been surveying these suckers for ten years. I knew some of them were better than others. I didn't know how bad the bad ones were.

Carol: Oh?

Karen: I have learned, were I still surveying, where to look. I am finding things that I didn't know to look for. I would have looked more thoroughly at infection control. I would have sure looked . . .

Carol: You think that's a problem here?

Karen: I think that cleanliness is a problem. I think here roaches are a problem. We are having a roach war here, okay? They are trying to kill the roaches. I myself am not a roach person. I don't like them. I used to write out nursing homes for roaches all over. And this place has probably got as good roaches as I have ever run into.

Carol: Ugh.

Karen: I mean, I was sitting with Harry [another resident] last night talking and one of them walks up the leg of the chair. In my room, one of them walks up the back of my dresser. I do not keep loose food in my room, okay? An experienced surveyor knows this. We have got a really, truly, serious, bad roach problem. We have, you know, the age group that hoards, like food, and we have some real hoarders here and they cleaned them out a couple of weeks ago and hopefully things are better. That's what you've got to do in these places if you're going to keep the roaches down. I've seen it in all these nursing homes.

Carol: They're all like that?

Karen: Well, really, yeah. I would look at bathtubs, too, because I got bathed this morning and you know that funny scaly stuff in bathtubs? Yeah, and were I surveying, I would run my finger in every damn bathtub. I wasn't smart enough to do that back then. But now that I've lived in them, you'd look at stuff like that.

Carol: I see. So you generally knew what you were getting into, for the most part though, when you moved here?

Karen: For the most part.

Carol: So you're not surprised living in 'em now, relative to what you thought when you were surveying them?

Karen: I am sort of repulsed. I have been in facilities better than this for sure. The rudeness and the ignorance of the aides, I have now experienced. As a surveyor walking into a facility, everybody is always so nice and polite and lovely. And everybody is always busy taking care of patients and, believe me, that ain't the way it is. They need to walk in on [shift] three to eleven and you'll find the nurse out somewheres and you'll have three aides sitting at the nurse's station. I'm sure they can cough up a good excuse of why they're doing that. That's the way these places are. The lack of caring. The lack of involvement. The lack of a place for me. I've made friends with other nursing services. This particular one is very remote and exclusive. I don't really know what's going on internally, but we practically never get the same three to eleven nurse. We have some consistency. I think I've had three or four baths since I have been here, by choice, but I think that a different person is doing it every time.

Nobody knows my routine. They are terribly rude about moving your crap around so that they can paint or paper or whatever they want to do and not putting it back. Then when they put it back, everything's out of place. I need some accommodation, you know, with a wheelchair and the transfers and all that stuff. Nobody knows my routine.

We had a care planning conference and they were kind enough to invite me, which is one of the federal regs, that if you are able, you are supposed to be included. They did do that here. But the little girl that was doing the conference was concerned with my hemorrhoids, which were a problem prior to my surgery a year ago, and I've got some needs that are really a lot greater than that . . . the fact that I have a catheter and really don't want to pick up any more strange bacteria; the fact that I've got a bowel problem related to my illness. The bowel problem is important to me because I don't want to be in the position where I shit in public, excuse me.

Carol: Right.

Karen: So I'm very compulsive about the darn thing because I know if I am taken care of in the morning, I will probably not have a boo-boo in the afternoon, and I have done this on occasion. These are the things that are important to me. And they're talking about my hemorrhoids!

Carol: I see what you mean.

Karen: I think that I need some recognition as an individual. Any patient does. I think that people should be aware of my needs and fit them into the routine. I think that if we had the same staff working, with all in the same way, basically every day, we could get a routine. These things would help these suckers.

Carol: Do you think of this place is part of your life or separate from it?

Karen: Basically, it is part of my life . . . because I worked with nursing homes so intensively for the ten years prior. I worked for ten years with them and then I ended up in them. I don't feel it's that hard. I feel like I got a lot to contribute. I'm frustrated because they have their system and I have no input.

Carol: Is there anyone in here that you feel close to?

Karen: At this point, not particularly. We've got a couple of older gentlemen that have a little bit of sense. I sort of assume almost a professional role with at least one of them, Alec. He is telling me about his sexual problems and I'm sitting there studiously not being turned off and I really don't care whether he can have a hard-on or not, you know.

But he's gonna have a [penile] implant and he's gonna tell me about the implant. It makes him happy. So, you know, what the hell.

I find it frustrating here because I've got more desires than I can physically accommodate. You know, I would be retiring in ten years and I could, you know, get loose and do some really neat things. I was thinking that Jake and I could travel and do things. Of course, he and Kitty [Jake's present wife] are traveling and doing things. 'Course he had a stroke. This is not a 100% great existence.

Carol: But you can still read and everything.

Karen: But you need a little more than that. You need some serious personal contact, besides listening to Alec's problems. You know what I'm saying? I guess I'm sorta getting personal now. Let's change the subject.

THE SECOND INTERVIEW

Six months later, discharged to an apartment, Gray feels isolated. The loneliness calls out a different persona, not the straightforward, professional surveyor of health care settings, but the sedentary, disabled woman whose personal hat now frames daily living. Speaking of Fairhaven, the framing serves to contrastingly portray the quality of the facility's care at the time she was resident.

Carol: Looking back at where you were when we last talked, how do you feel about it?

Karen: It's been an interesting experience. There've been a lot of problems. Discharge planning is not something that I think any facility is good at, and we made a bunch of mistakes.

Carol: Like what?

Karen: I did not manufacture an adequate support system. I have imposed on my daughter enough that we are now estranged. I have gone through a period of real insecurity. I didn't like a lot of reg stuff that was going on at Fairhaven, but at least I felt secure there. I guess you might say that there's more to life than regs. I haven't gotten enough help, I think, from the home health agency. I should have probably signed up for the aide services with those people. Except, basically, I'm able to pay for it and I feel like I'm cheating the government if I take something at the price they charge. I can hire it for a third on my own.

Actually, I'm planning to move back to Mississippi. I have an old lover there, Jerry, who has got a lot of physical and emotional problems. I think that if I say I want something, that he will manage to get it for me. I've got another friend, too, who's a nurse practitioner and I'm planning on using her general practice group. I feel like I can ask Sharon for anything.

Carol: How does living here compare with being at Fairhaven, where we talked last time?

Karen: Different.

Carol: Would you say better or worse or anything like a value judgment of any kind?

Karen: Oh golly. There are pluses there. It wasn't all that bad. Basically, in a nursing home, you have three hots and a cot. You didn't have to worry about that sort of thing. Over there, there were families coming in that you could chat with. There were staff members that were pretty yucky, but you pretty well avoided those. There were others that I really got to be pretty fond of. You could complain a lot, you know, professionally, which I did, but it was more secure in a certain sense. And there was some companionship. The isolation here has been real bad. I guess I didn't perceive my disability as great as I now know it is.

The conversation turns into a lengthy discussion of Gray's cat, which she adores, and Gray's relations with her daughter. Evidently, living in the apartment would not be half as bad if relations with the daughter weren't strained. Gray remarks that while "a lot of little things" sparked the estrangement, much of it can be attributed to the fact that Lynne can't fathom the extent of Gray's helplessness. Gray explains didactically what she means in the following extract, ending the lesson with a positive reference to her most recent nursing home stint at Fairhaven.

While I was visiting in Mississippi, there was an MS support group that had probably about a dozen people. I was just sort of sitting in. It was a little, local group, you know, and they sorta knew each other. I was there for just one meeting, so I mostly listened. The thing I heard over and over again was that their kids wanted them to be normal. One lady had two little stepsons and, you know, it was, "Where ya going? Why are you doing that? Why aren't you? Why? Why?" They didn't understand. There was a lovely Dutch lady who writes letters, apparently to everybody, and the kids are saying, "But Mom, we can't read it." And she says, "It's not my writing. It's . . . I mean it's not my MS. It's the way I learned to write in Holland." A younger woman was saying that she finally made it over to the couch and she laid down, and her little kid wanted a glass of water. She says to him, "Run and look and see if there's one in the refrigerator. I knew there wasn't, but at least he could leave me alone while he went and looked." And then he comes back and he says, "It's not there." There was a young girl who looked as good as you look, I promise you, wearing a sweatsuit. Believe me, any MS person with a sweatsuit is pretty all right. Heat tolerance is limited. And her mother is saying to her, "But Carrie, you would feel so much better when you came home from work if you didn't go to bed and if you got up and got out with your friends like you used to." And Carrie is saying, "And I'm dead at the end of the day." Things like that that Lynne can't seem to get, like you didn't have to think twice about at Fairhaven. At least there they understood dependency.

Mention of Fairhaven leads Gray to recollect her father's death in a nursing home and her move there to be with him. Gray wears her personal hat as she recounts her experiences there and in other facilities. In the process, she speaks of what nursing home life is like in general, despite differences in the quality of care.

Carol: You were in the home with him [Gray's father]?

Karen: Yeah. That was after the other two.

Carol: And how long did that last? The one you were in with your father.

Karen: December until he expired, like the end of either April or May. I've forgotten. I'm bad on times. We lost him in April. After that, Lynne brought me down here.

Carol: I'm curious about the experience with your father. How was that, living in the same place? Did it make being in a nursing home easier for you, him being there and all, or more difficult?

Karen: I don't think it made much difference either way. It was as good as any other for me. A nursing home is a nursing home. There was some nice people there. The food was particularly good. The care was not bad. Some of his friends visited, which tended to make it easier. The fact that he was down the hall dying was just one of those things. It really didn't make that much difference to me, except that I could look in on him every so often. When you live in those places . . . well, there are the differences you can list out, like that . . . but it's still a nursing home, right? You take the bad with the good, you know what I mean? It's like living any other place. Shit happens wherever.

Carol: He was aware of you and everything?

Karen: Yes, he knew I came. Yes, at times, he knew I was there. But I remember, one day, he was insisting that I was not his daughter, you know, just off-the-wall sort of crap. Initially, he was maybe aware that I was there. He didn't regard my presence as a love offering, which was basically what it was. For the first time in my life, I realized what a really egocentric, self-centered person he was. I mean just a lot of kinda pointless self-pride. I was really, really upset . . . excuse me . . . to find out what a son-of-a-bitch he was, 'cause I always thought he was great. He not only was not so great, but he wouldn't ask for help when he needed it. [Elaborates] They're still trying to straighten out his taxes, which he messed up so bad because he thought he could do everything himself.

Carol: So it had more to do with him than that place.

Karen: Oh sure. Ya got a lot on your mind anywhere you are, right? I had a lot on my mind: him, him dyin' and all, and what he got to be like.

Carol: So those kinds of things affect your judgment about these places?

Karen: Sure they do. Hell, you've got a life, too. Don't get me wrong. That last place [Fairhaven] I was in wasn't all that bad. Yeah, they had roaches, but you name any place down here and it's got roaches.

Carol: So how does life look like to you from where you're at now?

Karen: Well, I'm looking ahead to moving back to Mississippi. I see my life as a pretty knotty situation at this point. I don't really have a place to live that suits my needs. I'm walking away from this soon and walking into a new situation. I don't know what I'm gonna be dealing with. I don't know if we're gonna find digs that are appropriate. I don't know if I'm gonna get a bed in a nursing home. I don't know a lot of things. If worse comes to worse and I can't make it out of here, I can go back and live in that nursing home [Fairhaven]. Personally speaking, it was not *that* bad. I think I can survive it. I've survived others.

Carol: What do you think you're life will look like a year from now?

Karen: Hopefully, I'll be in Mississippi. I've got friends there. Jerry's there [the old lover]. I'll have some sort of assisted independent living facility or a nursing home. At least I won't have the isolation I've got here. I maybe can lean on somebody for a ride to church, you know, to help me out and feel like he's getting brownie points with God. And I'll have the pleasure of being out with some people. I'm not sure whether that's an appropriate or inappropriate use of the church.

The interview moves back and forth between Gray's present living situation, being resident at Fairhaven, and future options. Gray recounts her life story chronologically, but comments that it might have been better told thematically. Certain themes "really" stand out, she remarks, such as MS, her childhood, and nursing homes. As the interview winds down, Gray's current living situation is considered. Gray speaks of it metaphorically and eventually uses the metaphor to convey the meaning of her Fairhaven experience. While Gray's comments might be interpreted as retrospective nostalgia, embellished by her present situation, one thing is nonetheless clear: The subjective meaning of her nursing home experience is drawn from the different linkages that articulate narrative, from her two hats to her past and current troubles.

Carol: Living here. Is it part of your life or separate from it?

Karen: Well, personally, it's part of the continuum, but it's like a narrow place on the ribbon, if you will.

Carol: A narrow place on the ribbon?

Karen: A detour on the highway, if you will.

Carol: I'm not sure I'm picking up that metaphor. It's a detour on the ribbon or a narrowing of the ribbon? Which or what?

Karen: I think that life is a continuum.

Carol: Uh huh.

Karen: And I think that a continuum, that ribbon, has got a certain width as well as an unknown length.

Carol: Right.

Karen: I think there are times in your life when it isn't very rich and the ribbon is pretty narrow, although it continues.

Carol: Uh huh.

Karen: And the ribbon can spread out. It's like you're knitting a sweater and you get real tense and it gets real tight in that particular area.

Carol: And narrows.

Karen: Uh huh. You're with me. So now we're in one of the tight places.

Carol: So was living at Fairhaven in one of those spots?

Karen: It was part of the continuum.

Carol: Was that tighter than this part?

Karen: No, no. It's different, because, you see, there were people in and out, and there were families, and there were patients that were . . . that you could talk to.

Carol: So the ribbon was wider there, looser knit?

Karen: Yeah, sure. This here is the tightest.

Carol: Because of the isolation?

Karen: Yeah and the estrangement from Lynne. So I'm looking for it to loosen up, either here or in Mississippi or back in that nursing home.

* * * * *

Being knowledgeable as Karen Gray is, is fairly rare among nursing home residents. But rarity does not detract from the fact that an additional horizon serves to articulate the subjective meaning of the qualities of her nursing home's care and life. The horizon informs her comments in complex ways, narratively linked with the role (hat) she chooses to take in making comparisons and offering judgments, as well as with the MS and her history of interpersonal relations with her daughter, her former husband, friends, and her parents. From Gray, we learn how fine-grained the meaning of the qualities of care and life can be, actively linked as the latter are with contrasting biographical categories.

CHAPTER

12

Lessons

The narratives presented in the preceding chapters are a slice of those collected in the study. There were other residents whose orientations to the quality of life only hinted at being worried to death, possibly making a new home, or "taking no lip" only if push actually came to shove. There were some who seemed to make a frenzied job of being worried, who were so emotionally distraught that they were hardly interviewable. Some residents combined these horizons, such as making a new home and taking no lip from family members about the life they had formed in their new environs. A few linked being worried to death with "lovin' the Lord," aching for the afterlife as a way of leaving dire straits behind.

Other special circumstances also presented themselves. Some spouses and siblings resided in the same nursing home but not the same room, as Karen Gray from the last chapter did in the facility she moved into to be with her dying father. There were residents who had relatives, sometimes a husband, a wife, or a parent, living in nursing homes distant from their own. Some pined for the relative whom they felt might never again be seen alive; others seemed to care less, not knowing whether the relative were alive or dead. There were those whose special circumstance was that they could not speak English or who were otherwise incommunicable, but who were nonetheless alert, ambulatory, and available for interaction.

That there are horizons and diverse narrative linkages across the variety conveys general lessons about subjective meaning. Some lessons are conceptual and instruct us about how to understand the subjective contours of lives. Some are methodological and offer guidelines for studying subjective meaning and, specifically, its relationship to the quality of care and the quality of life. There also are lessons for us as fellow persons, about what any one of us might very well become in years to come—nursing home residents. This concluding chapter presents the lessons, returning us to matters raised at the start.

177

CONCEPTUAL LESSONS

As a way of orienting the reader to the interview material at the end of Chapter 1, I distinguished the life history from the life narrative, noting that the life history is an objective record of the person's past, while the life narrative is the subjectively constructed life. Life narratives are offered in response to what sociologist Brandon Wallace (1992, 1993) calls "narrative challenges" or occasioned requests to recount life. When Carol Ronai and I asked our respondents to tell us their stories and subsequently discussed with them their pasts, presents, and futures, together with related matters of home, family, and the qualities of institutional life, the narrative challenge was for residents to offer up accounts in response to the requests. The occasion itself—the interview, its participants, and the topics—was part of what ensued, making residents' stories narrative collaborations.

One lesson of this regards how to conceive of the way in which the lives that are the subject of narration fit in the flow of experience. The life is not something distantly set in stone, which the researcher more or less accurately retrieves and records. Rather, the life is a narrated entity, a constructed whole served up against horizons, in relation to which matters of various kinds such as the quality of care are given voice. The narrated entity that is a life is current and practical. When Roland Snyder, Jake Bellows, Lula Burton, Grace Wheeler, and others speak of life, linking it with particular versions of home and institutional living, it is life articulated out of its narrators' present situation as nursing home residents. Yet the situation is not subjectively homogeneous, complicated as its meanings are by different orientations and special circumstances. "Distant" lives are as recent as the present and its perspectives.

The constructed life informs us that what is told is pertinent to the here-and-now, indeed cannot be separated from the here-and-now (Gubrium et al. 1994). The constructed life only makes sense when we consider it in relation to the situation in which it is conveyed. In a manner of speaking (or writing), the constructed lives of nursing home residents Snyder, Bellows, Burton, Wheeler, and others are conceptually hyphenated lives: versions-of-life-subjectively-pertinent-to-the-nursing-home-situation. How the lives and their linkages would be articulated in other situations would need to take the situations' respective orientations and special circumstances into account.

The meaning of the past in relation to the present is neither narratively uniform nor unilinear. As travelers, Jake Bellows and Peter Rinehart orient to their nursing homes as hotels, the facilities virtually being two more resting places along well-traveled roads. Lovin' their Lord, Julia McCall and Mary Carter orient to an altogether different world, marginally concerned with the comforts or discomforts of the present. Bellows, Rinehart, McCall, and Carter hardly accord to the quality of care the significance that, say, Bea Lindstrom does, who is vigilantly attuned to the quality of care and will "take no lip" from her caregivers. Moreover, as the longitudinal aspect of the project showed, narrative linkages change in a complex manner over time. The change is not stepwise or generally unilinear, akin, say, to a process of adjustment, but change that relates to the shifting and varied linkages of the present in relation to life as a whole.

Another conceptual lesson concerns how to think about the related roles of everyday life. Pertinent here is the role of the nursing home resident, although other roles such as family caregiver and significant other are implicated. The life narratives of residents indicate that the role of nursing home resident cannot be defined separately from the horizons of meaning brought to the definition. The role means something personally positive for Martha Gilbert, who admittedly never had a home to speak of. It means something quite the opposite to Rebecca Bourdeau, who left a lovely home to recover at Oakmont, the nursing home in which she now resides. For spouses Amy and Tom Malinger, home is wherever they are together. Fairhaven finds them as much household occupants as registered residents. Twins Lula Burton and Lily Robinson continue the sisterly conversation at Florida Manor they have had all of their lives residing and working a mere stone's throw from each other.

The category "role" does not stand isolated from biographical activity (Gubrium 1988). Knowing that Martha Gilbert and the others are nursing home residents gives us a certain, broad fix on their lives, but it does not inform us of subjective meaning. For that, we need to turn to narrative, in which, say, Myrtle Johnson, a resident of Westside Nursing Center, wonders audibly how it could possibly have come to this, referring to how the meaning of life and destiny could be reduced, day in and day out, to forever being sick, incapacitated, and staring at four institutional walls.

A third conceptual lesson derives from the contrast between the biographically active idea of role and its official organizational understanding. Officially, there are relatively few roles in nursing homes. There are staff roles, administratively distinguished into aides, nurses, dietitians, social workers, and physical therapists. There are resident roles, which are commonly classified into personal-, intermediate-, and skilled-care. In some nursing homes, certain residents are called "patients" to differentiate them from the more able-bodied or "residents." There also are family roles, although they border on the unofficial.

The workings of organizations, evident in their daily shifts and rhythms, job descriptions, and surveillance functions, tend to homogenize the lives within them into official classifications. Residents who orient to the nursing home experience in dramatically different ways, or whose special circumstances articulate particular horizons, officially are more or less simply residents, albeit with varied care needs. While the aide has a past, a home life of her own, and distinct ambitions, she is officially just an aide. As Diamond (1993) shows in his book *Making Gray Gold*, if anything, these subjective matters intrude on organizational rationality, which, as Diamond argues, shortchanges the profit motive.

From a formal organizational perspective, official roles fully penetrate the nursing home experiences of staff and residents. As far as "the" resident is concerned, he or she not only is housed in a room, has a bed, and is served three meals a day, but thinks and feels like a resident. The subjective contours of the resident's past and future are relevant only to the extent they are periods of life pertinent to the official present. Biographical particulars, such as the residents' view of life, are ultimately marginalized in organizational processing, even while enlightened administrators and staff try to take them into account. In the care planning conference, for example, short- and long-term care goals are set and biographical particulars mainly accorded meaning in terms of care needs and service provision (Gubrium 1975).

The idea of the biographically active resident is a conceptual defense against this. Residents are viewed as articulating their roles in different ways, only some of which convey thoughts and feelings appropriate to official concerns. The idea allows us to recognize that, within the parameters of their situations, residents construct and live in worlds of their own making as much as they participate in or forebear the official nursing home world and its roles. Conceiving of residents in this way could provide the rationale for establishing institutional structures for displaying and regularly affirming subjective meaning.

METHODOLOGICAL LESSONS

Methodological lessons relate to the study of subjective meaning, particularly researching the quality of care and the quality of life. I put these in the context of the interview as a research tool, considering interviewing as a narrative collaboration with the respondent.

Social research methods books commonly describe the interview as a technique for gathering information from individuals about their thoughts, sentiments, and activities. The interview involves someone called the interviewer asking questions of someone else called the respondent, who in turn answers the questions out of his or her experience. The ideal interview is one in which respondents' answers convey what was in the respondents' experiences "all along," as it were.

The life narratives presented here warrant another approach. Its point of departure is that the interview is a meaning-making occasion; results cannot be conceived as completely separate from the occasion's narrative challenges. The interviewer is not a passive inquirer. While the interviewer may work from a set of orienting questions such as those contained in our interview guide, he or she participates with the respondent in considering the kinds and versions of questions the respondent deems pertinent to particular concerns. The interviewer attends to how the respondent narratively organizes experience in the process of linking elements of the past, the present, and the future, and from that targets meaning. This allows the respondent to set his or her own horizons of meaning for the matters under consideration.

Not just anything goes. The interviewer encourages the respondent to construct a sense of experience based on the assumption that horizons organize subjective meaning and a working commitment to trace linkages from the broader context of the respondent's life as a whole. This is not an interviewer who passively inquires from an interview schedule or is bound by the topics of an interview guide, but someone who nonetheless remains assiduously sensitive to the respondent's biographical activity. The procedural understanding is that horizons and their narrative linkages guide the active interviewer.

Research methods books commonly assume that the respondent is whoever he or she is designated to be, in our case, a nursing home resident. In the research process, designated respondents remain narratively fixed from start to finish. A sample of nursing home residents is taken to respond as nursing home residents. They are not viewed as differing so much in orientation as to lead the researcher to raise questions about the subjective relevance of the role of nursing home resident. Nor do respondents shift identities in the course of their interviews. The idea that the respondent puts on different hats during an interview, as Karen Gray did in hers, confounds the assumption.

Yet this is precisely what horizons of meaning and their narrative linkages do from respondent to respondent or during a single respondent's interview. In my experience as a field-worker doing both participant observation and ethnographic interviewing, it wasn't unusual for respondents to specify the capacity in which they were addressing a particular question or topic. Sometimes, they simply stated the capacity. For example, in field research on Alzheimer's disease caregiver support groups (Gubrium 1986), caregivers prefaced remarks about their home care experiences with statements such as "Speaking as a wife, I feel [such and such]" and "Putting my caregiver's hat on, I think [thus and so]." They then went on to describe how they felt or what they thought, in those capacities. Some would turn about midresponse to convey sentiments and thoughts from another vantage point. Capacities could even represent preferred thoughts and feelings, as when a caregiver stated, "Right now, I prefer to think of myself as a wife, not his caregiver, because a wife naturally feels more."

The contrast between the designated respondent and narrative capacity presented itself poignantly in one field site. Caregivers had completed a standard burden-of-care questionnaire as part of their participation in a hospital-based study of related stresses. A few days later, in a support group, the caregivers recalled their thoughts and feelings in completing the questionnaire. Some mentioned that they didn't think of themselves as being burdened, but just doing, as one of them put it, "what I feel I have to do." According to a caregiving adult daughter, it hadn't even crossed her mind that caring for her mother should be framed in those terms—burden, stress, strain. The daughter always considered what she was doing for her mother as part of what the daughter owed to her mother in return for the mother's devotion to her daughter over the years. The daughter had come to the support group to learn how to be a grateful daughter, as it were. In contrast, other caregivers felt that the tone of the questionnaire captured matters well, clarifying for them what had been vague thoughts and mixed emotions. In their case, the tone served to crystallize the narrative capacities required to make responses meaningfully those of *caregivers*. Unbeknownst to the administrators of the questionnaire, the questionnaire itself was biographically active, which also remains unrecognized in nursing home quality assurance assessments.

Using a questionnaire, interview schedule, or interview guide for purposes of inquiring about the thoughts and feelings of the respondent without attending to the capacity in which the respondent gives voice to experience puts the procedural cart before the horse. As we try to understand respondents' experiences, we must make sure whose voices speak to us. Nursing home residents' life stories and related responses suggest that narrative horizons must be discerned in order to sort the variety.

There are specific methodological lessons about quality-of-care and quality-of-life assessment in the nursing home. While research on quality of care and quality of life has burgeoned in the last decade, especially as applied to frail elderly, the concepts' methodological underpinnings remain muddled and tentative (Birren et al. 1991).

As far as the nursing home is concerned, quality of care usually has referred to the cleanliness of the premises; the kinds of nursing, medical, therapeutic, domiciliary, and ancillary services offered; staffing patterns; the physical and psychosocial status of residents; and compliance with regulations. Emphasis is on the actual care given, the availability and qualifications of professional caregivers, and care and treatment outcomes, all of which are taken to be objectively assessable conditions.

At the same time, it has been noted that there is more to quality than concrete care provision, especially in the context of the nursing home (Estes and Binney 1989; Kane 1989; Institute of Medicine 1986). In contrast to the nursing home, hospital stays are relatively short and pose fewer problems of life-style adjustment for patients. Short stays mean that patients can virtually put their lives on hold or temporarily leave their lives behind as they undergo treatment and initial recovery. In nursing homes, except for brief periods of convalescence following acute care or physical rehabilitation, stays are lengthy and present significant life-style challenges to residents. The term *nursing home* not only connotes a hospitallike venue providing nursing cares, but a homelike setting offering shelter and sustenance, in many cases for years or for the rest of one's life.

Long-term stays bring lives along as well as ills and disabilities. For some, such as those who are worried to death, what is brought along figures distressingly into personal outcomes. For others, such as those who love their Lord, personal outcomes are subordinated to something of much greater value. A variety of lifelong concerns is at stake in the nursing home experience and affects adjustment. These subjective concerns are a diverse configuration, far broader, more complex, and less immediately concrete than the specifications regularly taken to make up the quality of care.

Psychologist Powell Lawton (1983) has written that quality assurance, especially in the nursing home setting, includes residents' life-styles and perceptions of the value of life—features of what Lawton calls the "good life." He explains that quality of life is a general, multidimensional concept and suggests that what it means to be a long-stay nursing home resident cannot be understood without taking this into account. Most researchers agree that quality of life is a key ingredient of quality assurance and many, but not all, think of it as something distinct from, if not unconnected with, standardized quality of care (see Birren et al. 1991; Institute of Medicine 1986).

Significant as quality of life is considered to be, the concept is not easily rendered into the restricted operations of measurement. Psychologists James Birren and Lisa Dieckmann state that

> for many years the concept of quality of life was viewed as abstract, "soft," and difficult to operationalize. Consequently, this concept was overlooked, particularly by psychology and other disciplines intent on achieving "hard science" status. More concrete health measures, such as

mortality, morbidity, restricted activity days, and functional status typically have been used to evaluate the cost-effectiveness of interventions or
to assess quality of care, and social scientists have relied on related but less
complex concepts, such as life satisfaction, to elucidate the subjective aspects of life. (1991, p. 344)

The statement conveys a disturbing irony. On the one hand, it is
agreed that, while abstract, quality of life is highly significant in its own
right, if not also in connection with the quality of care. On the other
hand, there is notable handwringing over how to measure it. Because
the concept is recalcitrant to "hard science" operationalization (which
confuses science with technology), the concept either has been ignored
or thought too methodologically complicated to research, something like
starving for lack of a particular eating utensil and not thinking to use
one's hands. As the front-page article entitled "Quality of Life" states in
a recent issue of the newsletter *Network*, published by the New England
Research Institute, the specific instance of "health-related quality of life"
or HQL

> generally denotes aspects of life most likely to be affected by health, such
> as physical functioning, physical health, mental health, cognitive func-
> tioning, social functioning, intimacy or sexual functioning, and productivi-
> ty. Although HQL has gained widespread acceptance as an important
> medical outcome, its measurement is riddled with conceptual and meth-
> odological issues. What constitutes HQL? What factors moderate HQL?
> Should HQL be represented by a single overall score or by scores on
> different dimensions of functioning? Should measures be generic or
> disease-specific? Should measures reflect patients' perceptions of HQL or
> objective assessments of functioning? The array of instruments and com-
> plexity of approaches to measuring quality of life can seem overwhelming,
> even to those in the field. (1992, p. 1)

The preference is for measurement scales, quality of life scores, or the
like, the idea being that life and its qualities can be described arithme-
tically. The article goes on to list criteria for the ideal instrument, among
which are that it should "require less than 15 minutes to complete" and
be suitable for telephone as well as other forms of administration (p. 2).
It is explained that some existing instruments are completed by the
physician, which assumes that the physician or, as is more often the case
in nursing homes, a nurse can effectively assess that "holistic" entity
called quality of life. This is the way in which information in minimum
data sets is to be collected (see Morris et al. 1990). While lip service is
paid here and elsewhere to the validity of assessment—namely, that
assessment be about that which it claims to be, in this case quality of
life—efficiency is the name of the game.

The idea of efficiency bandied about in such discussions centers on four criteria. First, measurement or, more broadly, assessment is efficient if it can be completed in short order, such as in ten to fifteen minutes. A quality of life assessment instrument that would take longer to complete would be considered inefficient because, among other things, it would take too much time away from other activities for which those who administer the instrument are responsible. Second, assessment is efficient if the information gathered can be readily coded for data processing. On this criterion, the precoded response categories of a staff-administered, survey instrument would be more efficient than the transcribed narrative of an open-ended interview. Third, efficiency is productive of concise data, usually meaning numeric data. Results reportable in the form of a single, overall score or individual scores for particular components of quality of life are preferred. Fourth, efficiency has a scientistic tenor. Assessment that sounds "scientific," presented in a vocabulary replete with terms such as measurement, reliability, statistical analysis, and indexes, is more acceptable than the so-called soft and "unscientific" vocabulary of narrative. The criterion is scientistic because it capitalizes as much on the rhetoric of popular science as on scientific rigor.

But rigor in science would seem to center ideally on the relationship between method and subject matter. If quality of life concerns the qualities of the subject's life, the concept ostensibly would pertain to whatever might be included and evaluated in the life by the experiencing subject whose life it is. Psychologist Torbjörn Svensson specifies what he would take this to mean.

> There seems to be general agreement that quality of life is a global measure or concept. At the same time, it is agreed that quality of life is built upon other concepts, which have been described as domains or attributes. . . . [I]t is proposed that these domains are qualities *in* life. Qualities in life are defined as the specific areas a person perceives to be vital to the ability to enjoy life and to feel that it has meaning. It can also be said that these qualities are areas into which an individual puts high meaning and involvement. As such, involvement and meaning are important aspects for measurements that seek to discern what is perceived as a quality in life. Meaning in life particularly must be considered since it involves a global evaluation of the entire life situation, with former, present, future, and perhaps transcendent aspects of the individual's life content. (1991, p. 257)

The last sentence, especially, not only would extend the concept to the life and the qualities described by nursing home residents Karen Gray, Rita Vandenberg, and Jane Nesbit, but also to those conveyed by Myrtle Johnson, Alice Stern, Julia McCall, and Mary Carter, whose narrated lives have borders and qualities taking them beyond the official parameters of their immediate situation and its time frame.

Truly rigorous assessment requires a different sense of efficiency, one directing us to draw out and convey whatever a concept validly references, however resistant to arithmetic representation that might be. This expressly links efficiency with validity, enhancing efficiency's scientific status even while reducing its scientistic tenor, which in part has motivated the narrative character of the research reported in this book.

A lesson to be drawn from this is that quality of life can be revealed to be something quite distinct from the quality of care, even while some narrative linkages, such as Bea Lindstrom's, immerse the quality of life in the quality of care. This does *not* mean that, in the context of some horizons, the quality of care provided by the nursing home doesn't need to matter. What it does mean is that lives and care are not necessarily understood by their subjects in terms of the administratively defined or scientistically attributed conditions of immediate situations. As the horizons, narrative linkages, orientations, and special circumstances of our nursing home residents show, there is far more to life and its qualities than the multidimensional components of a measurement scale.

A related lesson is that we need to take on board entirely different methods of procedure to study the subjective meaning of the quality of life and the quality of care than those customarily used in assessment. Required is a methodology attuned to life as a broad and narratively assembled entity, guided by an analytic orientation that recognizes stories to be invariably situated. It is a methodology centered on subjects as active agents in determining whatever is meaningful and valued in life, a methodology whose narrative purview extends beyond the immediate present because subjects make meaning from lifelong experience.

I don't mean to suggest that standardized quality assessment is irrelevant. Such assessment is useful for helping to maintain minimum levels of care for what might be called the "objective" conditions of residents' daily lives. But we need to remind ourselves, too, that residents live as much in subjective worlds as in relation to objective conditions. Indeed, while I have argued that horizons and narrative linkages meaningfully and collaboratively assemble the subjective qualities of care and nursing home life, minimum data sets and the like are also meaningful collaborations in that they are constructed out of what we as a society believe objective standards of care should be (Pifer and Bronte 1986) and their facts are generated out of the descriptive contingencies of assessment occasions (see Cicourel 1964). It all suggests, on the contrary, that methodologies pertaining to the study of lives and their qualities need to be most inclusive.

PERSONAL LESSONS

I have been personally instructed by the narratives. One lesson, precious to me, is how narratively rich lives can be even as their subjects suffer from pain, are severely restricted by disabilities, have lost most if not all of their loved ones, and have little or no chance for recovery. Theirs are faces *with* stories, who under the most trying bodily conditions are still able to make meaning, to link together semblances of explanation and understanding for life and living. Their stories have taught me that, even with dreadful insults to one's body or being near death, varied horizons communicate meaningful differences. Experience does not necessarily coalesce around immediate afflictions, their cares, their trials, or dying.

I cherish the memory of the many residents who readily spoke of their lives, who in many instances I actually could see breathing with difficulty or aching from pains in their backs, chests, legs, and elsewhere as we talked. Most went on, wanted to go on, despite the difficulties. Their will and stamina amazed me. In a few cases, it was more than I could bear, knowing that they were succeeding in presenting to me what their lives had been like, what life had become, and, perhaps most significant, what a life could still be.

Here I was, a man in his midforties at the time of the research, concerned with the completion of the interviews, the management of the narrative material, and the emerging results. And here in front of me during the interviews were persons near the end of their lives or in intractable pain. What was I hearing as they conveyed their experience? Data? Stories? Responses? Meanings? Interviewees? Narratives? I was hearing all of this, of course, but placed side by side, the resulting polarities shocked me. Data versus stories. Responses versus meaning. Interviewees versus storytellers. It shocked me because, on the one side, I was aiming to complete a study and, on the other, I was witnessing what the suffering and dying were telling me, were conveying *for me*. It was a gift, really, and it shocked me that I had to remain committed at the time to listening, recording, and going about research business, respondent after respondent. It was a gift I could not return then, having to remain satisfied that only later could I give something in return by telling their stories in the best way I could.

Another lesson relates to the idea of the end of life. Residents Julia McCall, Mary Carter, and others seemed ready to die, but only bodily. They loved their Lord and were set to go on to another world, a life they imagined in the beyond. For them, the end of life signified the end of life in this world, not the end of life altogether. Roland Snyder, Rita Vandenberg, and Rebecca Bourdeau were worried enough to want to die, because this world was too bodily or spiritually painful. Spouses Amy and Tom Malinger and Sue and Don Hughes were in it together until the end, which would seem to come when a spouse died. Other residents construed death in still different ways: as the eclipse of security, the demise of imagination, the loss of home and significant others, or in terms of the unfathomable place of fate in life.

In their narratives of life and death, living and dying, the residents taught me that endings are made, constructed, and reconstructed, even at the very end, as it were. Having heard their stories, their thoughts and feelings about living in relation to dying and to pasts, present conditions, and futures, I am hard pressed to think of the final years of life as years of "life review," as psychiatrist Robert Butler (1963; Butler and Lewis 1977) puts it, that is, as a time of final reckoning or stocktaking. The longitudinal material gathered from residents interviewed more than once indicates that the very idea of a course of adjustment at the end of life shortchanges its variety, complexity, improvisations. There is little overall evidence that affairs are ultimately settled, sundered ties finally repaired, transgressions at last righted or accounted for, or preparations for the future or afterlife completed. While some residents, of course, do speak of waiting for heaven, buying cemetery plots, and making funeral arrangements—points of information that indeed may hold considerable value for them—these do not necessarily signify terminal horizons.

Finally, I draw a lesson from reflecting on certain aspects of my own life. As I look over the residents' stories, I read about significant others. I have twin daughters, now college sophomores. As I read the transcripts of twin sisters Lula Burton's and Lily Robinson's remarks about the lifelong conversation that continues to sustain them at Florida Manor, do I hear what my own daughters, fifty years hence, might call upon to give meaning to those years? Looking back on my own, still developing research career—seemingly filled with important research, momentous decisions, and academic achievement—what do Myrtle Johnson and Alice Stern tell me about destiny? That it all could come to "this"? And what is "this" in any case? Certainly "this" could be part of a new life or the life to come, even a life that isn't so bad after all if one removes a professional hat. The stories and narratives are about *our* lives, whose horizons and linkages can form in many directions to give meaning to the years ahead.

Appendix

LIFE NARRATIVE PROJECT—INTERVIEW GUIDE
(Probe for Thoughts and Sentiments)

Life in General

1. Everyone has a life story. Tell me about your life, in about twenty minutes or so if you can. Begin wherever you'd like and include whatever you wish.
2. What were the most important turning points in your life?
3. Tell me about the happiest points in your life.
4. What about the saddest points?
5. Who've been the most important people in your life?
6. Who are you closest to now?
7. What does your life look like from where you're at now?
8. If you could live your life over, what would you do differently?
9. How do you explain what's happened to you over your life?
10. If had the opportunity to write the story of your life, what would the chapters be about? Chapter 1? Chapter 2? . . . What about the last chapter?

Daily Life

11. Describe a typical day in your life now. People here. Others. Quality of care/life.
12. How is a typical day now different from before you came to live here?
13. What do you think your daily life will look like a year from now?
14. Before you came to live here, what did you think it would be like?

Home

15. What does the word *home* mean to you?
16. Now that you've been here for _____, does it feel like home?

17. What would it have to be like here for it to be like home?
18. Do you feel this place/living here is part of your life or separate from it? Why is that?

Family

19. What does the word *family* mean to you?
20. Right now, in this place, is there anybody who's like family to you?

Self

21. How would you describe yourself when you were younger?
22. How would you describe yourself now?
23. Have you changed much over the years? How?
24. What is your philosophy of life? Overall, what is the meaning of life to you?

Aging

25. How do you feel about growing older?
26. What do you like about being your age?
27. What do you dislike about being your age?
28. Do you think about the future? Make plans?
29. What do you look forward to now?
30. Do you think about death?

References

Atkinson, Paul. 1990. *The Ethnographic Imagination*. London: Routledge.

Bauman, Richard. 1986. *Story, Performance and Event: Contextual Studies of Oral Narrative*. New York: Cambridge University Press.

Berger, Peter and Hansfried Kellner. 1970. "Marriage and the Construction of Reality." Pp. 50–72 in *Recent Sociology No. 2*, edited by Hans Peter Dreitzel. New York: Macmillan.

Bertaux, Daniel (ed.). 1981. *Biography and Society*. Newbury Park, CA: Sage.

Bertaux, Daniel and Martin Kohli. 1984. "The Life Story Approach: A Continental View." *Annual Review of Sociology* 10:215–37.

Birren, James E. and Lisa Dieckmann. 1991. "Concepts and Content of Quality of Life in the Later Years: An Overview." Pp. 344–60 in *The Concept and Measurement of Quality of Life in the Frail Elderly*, edited by James E. Birren et al. New York: Academic Press.

Birren, James E., James E. Lubben, Janice Cichowlas Rowe, and Donna E. Deutchman (eds.). 1991. *The Concept and Measurement of Quality of Life in the Frail Elderly*. New York: Academic Press.

Blumer, Herbert. 1969. "Science without Concepts." Pp. 153–70 in *Symbolic Interactionism*, Herbert Blumer. Englewood Cliffs, NJ: Prentice-Hall.

Bruner, Jerome. 1986. *Actual Minds, Possible Worlds*. Cambridge, MA: Harvard University Press.

Butler, Robert N. 1963. "The Life Review: An Interpretation of Reminiscence in the Aged." *Psychiatry* 26:65–76.

Butler, Robert N. and Myrna I. Lewis. 1977. *Aging and Mental Health*. St. Louis: C.V. Mosby.

Charmaz, Kathy. 1991. *Good Days, Bad Days: The Self in Chronic Illness and Time*. New Brunswick, NJ: Rutgers University Press.

Cicourel, Aaron V. 1964. *Method and Measurement in Sociology*. New York: Free Press.

Clifford, James and George E. Marcus (eds.). 1986. *Writing Culture*. Berkeley: University of California Press.

Clough, Patricia Ticineto. 1992. *The Ends of Ethnography*. Newbury Park, CA: Sage.

Coe, Rodney. 1965. "Self-Conception and Institutionalization." Pp. 225–43 in *Older People and Their Social World*, edited by Arnold M. Rose and Warren A. Peterson. Philadelphia: F.A. Davis.

Diamond, Tim. 1993. *Making Gray Gold*. Chicago: University of Chicago Press.

Estes, Carroll L. and Elisabeth A. Binney. 1989. "The Biomedicalization of Aging: Dangers and Dilemmas." *The Gerontologist* 29:587–96.

Frank, Gelya. 1980. "Life Histories in Gerontology: The Subjective Side to Aging." Pp. 155–76 in *New Methods for Old Age Research*, edited by Christine L. Fry and Jennie Keith. Chicago: Loyola University Center for Urban Policy.

Gadamer, Hans-Georg. 1993. *Truth and Method*. New York: Continuum.

Garfinkel, Harold. 1967. *Studies in Ethnomethodology*. Englewood Cliffs, NJ: Prentice-Hall.

Geertz, Clifford. 1988. *Works and Lives: The Anthropologist as Author*. Stanford, CA: Stanford University Press.

Goffman, Erving. 1961. *Asylums*. Garden City, NY: Anchor.

————. 1974. *Frame Analysis*. New York: Harper and Row.

Gottesman, L. E. and N. C. Bourstrom. 1974. "Why Nursing Homes Do What They Do." *The Gerontologist* 14:501–6.

Gubrium, Jaber F. 1975. *Living and Dying at Murray Manor*. New York: St. Martin's.

————. 1986. *Oldtimers and Alzheimer's: The Descriptive Organization of Senility*. Greenwich, CT: JAI Press.

————. 1988. *Analyzing Field Reality*. Newbury Park, CA: Sage.

————. 1991. *The Mosaic of Care: Frail Elderly and Their Families in the Real World*. New York: Springer.

Gubrium, Jaber F., James A. Holstein, and David R. Buckholdt. 1994. *Constructing the Life Course*. Dix Hills, NY: General Hall.

Gubrium, Jaber F. and Robert J. Lynott. 1985. "Alzheimer's Disease as Biographical Work." Pp. 349–67 in *Social Bonds in Later Life*, edited by Warren A. Peterson and Jill Quadagno. Newbury Park, CA: Sage.

Gustafson, Elisabeth. 1972. "Dying: The Career of the Nursing Home Patient." *Journal of Health and Social Behavior* 13:226–35.

Henry, Jules. 1963. *Culture Against Man*. New York: Vintage.

Institute of Medicine. 1986. *Improving the Quality of Care in Nursing Homes*. Washington, DC: National Academy Press.

Johnson, Colleen L. and Leslie A. Grant. 1985. *The Nursing Home in American Society*. Baltimore: Johns Hopkins University Press.

Kane, Robert L. 1989. "The Biomedical Blues." *The Gerontologist* 29:583.

Kane, Rosalie A. and Robert L. Kane. 1981. *Assessing the Elderly*. Lexington, MA: Lexington Books.

Kaufman, Sharon R. 1986. *The Ageless Self*. Madison: University of Wisconsin Press.

Kayser-Jones, Jeanie. 1981. *Old, Alone, and Neglected*. Berkeley: University of California Press.

Lawton, M. Powell. 1983. "Environments and Other Determinants of Well-Being in Older People." *Environment and Behavior* 17:501–19.

Maines, David R. 1993. "Narrative's Moment and Sociology's Phenomena: Toward a Narrative Sociology." *Sociological Quarterly* 34:17–38.

Maines, David R. and Jeffrey T. Ulmer. 1993. "The Relevance of Narrative for Interactionist Thought." *Studies in Symbolic Interaction* 14:109–24.

Morris, John N., et al. 1990. "Designing the National Resident Assessment Instrument for Nursing Homes." *The Gerontologist* 30:293–307.

New England Research Institute. 1992. "Quality of Life." *Network* (Winter):1–3. Watertown, MA: Author.

NHCMQ Training Manual. 1991. Natick, MA: Eliot Press.

Pastalan, Leon. 1970. "Privacy as an Expression of Human Territoriality." Pp. 37–46 in *Spatial Behavior of Older People,* edited by Leon Pastalan and Daniel Carson. Ann Arbor: Institute of Gerontology, University of Michigan.

Pifer, Alan and Lydia Bronte (eds.). 1986. *Our Aging Society.* New York: Norton.

Rubinstein, Robert L. 1988. "Stories Told: In-Depth Interviewing and the Structure of Its Insights." Pp. 128–46 in *Qualitative Gerontology,* edited by Shulamit Reinharz and Graham D. Rowles. New York: Springer.

_____. 1989. "The Home Environment of Older People: A Description of the Psychosocial Processes Linking Person to Place." *Journal of Gerontology* 44:S45–S53.

_____. 1990. "Personal Identity and Environmental Meaning in Later Life." *Journal of Aging Studies* 4:131–47.

_____. 1992. "Personal Meaning and Acts of Interpretation." Paper presented at the annual conference of the Gerontological Society of America, Washington, DC.

Sarton, May. 1973. *As We Are Now.* New York: Norton.

Savishinsky, Joel S. 1991. *The Ends of Time: Life and Work in a Nursing Home.* New York: Bergen and Garvey.

Schutz, Alfred. 1967. *The Phenomenology of the Social World.* Evanston, IL: Northwestern University Press.

Shield, Renee Rose. 1988. *Uneasy Endings: Daily Life in an American Nursing Home.* Ithaca, NY: Cornell University Press.

Skolnick, Arlene S. 1983. *The Intimate Environment.* Boston: Little, Brown.

Stannard, Charles I. 1973. "Old Folks and Dirty Work: The Social Conditions for Patient Abuse in a Nursing Home." *Social Problems* 20:329–42.

Svensson, Torbjörn. 1991. "Intellectual Exercise and Quality of Life in the Frail Elderly." Pp. 256–75 in *The Concept and Measurement of Quality of Life in the Frail Elderly,* edited by James E. Birren et al. New York: Academic Press.

Van Maanen, John. 1988. *Tales of the Field: On Writing Ethnography.* Chicago: University of Chicago Press.

Vourlekis, Betsy S., Donald E. Gelfand and Roberta R. Greene. 1992. "Psychosocial Needs and Care in Nursing Homes: Comparison of Views of Social Workers and Home Administrators." *The Gerontologist* 32:113–19.

Wallace, J. Brandon. 1992. "Reconsidering the Life Review: The Social Construction of Talk about the Past." *The Gerontologist* 32:120–25.

Wallace, J. Brandon. 1993. "Life Stories." In *Qualitative Methods in Aging Research,* edited by Jaber F. Gubrium and Andrea Sankar. Newbury Park, CA: Sage.

Ward, Russell. 1979. *The Aging Experience.* New York: Lippincott.

Watson, Wilbur and Robert Maxwell. 1977. *Human Aging and Dying*. New York: St. Martin's.
Zusman, Joseph. 1966. "Some Explanations of the Changing Appearance of Psychotic Patients: Antecedents of the Social Breakdown Syndrome Concept." *Milbank Memorial Fund Quarterly* 64:363–94.

Index